EARLY DIAGNOSIS AND TREATMENT

OF ENDOCRINE DISORDERS

CONTEMPORARY ENDOCRINOLOGY

P. Michael Conn, SERIES EDITOR

EARLY DIAGNOSIS
AND TREATMENT OF
ENDOCRINE DISORDERS

Edited by

ROBERT S. BAR, MD

Division of Endocrinology and Metabolism
Department of Internal Medicine
The University of Iowa School of Medicine
Iowa City, IA

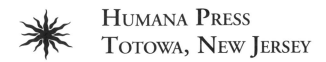

HUMANA PRESS
TOTOWA, NEW JERSEY

Library of Congress Cataloging-in-Publication Data
Early diagnosis and treatment of endocrine disorders / edited by Robert S. Bar.
      p. ; cm. -- (Contemporary endocrinology)
    Includes bibliographical references and index.
    ISBN 1-58829-193-6 (alk. paper); E-ISBN: 1-59259-378-X
    1. Endocrine glands--Diseases. I. Bar, Robert S. II. Contemporary endocrinology (Totowa, N.J.)
    [DNLM: 1. Endocrine Diseases--pathophysiology. 2. Endocrine Diseases--diagnosis. 3. Endocrine Diseases--therapy. WK 140 E12 2003]
    RC648 .E274 2003
    616.4--dc21

                                                  2002035284

8/27/04

PREFACE

Most endocrine diseases can be treated successfully, and the patient's state of well-being can usually be improved. Not surprisingly, the earlier the diagnosis is made the more positive the clinical response. *Early Diagnosis and Treatment of Endocrine Disorders* focuses on early signs and symptoms of endocrine disorders and surveys the appropriate tests to document the diseases as well as current recommendations for therapy. Each chapter reviews the pathophysiology of the endocrine disease—important for understanding each disorder as well as the rationale for early therapy—and the basis for the early recognition and treatment of each condition.

Although the practicing endocrinologist is likely to be quite knowledgeable regarding many of these diseases, *Early Diagnosis and Treatment of Endocrine Disorders* includes treatment of those conditions only recently classified as endocrine disorders, such as polycystic ovarian syndrome, obesity, and hypogonadism. The book also provides new approaches that are urgently needed to slow the epidemic of type 2 diabetes, which should be an overriding concern for all clinicians.

Until now, no other endocrinology text has focused primarily on the details of early recognition and therapy of endocrine disorders. The information in *Early Diagnosis and Treatment of Endocrine Disorders* is presented in an orderly and easy-to-follow manner, which should greatly facilitate the early recognition of endocrine diseases by medical students, house staff, primary care physicians, and endocrinologists, the four groups of clinical personnel to which this book is specifically directed.

Robert S. Bar, MD

CONTENTS

CONTRIBUTORS

ROBERT S. BAR, MD, *Division of Endocrinology and Metabolism, Department of Internal Medicine, The University of Iowa College of Medicine; VA Medical Center, Iowa City, IA*

RITA BASU, MD, *Division of Endocrinology and Metabolism, Mayo Clinic, Rochester, MN*

RUTH M. BELIN, MD, *Division of Endocrinology and Metabolism, Johns Hopkins University School of Medicine, Baltimore MD*

VIVIEN BONERT, MD, *Cedars-Sinai Medical Center, University of California–Los Angeles School of Medicine, Los Angeles, CA*

LEWIS E. BRAVERMAN, MD, *Section of Endocrinology, Diabetes and Nutrition, Boston Medical Center, Boston, MA*

NICHOLAS CLARKE, MD, *Division of Endocrinology and Metabolism, Department of Internal Medicine, The University of Iowa College of Medicine, Iowa City, IA*

JOSEPH S. DILLON, MD, *Division of Endocrinology and Metabolism, Department of Internal Medicine, The University of Iowa College of Medicine; VA Medical Center, Iowa City, IA*

GREGORY DOELLE, MD, *Division of Endocrinology and Metabolism, Department of Internal Medicine, The University of Iowa College of Medicine, Iowa City, IA*

ANUJA DOKRAS, MD, PhD, *Division of Reproductive Endocrinology, Department of Obstetrics and Gynecology, The University of Iowa College of Medicine, Iowa City, IA*

GRAEME EISENHOFER, PhD, *Clinical Neurocardiology Section, National Institute of Neurological Disorders and Stroke, National Institutes of Health, Bethesda, MD*

NGOZI E. ERONDU, MD, PhD, *Clinical Research, Endocrinology and Metabolism, Merck & Company, Inc., Rahway, NJ*

WHITNEY S. GOLDNER, MD, *Division of Endocrinology and Metabolism, Department of Internal Medicine, University of Iowa College of Medicine; VA Medical Center, Iowa City, IA*

ARNA GUDMUNDSDOTTIR, MD, *Division of Endocrinology and Metabolism, Department of Internal Medicine, The University of Iowa College of Medicine, Iowa City, IA*

WILLA HSUEH, MD, *Diabetes, Hypertension, and Nutrition, Division of Endocrinology, University of California–Los Angeles School of Medicine, Los Angeles, CA*

UDAYA M. KABADI, MD, FRCP(C), FACP, FACE, *Division of Endocrinology and Metabolism, Department of Internal Medicine, The University of Iowa College of Medicine, Iowa, City, IA*

CHRISTIAN A. KOCH, MD, FACE, FACP, *Pediatric and Reproductive Endocrinology Branch, National Institute of Child Health and Human Development, National Institutes of Health, Bethesda, MD; Department of Endocrinology and Nephrology, University of Leipzig, Germany*

YOGISH C. KUDVA, MB BS, *Division of Endocrinology and Metabolism, Mayo Clinic, Rochester, MN*

PAUL W. LADENSON, MD, *Division of Endocrinology and Metabolism, Johns Hopkins University School of Medicine, Baltimore MD*

JACQUES W.M. LENDERS, MD, PhD, *Department of Medicine, St. Radbound University Medical Center, Nijmegen, The Netherlands*

D. LYNN LORIAUX, MD, PhD, *Department of Medicine, Oregon Health and Sciences University, Portland, OR*

JOHN H. MACINDOE, MD, *Department of Endocrinology, HealthPartners Medical Group and Clinics; Department of Internal Medicine, University of Minnesota School of Medicine, Minneapolis, MN*

DOROTHY MARTINEZ, MD, *Diabetes, Hypertension and Nutrition, Division of Endocrinology, University of California–Los Angeles School of Medicine, Los Angeles, CA*

ERNEST L. MAZZAFERRI, MD, MACP, *Department of Internal Medicine, University of Florida, Gainesville, FL; Center for Health Outcome Policy Evaluation Studies, The Ohio State University, Columbus, OH*

SHLOMO MELMED, MD, *Cedars-Sinai Medical Center, University of California–Los Angeles School of Medicine, Los Angeles, CA*

THOMAS O'DORISIO, MD, *Division of Endocrinology and Metabolism, Department of Internal Medicine, The University of Iowa College of Medicine, Iowa City, IA*

CHRISTINA ORR, MD, *Division of Endocrinology and Metabolism, Department of Internal Medicine, The University of Iowa College of Medicine, Iowa City, IA*

KAREL PACAK, MD, PhD, DSc, *Pediatric and Reproductive Endocrinology Branch, National Institute of Child Health and Human Development, National Institutes of Health, Bethesda, MD*

ELIZABETH N. PEARCE, MD, *Section of Endocrinology, Diabetes and Nutrition, Boston Medical Center, Boston, MA*

JEFFREY E. PESSIN, PhD, *Department of Physiology and Biophysics, The University of Iowa, Iowa City, IA*

DARCY PUTZ, MD, *Division of Endocrinology and Metabolism, Department of Internal Medicine, The University of Iowa College of Medicine, Iowa City, IA*

ROBERT A. RIZZA, MD, *Division of Endocrinology and Metabolism, Mayo Clinic, Rochester, MN*

WILLIAM I. SIVITZ, MD, *Division of Endocrinology and Metabolism, Department of Internal Medicine, The University of Iowa College of Medicine; VA Medical Center, Iowa City, IA*

ROBERT G. SPANHEIMER, MD, *Division of Endocrinology and Metabolism, Department of Internal Medicine, The University of Iowa College of Medicine, Iowa City, IA*

PREETHI SRIKANTHAN, MD, *Department of Internal Medicine, The University of Iowa College of Medicine, Iowa City, IA*

1

Thyroid Cancer

Ernest L. Mazzaferri, MD, MACP

INTRODUCTION

Multiple factors affect the long-term prognosis of thyroid malignancies *(1)*, but outcome is mainly decided by an interplay between the patient and tumor and by the impact of therapy, which must be applied early when tumor mass is small in order to eradicate the malignancy or slow its growth substantially. An elderly man, for example, with a long-standing undiagnosed 5-cm thyroid nodule found to be papillary cancer is at high risk of death from it within a relatively short time, even though the tumor might initially appear to be confined to the thyroid (2). A young girl, on the other hand, with lung metastases from papillary cancer found when the cancer was first diagnosed might live for decades (2), underscoring the primacy of a person's age and the influence of early diagnosis on outcome (Here and elsewhere age refers to age at the time of diagnosis.)

Therapy has an important impact on the prognosis of thyroid malignancies *(2)*. Outcome is especially favorable for papillary, follicular, and medullary thyroid cancers and for thyroid lymphoma treated at an early stage. Anaplastic thyroid cancer (ATC), a tumor evolving from benign thyroid neoplasms or more differentiated thyroid cancers, poses major therapeutic challenges *(3,4)*. Nonetheless,

From: *Contemporary Endocrinology: Early Diagnosis and Treatment of Endocrine Disorders*
Edited by: R. S. Bar © Humana Press Inc., Totowa, NJ

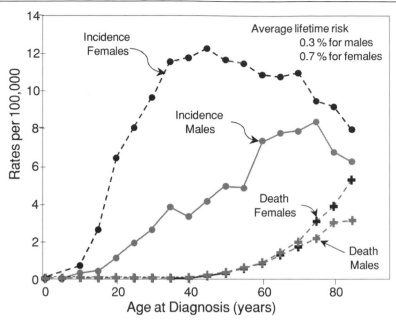

Fig. 1. Incidence and cancer-specific mortality rates for thyroid carcinoma in men and women by decade of diagnosis. (Data from the SEER [1993–1997] database *[37]*.)

early removal of benign follicular cell adenomas and low-grade thyroid cancers has undoubtedly contributed to the declining incidence of ATC in the past four decades *(5)*.

INCIDENCE AND DEATH RATES
OF THYROID CANCER AND LYMPHOMA

About 17,000 new cases of thyroid cancer are diagnosed annually in the United States, making it about 14th in incidence among malignancies *(6)*. It occurs at all ages but is most common among middle-aged and postmenopausal women (Fig. 1). The lifetime risk of developing thyroid cancer is about 1% (0.65% for women and 0.25% for men) *(7)*, and death rates are less than 10% (1200 deaths occurred among 135,000 thyroid cancer patients in 1998) *(6)*. However, both the incidence and mortality rates vary substantially among the different forms of thyroid cancer (Table 1) *(8)*.

To appreciate the impact of early treatment, one must know the survival rates with different types of thyroid malignancy. Although death rates are usually low, cell type and tumor stage substantially alter outcome (Table 1). Prognosis is determined by many variables, but a patient's fate largely depends on three things: the gross and histologic characteristics of the tumor, the patient's age and general health, and prompt therapy *(9)*.

Table 1
Incidence and 10-Year Relative Survival of 53,856 Patients with Thyroid Cancer

Type of thyroid cancer	Incidence (%)	10-yr relative survival (%)	Proportion of all cancer deaths (%)
Papillary	80	93	53
Follicular	11	85	16
Hürthle	3	76	7
Medullary	4	75	10
Anaplastic	2	14	14

Data from ref. 8.

Papillary and Follicular Thyroid Cancer

Derived from follicular epithelial cells, papillary and follicular thyroid cancers comprise the majority of thyroid malignancies and have the best prognosis of the various thyroid cancers; however, they account for nearly 70% of all thyroid cancer deaths (Table 1) (8). They are the only tumors that respond to radioiodine (^{131}I) therapy and that synthesize and secrete thyroglobulin (Tg), a sensitive tumor marker, which in the absence of normal thyroid tissue identifies small amounts of persistent tumor that can be promptly treated.

FAMILIAL PAPILLARY CANCER

About 5% of papillary cancers are inherited as an autosomal dominant trait, the gene for which is still unknown (10,11). They have a less favorable prognosis than sporadic papillary cancer (12,13), unless they occur in the setting of certain syndromes such as familial adenomatous polyposis (Gardner's syndrome), for example, in which thyroid cancer occurs at a young age as bilateral, multicentric tumors with an excellent prognosis, particularly those with ret-PTC activation (14,15). Likewise, thyroid cancers occurring in Cowden's disease (an autosomal dominant disease with mucocutaneous hamartomas and breast cancer) have a good prognosis (16,17). Another familial syndrome, Carney's complex (spotty skin pigmentation, myxomas, schwannomas, and multiple neoplasias affecting multiple glands) is also associated with thyroid cancer that has a good prognosis (18). Once recognized as familial, these thyroid cancers lend themselves to early diagnosis and treatment at an early stage.

Hürthle Cell Follicular Cancer

Oxyphilic cells, termed Hürthle cells, which contain large amounts of acidophilic cytoplasm with numerous mitochondria, may constitute most of a follicular cancer. Some think this is a distinct entity; and others believe it is a variant of follicular cancer (19), it has an unfavorable prognosis (Table 1) (20).

Hürthle Cell Papillary Cancer

About 2% of papillary cancers have Hürthle cells *(21)*, which in some cases are familial *(22)*. Compared with typical papillary cancers, they have higher recurrence and mortality rates, similar to oxyphilic follicular cancer *(21,23)*.

Medullary Thyroid Cancer

First recognized in 1959 as a pleomorphic neoplasm with amyloid struma, medullary thyroid cancer (MTC) arises from thyroidal calcitonin-secreting C-cells. It accounts for about 4% of all thyroid malignancies *(8)*, up to 40% of which are familial tumors transmitted as an autosomal dominant trait. Ten-year relative survival rates for MTC are about 75% (Table 1), but this statistic fails to take into account major differences in prognosis among sporadic and familial tumors.

Anaplastic Thyroid Cancer

In the past, ATC comprised about 5–10% of thyroid cancers *(24)* but in recent years has accounted for about 2% of all thyroid cancers *(8)*. In a review of 475 patients with this disease reported in six large studies, the mean age was 65 yr, with only a slight female predominance *(24)*. ATC is almost never seen before age 20 yr. It evolves from well-differentiated tumors *(24)* which may slowly transform into ATC *(25)*. One report, for example, described a 61-yr-old man who developed follicular cancer pulmonary metastases 12 yr after initial surgery, which transformed over several years into ATC (as shown by serial biopsies) *(26)*. Some appear to arise *de novo (27)*, but many are well-differentiated tumors that slowly transform into ATC *(24)*. One study *(28)* found elements of differentiated cancer in almost 90% of ATC specimens, which often came from persons previously treated for well-differentiated thyroid cancer, underscoring an important adverse effect of late or incomplete treatment of differentiated thyroid cancer.

Thyroid Lymphoma

The annual incidence of thyroid lymphoma in the United States is less than 1 in 2 million persons *(29)*. Thus the likelihood that a thyroid nodule is a primary thyroid lymphoma is less than 1 in 1000; it is much more likely to be a manifestation of systemic lymphoma, which affects the thyroid in about 10% of those who die of the disease *(29)*. However, the incidence of thyroid lymphoma has been rising significantly and now constitutes about 5% of all thyroid malignancies *(29)*. The reason for this is uncertain, but many in the past were incorrectly diagnosed as small cell ATCs *(29)*; however, pathologists are now more adept at recognizing thyroid lymphoma *(29)*. Some of the change in incidence may be related to increased use of fine-needle aspiration (FNA) evaluation of thyroid nodules, but the increasing frequency of thyroid lymphoma has paralleled the rising incidence of Hashimoto's thyroiditis in the United States in the past few decades.

The Role of Thyroid Radiation in Causing Thyroid Cancer

EXTERNAL IRRADIATION

The only environmental factor known to increase the risk of thyroid cancer is irradiation. The risk of developing papillary thyroid cancer after therapeutic external radiation, used in the past to treat children with benign head and neck conditions, is well known *(30)*. Exposure before the age of 15 yr poses a major risk that becomes progressively larger with increasing doses of radiation between 0.10 Gy (10 rad) and 10 Gy (1000 rad). The incidence of thyroid cancer begins increasing within 5 yr of exposure and continues unabated for 30 yr, after which it begins to decline *(30)*. After thyroid radiation exposure, females are more likely than males to develop thyroid cancer, and it is more prevalent among those with a family history of thyroid cancer *(30)*.

RADIOIODINE-INDUCED THYROID CANCER

Most early studies suggested that ^{131}I was unlikely to induce thyroid cancer *(31)*. A large U.S. study, for example, reported a slight elevation of thyroid cancer mortality following treatment of hyperthyroidism with ^{131}I, but the absolute risk was small and the underlying thyroid disease appeared to play a role *(32)*. Most studies in the past of the risk of thyroid cancer following exposure to ^{131}I involved adults in whom the risk appears small or nonexistent. However, when a large number of Chernobyl children developed thyroid cancer after being exposed to radioiodine fallout from a nuclear reactor accident in 1986, it became evident that ^{131}I and other short-lived iodine isotopes were potent thyroid carcinogens in children, particularly those exposed under the age of 10 yr *(33)*.

NUCLEAR WEAPONS FALLOUT

Above-ground nuclear weapons testing in Nevada between 1951 and 1963 released radioactive particles into the atmosphere that exposed thousands of individuals across the continental United States to radioiodine fallout. Exposure was highest for children who drank milk from a "backyard" cow or goat that had ingested grass contaminated with radioiodine. A study from the National Cancer Institute *(34)* concluded that nuclear weapons fallout had resulted in an average cumulative thyroid dose of 0.02 Gy (2 rad) in Americans, but for those under age 20 it was 0.1 Gy (10 rad), within the range known to cause thyroid cancer in children *(30)*. The National Academy of Sciences *(35)* reported that about 50,000 excess cases of thyroid cancer would result from these exposures, but these are highly uncertain estimates. Another study established an association between thyroid cancer and radioiodine fallout among children exposed at less than 1 yr of age and those born between 1950 and 1959 *(36)*. The Institute of Medicine *(35)*, however, recommended against mass screening for thyroid disease because there are many small benign thyroid nodules in the population.

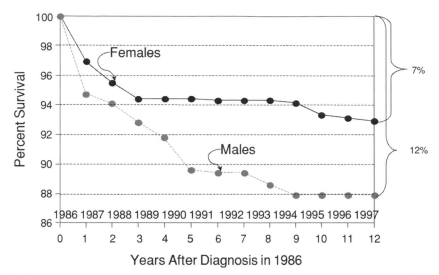

Fig. 2. Ten-year relative survival rates in men and women. (Data from the SEER database *[37].*)

Changing Incidence and Mortality Rates of Thyroid Cancer

THYROID CANCER INCIDENCE AND MORTALITY RATES AMONG MEN AND WOMEN

The incidence and mortality rates of thyroid cancer differ strikingly between men and women and among patients of different ages, but the incidence is more than twice as high in women (Fig. 1). (37) Occurring throughout life, its incidence peaks around age 40 in women and age 70 in men (Fig. 1) *(37)*, in whom mortality rates are twice those of women (Fig. 2). Why men fare so poorly is uncertain, but the rates appear to be linked to late diagnosis and advanced tumor stage.

CHANGING INCIDENCE AND MORTALITY RATES

Since the early 1970s, the incidence rates of thyroid cancer in the United States have increased by 49.1% ($p < 0.5\%$), and thyroid cancer mortality rates have fallen by 19.7% ($p < 0.5$) *(37)*. Why this has happened is uncertain; however, early detection or screening typically leads to two types of statistical bias: lead-time bias and length bias. Tumors detected by screening are found at an earlier stage (lead-time bias) and tend to be more indolent and more slowly growing (length bias) than those detected in the usual way. Other potential biases include changing diagnostic criteria, technologic advances in diagnostic tests (e.g., FNA), and evolution of stage classification *(37)*. Multiple factors have probably caused the observed changes, but some are the result of radiation exposure of children, whereas better therapy has probably improved mortality rates. Further analysis gives important clues about what has caused these striking changes in incidence and mortality.

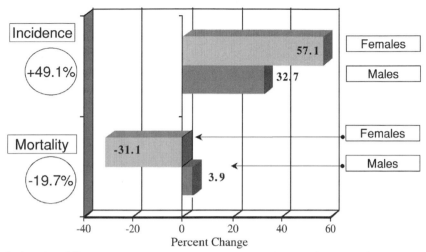

Fig. 3. Gender differences in incidence and mortality 1973–1996. [Data from the SEER database *(37)*.]

TUMOR STAGE IN MEN AND WOMEN

Of special note are the major differences in both the incidence and mortality rates of thyroid cancer among men and women during the past 30 yr: incidence rates have increased about 57% in women but only about 33% in men (almost a twofold greater rise in women than in men) whereas mortality rates have fallen 31% in women and have *increased* nearly 4% in men (about a tenfold difference between the sexes) (Fig. 3). Declining mortality rates have also occurred in black females but not in black males (Fig. 4). Compared with women, thyroid cancer in men is found at a later age (Fig. 1) and at a more advanced stage (Fig. 5), with about a 25% higher rate of regional metastases and a 100% higher rate of distant metastases (Fig. 5), supporting the notion that in women it is diagnosed earlier and at a much less advanced stage than it is in men, resulting in half the cancer mortality of men.

FNA AND OTHER TESTS

During the three decades during which the incidence and mortality rates of thyroid cancer have been changing, major shifts in diagnostic and therapeutic paradigms have also occurred: in the early 1970s, FNA of thyroid nodules was introduced and near-total thyroidectomy and ^{131}I ablation became more commonplace. These changing paradigms, which identify tumors earlier in their course and subject them to more aggressive treatment than had been the case previously, undoubtedly account for some of the changes seen during this period.

Contemporary use of Ultrasound and FNA. FNA has become widely accepted as the first-line test to diagnose cancer in thyroid nodules *(38,39)*,

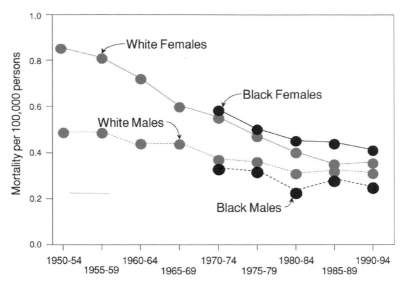

Fig. 4. Tumor mortality rates according to gender and race between 1950 and 1994. [Data from the SEER database *(37)*.

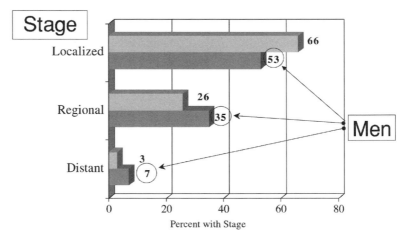

Fig. 5. Gender differences in tumor stage at the time of diagnosis 1973–1996. [Data from the SEER database *(37)*.]

mainly because of its high diagnostic accuracy. In one large study *(40)*, for example, of 1127 ultrasound-guided FNAs, the false-negative rate was 0%, the false-positive rate was 1.5%, the sensitivity was 100%, the specificity was 66.7%, the positive predictive value was 87.4%, and the negative predictive value was 100%. Global accuracy was 89.9%. The authors of this study compared their data with ten other series in which more than 100 ultrasound-guided FNAs were done on 12,961 patients with thyroid nodules, 2110 (16%) of when underwent surgery. The range of unsatisfactory cytology specimens ranged from 0.7 to 15%, averaging almost 5%. About 4% of the entire group had thyroid cancer. The sensitivity ranged from 87 to 100% and the specificity from 40.9 to 100%. This and many recent studies *(41)* show that ultrasound-guided FNA is clearly the best test to identify malignancy in a thyroid nodule. Nonetheless, there is wide variation in its use among different physician in the United States and Europe.

Approaches to Diagnosis of a Thyroid Nodule by Different Physician Groups. In a recent study *(42)* of 5583 patients who underwent surgery for thyroid cancer in 1500 hospitals in the United States, only 53% had thyroid FNA prior to surgery, and 7% had biopsy of a malignant cervical lymph node. Thus 40% of the patients underwent surgery for thyroid malignancy without benefit of FNA. In another study *(43)* however, of clinical members of the American Thyroid Association who responded to a questionnaire concerning a theoretical case of a 42-yr-old woman who had a solitary 3-cm nodule with no suggestion of malignancy, 87% opted for FNA of the nodule guided by palpation; moreover, when clinical features suggested malignancy, 50% disregarded FNA and referred the patient to surgery. Most euthyroid patients with a malignant thyroid nodule are asymptomatic without clinical evidence of malignancy; however, when the pretest probability of thyroid cancer is very high (for example, rapid growth of a nodule, or a nodule larger than 4 cm or with evidence of invasion, vocal cord paralysis, or large cervical lymph nodes), the likelihood of thyroid cancer is so great that a nondiagnostic FNA is probably a false-negative test *(44)*. This study shows that North American endocrinologists rely heavily on FNA after using their clinical judgment, employing scintigraphy, ultrasonography, and calcitonin levels less often than do european Endocrinologists in evaluating a thyroid nodule *(45)*.

DELAY IN DIAGNOSIS

Primary care physicians may manage thyroid nodules differently than do endocrinologists. For example, one study *(46)* of 70 patients independently reviewed by two endocrinologists found 87% concordance in diagnosis and 93% agreement in management between the two; however, only 25% of the patients targeted for surgery by the referring physician required it according to the endocrinologists' evaluations. Of greater concern, six patients (almost 10% of the group) not targeted for surgery by the referring physicians were sent to surgery by the endocrinologists; half of these patients had papillary cancer. Because primary care physicians used thyroid hormone suppression of the nodules in some cases, a practice no longer considered valid by most authorities *(38,39)*, 30% of the patients had a 12-mo or longer delay in diagnosis before referral to an endocrinologist, which has important consequences.

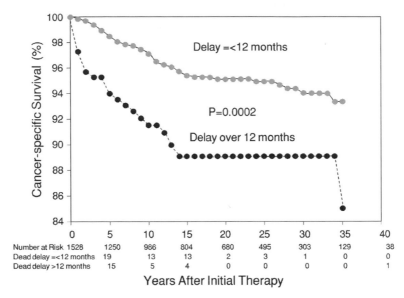

Fig. 6. Effects of delay in diagnosis of thyroid cancer on cancer deaths and persistent disease in patients with papillary and follicular thyroid cancer. (Data from ref. 9.)

We found the median time from the first manifestation of thyroid cancer—nearly always a neck mass—to initial therapy was 4 mo in patients who survived and 18 mo in those who died of cancer ($p < 0.001$) *(9)*. The 30-yr cancer mortality rates about doubled when therapy was delayed longer than a year (Fig. 6, 13% vs 6%, $p < 0001$) *(9)*. The greatest difference in outcome was in the first 15 yr after treatment (Fig. 6) *(9)*. Moreover, the TNM stage was more advanced when there was a delay of longer than 12 mo, with more than twice the frequency of distant metastases at the time of diagnosis (Table 2) *(9)*. In another study *(47)*, when completion thyroidectomy was delayed more than 6 mo, mortality rates were significantly higher than when it was done within 6 mo of initial surgery.

MORBIDITY AND MORTALITY

Despite low death rates, recurrence rates for thyroid cancer are very high, and many patients survive for decades with their tumor before succumbing to it. Analyses that only consider death as an endpoint thus fail to recognize the striking impact that tumor recurrence has on a person's life, especially the lingering effects of distant metastases that profoundly affect the quality of life, often for decades.

Causes of Death from Thyroid Cancer

Most patients who succumb to thyroid cancer die either from pulmonary metastases or local invasion of tumor. One large study *(48)* found a single cause

Table 2
Tumor Stage Relative to Time of Diagnosis [a]

Time to treatment	Stage 1	Stage 2	Stage 3	Stage 4	Total
≤12 months	802 (63%)	367 (29%)	89 (7%)	12 (1%)	1270 (100%)
>12 months	161 62%	63 (24%)	29 (11%)	5 (2%)	258 (100%)
Total	963 (63%)	430 (28%)	118 (8%)	17 (1%)	1528 (100%)

[a]Tumor stage in patients in whom diagnosis was delayed longer than 1 yr compared with those in whom the diagnosis was made within 12 mo of the presenting manifestations of papillary or follicular thyroid carcinoma.
Data from ref. 9.

of death in 106 fatal cases. The most common was respiratory insufficiency owing to lung metastases (43%), followed in frequency by circulatory failure owing to vena cava obstruction by extensive mediastinal or sternal metastases (15%) and massive hemorrhage (15%) or airway obstruction from local tumor. A search for pulmonary metastases or residual disease in the neck is thus a critical aspect of management after initial surgery.

PAPILLARY AND FOLLICULAR THYROID CANCER

Diagnosis

Most thyroid cancers are manifest by a lump in the neck. After obtaining a history that includes queries about familial thyroid cancer and exposure to radiation, FNA should be done immediately in a euthyroid patient. A history of head or neck radiation is important, but only 30% of such patients develop palpable thyroid nodules, about one-third of which are malignant (49). A family history of thyroid cancer should raise great suspicion. Nonetheless, evaluation of familial or radiation-induced tumors is similar to that of sporadically occurring nodules.

In the past, thyroid cancers were often diagnosed at a late stage when the tumor was large and invasive (50). Now more are identified at an earlier stage by FNA of asymptomatic small nodules—usually in the range of 2 cm—found on routine neck exam or discovered serendipitously with cervical imaging studies done for other reasons (20). A few come to attention as the result of pain, hoarseness, dysphagia or hemoptysis, or other signs of tissue infiltration or by rapid tumor growth, findings typically associated with a high probability of cancer (44) and higher than usual mortality rates (9). Sometimes palpably enlarged cervical lymph nodes are the only clue to the diagnosis.

FNA should be the first test done in a euthyroid patient, whether it is a single nodule or one of several in a multinodular goiter (38). Imaging studies are too nonspecific to be used as the first test. FNA identifies papillary cancer in nearly 100% of the cases; however, follicular and Hürthle cell cancers often cannot be differentiated from their benign counterparts by FNA or by large-needle aspiration or cutting-needle biopsies, which yield results similar to those of FNA but cause more complications *(38)*. Cytology showing sheets of normal or atypical follicular or Hürthle cells are often simply designated as follicular or Hürthle cell neoplasms because their malignant character cannot be determined until the final histologic sections are studied, and even then there may be difficulty separating malignant and benign tumors *(38)*. Patients with such cytology results should undergo a thyroid ^{123}I scan to eliminate hot nodules that are usually benign; the other nodules should be subjected to hemithyroidectomy. About 20% of such lesions are malignant and often require completion thyroidectomy, especially if they show vascular or complete tumor capsular invasion or are larger than 4 cm and completely encapsulated but with minimal capsular invasion and no vascular invasion *(39)*.

EARLY DIAGNOSIS

Tumor staging predicts tumor recurrence and mortality *(1)*. *Clinical staging systems*, however, combining *age* and tumor stage, do not predict tumor recurrence (*see* Mortality and Recurrence Rates Section below). Compared with adults, children typically have more advanced tumor stage at diagnosis; although their mortality rates are low, recurrence rates (including distant metastases) are higher than those in adults (Fig. 7) *(9)*; thus near-total thyroidectomy and ^{131}I ablation are usually preferred therapy for children. Late recurrences, including lung metastases, are a matter of record for papillary and follicular cancer *(1)*. Most are cases of persistent disease (often in children) that in the past fell below the detection limits of our tests, sometimes for decades. Now lung metastases, especially in children and young adults with high serum Tg levels and negative diagnostic whole-body scans (DxWBS), are often identified on posttreatment whole-body scans (RxWBS) after 100 mCi of [131]I *(1)*. A multicenter study found that metastases were detected by a serum Tg above 2 ng/mL in response to recombinant human TSH (rhTSH) administration. Treating lung metastases early in their course gives the best outcome.

Early Diagnosis of Lung Metastases. Schlumberger *(51)* reported that complete remission and 10-yr survival rates were, respectively, 96 and 100% when the metastases were detected by high Tg and positive RxWBS alone, 83 and 91% when the diagnosis was apparent on [131]I DxWBS, and 53 and 63% when micronodules were seen on chest x-ray. Discovering lung metastases only by high Tg and positive RxWBS is not uncommon. We identified *(1)* occult lung metastases by elevated serum Tg levels in 11 of 89 consecutive patients, 9 (75%) of which were seen only on RxWBS. Tumor bulk ranks second only to patient age as a predictor of death from thyroid cancer *(52)*, making a strong argument for early treatment of lung metastases. Early detection increases the likelihood that tumor will concentrate [131]I. One study *(52)* found ^{131}I uptake in 95% of

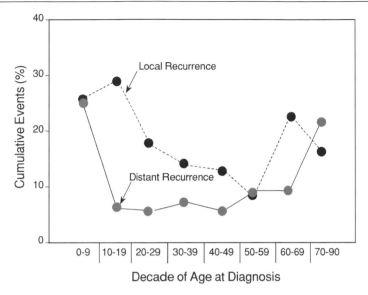

Fig. 7. Patient age at the time of diagnosis has an important impact upon subsequent tumor recurrence. (Data from ref. *9*.)

patients with pulmonary metastases and a normal chest x-ray, 88% of those with micronodular disease, and 37% of those with macronodular disease *(52)*. Complete responses to treatment occur in 82% of patients with lung or bone metastases and a normal radiograph compared with 15% of those with an abnormal radiograph *(52)*.

Mortality and Recurrence Rates

Mortality rates of differentiated thyroid cancer are low, less than 10% over three decades in our study *(9)*; however, recurrence rates were 30%, and distant metastases or serious local recurrences often occurred years after initial therapy (Fig. 8) *(9,20)*. Prognosis varies greatly, however, among subsets of patients.

PATIENT AGE AT TIME OF DIAGNOSIS

Age over 40 yr at the time of diagnosis is among the most important adverse prognostic factors that predict death from thyroid cancer. Mortality rates become progressively worse with advancing age, increasing at a particularly steep rate after age 60 yr (Fig. 1) *(9,20)*. The best outcomes are in younger patients whose tumors concentrate [131]I *(53–55)*.

PROGNOSIS IN CHILDREN

Survival rates are most favorable in children, although their tumors at diagnosis are typically more advanced, with more local and distant metastases than those in adults *(53,55–57)*. However, tumor recurrence rates over several decades

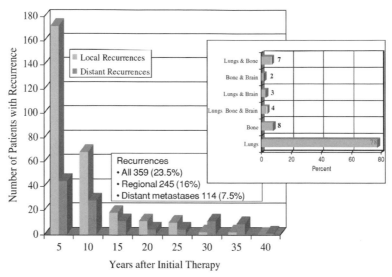

Fig. 8. Recurrence of differentiated thyroid cancer according to time after initial therapy. (Data from ref. 9.)

are about 40% in children, compared with 20% in adults (9,55); the rate of pulmonary metastases in children is over 20% in some series, almost twice that in adults (9,20,56). Prognosis for survival is nonetheless excellent in children with or without a history of irradiation, except among those under age 10 yr who have high mortality rates (53–55), which may be the reason that survival rates are lower among children with thyroid cancer compared with normal children (58).

PATIENT GENDER

Cancer-specific mortality rates in men are about twice those in women (Fig. 2), because at diagnosis men are older and have more advanced tumor stage compared with women (Figs. 2 and 3).

TUMOR HISTOLOGY

Outcome is less favorable with follicular cancer than it is with papillary cancer. Among 9744 patients whose average age was about 47 yr, 10-yr mortality rates were 29% for follicular and 12% for papillary cancer (20). In our study (9), 30-yr cancer-specific mortality rates for slightly younger patients were 5% for papillary and 13% for follicular cancer. Ten-year mortality rates for follicular cancer range from about 10% (59), to 50%, depending on the degree of tumor vascular and capsular invasion and the patient's age (20,59–61). Follicular cancer is more likely to have distant metastases at the time of diagnosis than is papillary cancer, which in our series occurred in 2.2% of the former and 5.3% of the latter (9). Tumor recurrence in distant sites is more frequent with follicular than papillary cancers, particularly with highly invasive tumors, or primary lesions larger than 4.5 cm, and in Hürthle cell cancers *(20,60,62,63)*. Marked cellular atypia or frank anaplastic transformation is also associated with a poor prognosis. Other tumor features that predict mortality are tumor size greater than 1 cm *(9)*, tumor penetrating the thyroid capsule *(9)*, vascular invasion [both follicular and papillary cancers *(64)*] and lymph node *(9)* or distant metastases *(20)*, and certain histologic variants, including Hürthle cell cancers, papillary tall cell or columnar cancers, and insular cancers *(1)*.

CLINICAL STAGING SYSTEMS THAT PREDICT PROGNOSIS

Clinical staging systems should not be confused with tumor staging such as that derived from the TNM (tumor, node, metastases) grading system. Clinical staging systems, which generally have been derived from multivariate analyses of large patient cohorts studied retrospectively, have been devised to predict thyroid cancer mortality rates. Unfortunately, most predict outcome using tumor and age (not therapy) and in so doing fail to predict recurrence rates or the impact of treatment. Using such a system, most patients in our study *(9)* are categorized as clinical stage 1, in which the largest number of tumor recurrences (75%) and cancer deaths (47%) occurred (Fig. 9). Providing minimal therapy (lobectomy without ^{131}I) for patients in clinical groups 1 and 2 fails to treat a large number of patients adequately, who subsequently develop tumor recurrences and die of their disease.

Impact of Therapy

Therapy generally comprises surgery, ^{131}I therapy, and TSH suppression with thyroid hormone. There are, however, differing opinions about the three principal aspects of treatment.

SURGERY

In our view, a preoperative diagnosis of papillary or follicular thyroid cancer *(1,39)* warrants near total or total thyroidectomy, with modified neck dissection for positive lateral neck nodes, and completion thyroidectomy for any patient with a tumor larger than 1 cm, or for tumor that is invading the thyroid capsule, that is incompletely resected, or that has recurred *(47)*. Although most *(39,47,65,66)* believe that this is optimal therapy when the diagnosis of papillary or follicular cancer is known preoperatively, a few *(67,68)* believe lobectomy alone is sufficient therapy for low-risk patients, variously defined as having TNM tumor stage 1 (size < 1 cm) or stage 2 (size 1–4) without metastases, invasion, or multifocality or TNM clinical stage 1 or 2 (Fig. 9), an opinion based on mortality rates alone that does not take into account the large number of recurrences and cancer deaths in patients classified as low risk (Figs. 7 and 9). A study *(47)* of 131 patients with differentiated thyroid cancer in which comple-

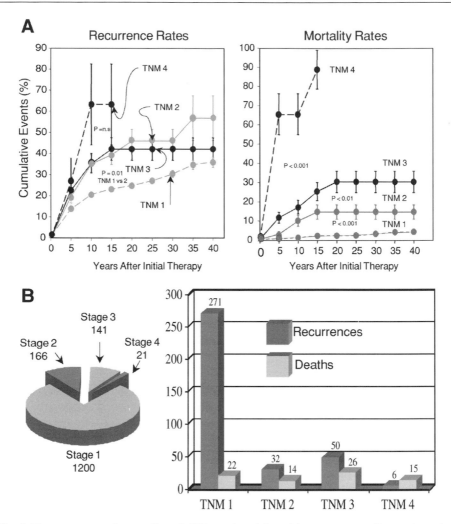

Fig. 9. Recurrence and mortality of differentiated thyroid cancer according to American Joint Committee on Cancer tumor stage applied to our patient cohort *(9).* TNM, pathologic grade of the tumor, node, and metastases. T is primary tumor: T1, <1 cm; T2, >1cm to 4 cm; T3, >4 cm; T4, extension beyond thyroid capsule. N is regional lymph nodes: N1, regional lymph node metastases (cervical and upper mediastinal nodes). M is distant metastases: M0, no distant metastases, M1, distant metastases. The clinical staging system is derived from the following: for patients under age 45 yr, stage 1 = M0, stage 2 = M1 (no stage 3 or 4); for patients aged 45 yr and older, stage 1 = T1, stage 2 = T2–3, stage 3 = T4 or N1, and stage 4 = M1. (**A**) Cumulative rates. This clinical staging system results in good prediction of cumulative mortality rates (left) but poor prediction of recurrence rates (right). (**B**) number of rates. Using this clinical staging system, most patients are categorized as stage 1 or 2 (pie chart), and most cancer deaths and recurrences occur in stage 1 and 2 patients.

tion thyroidectomy was done within 6 mo of the initial therapy for tumor stage more than T1 (i.e., > 1 cm, $n = 116$) or suspicion of persistent tumor ($n = 13$) or incompletely resected tumor ($n = 2$) found significantly longer survival than in patients in whom this was not done. Cox analysis of 1501 patients in our series showed that surgery more extensive than lobectomy was an independent variable that favorably affected cancer recurrence [hazard ratio (HR) 0.7, $p = 0.0001$)] and cancer mortality (HR 0.5, $p = 0.0001$).

RADIOIODINE (^{131}I) REMNANT ABLATION

Because most surgeons find it nearly impossible to remove all thyroid tissue routinely at surgery, uptake of ^{131}I is almost always seen in the thyroid bed postoperatively, which must be ablated before ^{131}I will optimally concentrate in metastatic deposits (69,70). Although there continues to be debate concerning the use of ^{131}I to ablate uptake in the thyroid bed after near-total thyroidectomy (71,72), there are several compelling reasons to do it. First, a thyroid remnant can obscure ^{131}I uptake in cervical or lung metastases (69,70). Second, high serum levels of TSH, which are necessary to enhance tumor ^{131}I uptake, cannot be achieved with a large thyroid remnant (73). Third, serum Tg is most sensitive in detecting cancer when measured during hypothyroidism or with rhTSH stimulation after thyroid bed uptake has been ablated (74). Fourth, there is evidence that recurrence and cancer mortality rates are lower after total thyroid ablation.

Recurrence after ^{131}I Ablation. Postoperative ^{131}I remnant ablation is done when the tumor has a potential for recurrence (72). A large number of studies demonstrate decreased recurrence and disease-specific mortality rates from differentiated thyroid cancer attributable to ^{131}I therapy (9,72,75–80). The lowest incidence of pulmonary metastases occurs after total thyroidectomy and ^{131}I. In one study, for example, recurrences in the form of pulmonary metastases, analyzed as a function of initial therapy for differentiated thyroid cancer, were reported to be as follows: thyroidectomy plus ^{131}I (ablation dose of 100 mCi), 1.3%; thyroidectomy alone, 3%; partial thyroidectomy plus ^{131}I, 5%; and partial thyroidectomy alone 11% (81). Cox analysis of 1501 patients in our series (9) showed that thyroid ^{131}I remnant ablation independently reduced cancer recurrence (HR 0.8, $p = 0.016$), the appearance of distant metastases (HR 0.6, $p = 0.002$), and cancer mortality (HR 0.5, $p = 0.0001$). The effect was greatest when ^{131}I was given after total or near-total thyroidectomy and thyroid hormone, after which 40-yr recurrence rates were lowest (23%) compared with subtotal thyroidectomy and ^{131}I (30%), or subtotal thyroidectomy and thyroid hormone therapy (36%) and total or near-total thyroidectomy and thyroid hormone therapy (43%) (1).

THYROID HORMONE SUPPRESSION OF TSH

Differentiated thyroid cancers contain TSH receptors, which when stimulated promote tumor growth and uptake of iodine. Thyroid hormone therapy significantly reduces recurrence rates and cancer-specific mortality rates *(9,72)*; however, the thyroid hormone dosage that is required to do this remains debatable. A French study found that a constantly suppressed TSH (≤0.05 µU/mL) was associated with a longer relapse-free survival than when serum TSH levels were consistently 1 µU/mL or greater and that the degree of TSH suppression was an independent predictor of recurrence *(82)*. However, a prospective U.S. study of 617 patients found that disease stage, patient age, and ^{131}I therapy independently predicted disease progression, whereas the degree of TSH suppression did not *(83)*. As a practical matter, the most appropriate dose of thyroid hormone for most patients with differentiated thyroid cancer is that which reduces the serum concentration to just below the lower limit of the normal range for the assay being used, unless the patient has active disease, in which case the TSH should be maintained at 0.1 µU/mL or lower.

Follow-Up of Papillary and Follicular Thyroid Cancer

Performing a whole-body scan and measuring serum Tg is the standard of care in the follow-up of patients with differentiated thyroid cancer *(1,84)*, although DxWBS before ^{131}I therapy is usually unnecessary. The panel of experts that formulated the National Cancer Center guidelines for thyroid cancer could not reach consensus on recommending a DxWBS in lieu of RxWBS during evaluation *(39)*. A retrospective study *(85)* of 76 patients undergoing follow-up after initial thyroid ablation found that two consecutive negative DxWBSs had a greater likelihood of predicting relapse-free survival than did one such study; however, serum Tg was not measured under TSH stimulation, which is a considerably more sensitive test than DxWBS *(86,87)*. A study of 256 patients *(88)* found that a 2–5-mCi [131]I DxWBS performed 6 mo to 1 yr after thyroid ablation did not correlate with the serum Tg but only confirmed the completeness of thyroid ablation, suggesting that DxWBS is unnecessary in this setting; patients with a Tg level exceeding 10 ng/mL after TH withdrawal were given 100 mCi of ^{131}I followed by RxWBS. Likewise, the paradigm of using rhTSH-stimulated Tg alone during follow-up is as successful as using rhTSH-stimulated Tg and DxWBS together *(86,87)*.

MEDULLARY THYROID CANCER

MTC accounts for about 4% of all thyroid malignancies *(8)*. Sporadic MTC is more frequent in women, with a female/male ratio of 1.5:1, whereas familial MTC occurs with equal frequency in both sexes. Only about 10–20% of MTC cases occur as familial tumors; the others are sporadic and may occur at any age but usually are detected later in life than familial MTC. The median age, for instance, of patients with sporadic MTC in one large study was 51 yr, compared with 21 yr for those with familial tumors *(89)*. The diagnosis is made even earlier now with genetic testing.

Sporadic MTC

Ranging from large bulky tumors to microscopic lesions, sporadic and familial tumors are histologically similar except sporadic MTC is typically unilateral and not associated with other somatic lesions. A wider spectrum of abnormalities is encountered in familial cases, ranging from isolated hypertrophied C-cells to large bilateral multicentric tumors in the superior portions of the thyroid lobes. MTC is typically composed of fusiform or polygonal cells surrounded by irregular masses of amyloid and abundant collagen. About half have calcifications that occasionally appear as trabecular bone formation. Calcitonin and carcinoembryonic antigen usually can be demonstrated in the tumors and metastases.

Metastases of MTC

Cervical lymph node metastases occur early in the disease and can be seen with primary lesions as small as a few millimeters. Tumors larger than 1.5 cm are more likely to metastasize to distant sites, especially to lung, bone, and liver, but also to the central nervous system.

Tumor Calcitonin

Immunohistochemical staining for calcitonin not only serves to identify MTC, but its pattern may differentiate virulent from less aggressive tumors. In one study, for example, patients with primary tumors that showed intense homogeneous calcitonin staining were clinically well on follow-up, whereas those with patchy localization of calcitonin in their tumors either developed metastatic disease or died of cancer within 6 mo to 5 yr of initial surgery *(90)*.

Familial MTC

The genes responsible for familial MTC are in the pericentromeric region of chromosome 10 *(91)*. The C-cells, which arc normally located in the upper and middle thirds of the lateral thyroid lobes, initially undergo hyperplasia in the multiple endocrine neoplasia (MEN) 2 syndromes before developing into MTC.

Multiple Endocrine Neoplasia Type 2 Syndromes

MTC occurs in four settings, three of which are familial syndromes transmitted as autosomal dominant traits.

MULTIPLE ENDOCRINE NEOPLASIA TYPE 2A

This familial syndrome comprises bilateral MTC associated with hyperparathyroidism and bilateral pheochromocytoma and is always inherited as an autosomal dominant trait.

MULTIPLE ENDOCRINE NEOPLASIA TYPE 2B

The MEN-2B syndrome comprises bilateral MTC, bilateral pheochromocytoma, an abnormal phenotype with multiple mucosal ganglioneuromas, and musculoskeletal abnormalities. It may be transmitted as an autosomal dominant trait or as a sporadic entity and is characterized by ganglioneuromas of the tarsal plates and the anterior third of the tongue and lips and a marfanoid habitus. Ganglioneuromas that occur in the alimentary tract may be associated with constipation, diarrhea, and megacolon. The marfanoid characteristics include long limbs, hyperextensible joints, scoliosis, and anterior chest deformities, but not the ectopic lens or cardiovascular abnormalities seen in Marfan's syndrome *(92)*.

FAMILIAL NON-MEN MTC

Familial non-MEN MTC (FMTC), an autosomal dominant trait, causes bilateral MTC with no other endocrine tumors or somatic abnormalities *(93)*. It is the least common form of MTC and manifests at a later age than the other familial syndromes *(93)*. FMTC occurs without other endocrine tumors and is usually detected later, around age 40–50 yr, compared with an average age of 20–30 yr for MEN-2A when detected by screening affected kindreds with calcitonin tests.

Diagnosis of MTC

SPORADIC AND UNRECOGNIZED FAMILIAL TUMORS

Patients with sporadic or unrecognized familial MTC have one or more painless nodules in an otherwise normal thyroid gland, although some experience dysphagia and hoarseness. The presenting feature may be enlarged cervical lymph nodes or occasionally distant metastases, most commonly to the lung, followed in frequency by metastases to the liver, bone, and brain. About half the patients with sporadic MTC have cervical lymph node metastases at the time of diagnosis. The thyroid nodule is usually solid on echography and malignant on FNA and may be cold or warm on ^{123}I imaging. Radiographs may show dense, irregular calcifications of the primary tumor and cervical nodes and mediastinal widening caused by metastases. Plasma calcitonin measurement is helpful in the early diagnosis of C-cell hyperplasia (CCH) and MTC. Elevated basal plasma calcitonin levels, which are almost always found once the MTC becomes palpable, correlate directly with tumor mass *(89)*. Basal calcitonin often is not elevated by small tumors and is almost invariably normal in those with CCH; however, calcium-stimulated calcitonin levels may be abnormally high.

FNA. Recognizing MTC on FNA specimens is often difficult, but when the diagnosis is suspected, immunocytologic staining for calcitonin should be performed. As a practical matter, the cellular pleomorphism and lack of follicles usually prompt referral for surgical excision, even when the diagnosis is not made by FNA cytology.

FAMILIAL TUMORS

The abnormal phenotype of MEN-2B may lead to the diagnosis. In most cases the diagnosis is established by testing the index case, since MTC often is not apparent in the family history.

Genetic Testing. All first-degree relatives of any patient who tests positive for a MEN-2 or FMTC mutation should be screened. However, the sensitivity of genetic screening for MEN-2A offered by diagnostic laboratories that limit *RET* analysis to exons 10 and 11 is about 83% *(94)*. Genetic testing that includes *RET* analysis of exon 14 results in a more complete and accurate analysis, with a sensitivity of nearly 95% *(94)*. It is recommended that clinicians confirm the comprehensiveness of a laboratory's genetic screening approach for MEN-2A to ensure thoroughness of sample analysis.

Factors Affecting Prognosis

AGE AND TUMOR STAGE

The cancer-specific mortality rate of MTC is about 10–20% at 10 yr *(8,59)*; however, pheochromocytoma causes a large number of the deaths in those with familial syndromes *(95)*. The mortality rate is substantially worse with sporadic tumors or when metastases are found at the time of diagnosis, and with the MEN-2B phenotype, and among patients older than 50 yr. Patients with familial MTC operated on during the first decade of life generally have no evidence of residual tumor postoperatively *(89)*; however, persistent MTC occurs in about one-third of patients undergoing surgery in the second decade of life, thereafter gradually increasing until the seventh decade, when about two-thirds have persistent disease *(89)*. This is largely owing to the combined effects of advancing age and tumor stage, which are the most powerful prognostic factors predicting outcome *(96,97)*.

FAMILIAL MTC

Prognosis is best with FMTC and MEN-2A. Early detection and treatment has a profound impact on the clinical course of MTC. When nodal metastases are not present, for example, the 10-yr survival rates are nearly similar to those in unaffected subjects, but they fall to about 45% when nodal metastases are present *(89)*. Before 1970, MTC was usually diagnosed in the fifth or sixth decade. For the next 20 yr biologic markers assumed a preeminent role in diagnosis. With periodic calcitonin screening, affected members of MEN kindreds were usually identified in the second decade of life or earlier, when they usually had CCH or microscopic MTC confined to the thyroid *(98)*. Nonetheless, the results of long-term studies using this approach are somewhat disappointing. One study comparing calcitonin measurement with genetic testing found 14 young gene carriers (18% of the 80 known gene carriers in the study) who had normal plasma calcitonin levels, 8 of whom had undergone thyroidectomy at the time their genetic defect was identified and were found to have foci of MTC *(99)*. Another study *(100)* reported long-term follow-up of 22 children in whom biologic screening studies were routinely performed once a year and thyroidectomy was recommended for any elevation in serum calcitonin levels. MTC developed in 17 children (77%), whereas only 5 had CCH. Thirteen of the 17 with MTC had macroscopic tumor, and recurrent disease developed in 4 of the children (24%) *(100)*.

Genotypes. There is growing awareness that genotypes may permit prognostication. In one study *(101)*, for example, *RET* mutations in exons 10, 11, 13, and 14 were associated, respectively, with different median ages at diagnosis: 38, 27, 52, and 62 yr ($p = 0.003$). Age differences became even more evident when the mutations were grouped by cysteine codons (exons 10 and 11 vs. exons 13 and 14) with median ages, respectively, of 30 and 56 yr ($p = 0.001$). Three risk groups were devised according to genotype. The high-risk group (codons 634 and 618) had the youngest ages of 3 and 7 yr at diagnosis. The intermediate-risk group (codons 790, 620, and 611) had ages of 12, 34, and 42 yr. A low-risk group (codons 768 and 804) had ages of 47 and 60 yr, respectively *(101)*, allowing for a more individualized approach to the timing and extent of prophylactic surgery. However, other studies describe unexpected differences in prognosis among patients with the same *RET* mutation *(102)*.

Treatment of MTC

Surgery offers the only chance for a cure and should be performed as soon as the disease is detected *(96,97)*. However, pheochromocytoma must be rigorously searched for and excised before thyroidectomy is performed. The treatment of MTC confined to the neck is total thyroidectomy because the disease is often bilateral, even with a negative family history, since patients are often unsuspected members of affected MEN-2 kindreds *(96,97)*. All patients with a palpable MTC or clinically occult disease that is visible on cut section of the thyroid should undergo routine dissection of lymph nodes in the central neck compartment because nodal metastases occur early and adversely influence survival. The lateral cervical lymph nodes should be dissected when they contain tumor, but radical neck dissection is not recommended unless the jugular vein, accessory nerve, or sternocleidomastoid muscle is invaded by tumor *(103)*. Multivariate analysis *(104)* shows that the best prognosis occurs in young patients undergoing total thyroidectomy and neck dissection. External beam radiotherapy (XRT) may significantly reduce local relapse in patients with limited nodal disease. In one study *(105)* there was no difference in local/regional relapse-free rates between patients receiving XRT and those that did not, but in 40 high-risk patients (microscopic residual disease, extraglandular invasion, or lymph node involvement), the local/regional relapse free rate was 86% at 10 yr with postoperative XRT (25 patients) and 52% for those with no postoperative XRT ($p = 0.049$). Some therefore advise external beam radiation in patients at high risk of local/regional relapse to optimize local/regional tumor control *(105)*.

TREATMENT OF FAMILIAL MTC

After 1993, when *RET* mutations were identified in hereditary MTC, surgeons had the opportunity to operate prophylactically on patients before MTC became manifest. Nonetheless, microscopic or grossly evident MTC is often present in the excised thyroid glands, and a few are metastatic to regional lymph nodes *(106)*. Almost all patients are biochemically cured with prophylactic total thyroidectomy, which can be performed safely at selected centers *(103)*. Prophylactic total thyroidectomy—done by an experienced surgeon—is recommended at age 6 yr for patients who test genetically positive for MEN 2A *(103,107)*. Thyroidectomy should be done at an even earlier age for children who test positive for MEN-2B, because its behavior is so aggressive *(108,109)*. It is recommended that central neck lymph node dissection be included when calcitonin levels are elevated or if patients are older than 10 yr *(103)*.

Delay in Diagnosis. One study found that without genetic testing, even when the mean age at the time of thyroidectomy was about 10 yr, a significant number of patients (21%) with MEN-2A or -2B developed persistent or recurrent MTC over a follow-up of about a decade *(108)*.

Follow-Up of MTC

Persistent or recurrent MTC is typically manifest by high postoperative calcitonin levels, which occurs commonly although survival is usually prolonged. A French study, for example, reported that 57% of 899 patients were not cured (57%), but that survival was 80% at 5 yr and 70% at 10 yr *(96)*. Reoperation in appropriately selected patients is thus appropriate because it is the only treatment that may reduce calcitonin levels and often results in excellent local disease control. Although the combined use of ^{111}In-octreotide and [99m]Tc (V) DMSA is the most sensitive imaging study for localized MTC, the combined use of computed tomography (CT) and magnetic resonance imaging (MRI) with radionuclide imaging methods may detect most metastatic tumor foci *(110)*. There is no curative therapy for widely metastatic disease, but neck microdissections may normalize calcitonin levels when persistent MTC is confined to regional lymph nodes. Improved results have been reported in recent years with the surgical management of persistent MTC, mainly through better preoperative selection of patients with routine laparoscopic liver examination or hepatic angiography *(111)* to identify hepatic metastases in patients with normal CT and MRI images *(112)*. Patients with widely metastatic MTC often live for years, but many develop symptoms from disease progression that may respond to palliative resection that removes discrete symptomatic lesions to provide symptomatic relief *(113)*.

ANAPLASTIC THYROID CANCER

Diagnosis

The diagnosis of malignancy is usually quite evident with anaplastic thyroid cancer because of the ominous symptoms and physical findings suggesting an aggressive and invasive tumor. The main diagnostic problems are differentiating

ATC from less aggressive undifferentiated thyroid tumors and delineating the extent of cervical disease.

CLINICAL PRESENTATION

ATC almost always causes a highly symptomatic neck mass that is rapidly enlarging in about two-thirds and causing symptoms of tracheal compression and invasion in one-third *(114,115)*. About one-third of patients have a history of a preexisting goiter, and about half have dyspnea at the time of diagnosis. Symptoms often appear abruptly, having been present for less than 3 mo in about half the patients *(115)*. Rapid tumor growth often causes neck pain that may mimic subacute thyroiditis, probably because of tumor necrosis and invasion of neck tissues. Hoarseness and cough with systemic symptoms such as fever or weight loss are usually present. Most patients have normal thyroid function, although thyrotoxicosis rarely occurs, probably from rapid thyroid tissue necrosis releasing thyroid hormone *(24)*.

On examination the tumor is typically hard, poorly circumscribed and fixed to surrounding structures. About two-thirds have a multinodular goiter *(115)*, another third have an isolated thyroid nodule, and only a few have diffuse thyromegaly. ATC is characteristically quite large and may be associated with palpable cervical lymph nodes. In one large series, about 80% were larger than 5 cm and half the patients had palpably enlarged cervical lymph nodes *(115)*. One-third of the patients in this same series had vocal cord paralysis *(115)*. Stridor that occurs when the patient's neck is extended heralds serious airway obstruction and should raise the question of elective tracheostomy to protect the airway. The tumor may cause a superior mediastinal syndrome with venous distention and edema of the face, arms, and neck.

FNA and Other Tests. Although a diagnosis of malignancy is almost always possible by thyroid FNA, anaplastic ATC may be difficult to distinguish from thyroid lymphoma, MTC, and other forms of undifferentiated thyroid cancer or cancers metastatic to the thyroid. Nonetheless, the giant and spindle cell patterns of anaplastic thyroid cancer usually predominate, sometimes with multinucleated giant cells, suggesting the correct diagnosis. MTC often shows a spindle cell population and usually can be identified by FNA cytology that may stain for amyloid or calcitonin *(24)*. Non-Hodgkin's thyroid lymphoma can be identified by FNA, usually by its small cells, but open biopsy and histochemical staining are necessary to differentiate it from ATC, especially when the lymphoma is composed of large cells. Poorly differentiated "insular" thyroid cancer may be mistaken for ATC. When diagnosed by FNA, open biopsy and immunohistochemical staining may be necessary confirmation of ATC.

Prognostic Factors

Although the prognosis of ATC is very poor, several large studies suggest that the patient's age and tumor stage are the two most important variables influencing prognosis; the younger the patient and the lower the tumor stage, the longer the survival *(114)*. In one study *(114)*, mean survival was 8.1 mo if the disease was confined to the neck compared with 3.3 mo when it was metastatic outside the neck. Relatively favorable prognostic features are unilateral tumors smaller than 5 cm without invasion of adjacent tissue or cervical nodal involvement *(115)*.

Mortality Rates

ATC has a dismal prognosis. In 1961, Woolner and associates *(50)* reported that 61% of 119 patients with ATC were dead within 6 mo and 77% had died within a year of diagnosis. Almost 30 yr later, another large study *(114)* reported a mean survival of 7 mo in patients with ATC. Only 8% (20 of 240 patients) from both series survived longer than a year. Median survival in a later series was only 4 mo *(115)*, which is within the 4–6 mo median survival range reported in most series in the past two decades *(24)*. Lymphomas and MTC that histologically resemble ATC have a much better prognosis and must be differentiated from ATC by immunohistochemical studies.

Treatment of Anaplastic Thyroid Cancer

THYROID SURGERY

Thyroidectomy with excision of the involved neck tissues and cervical lymph nodes should be done if possible, without resorting to radical surgery. In one large series *(115)*, 41% of the patients had surgical resection—mostly total lobectomy with subtotal resection of the contralateral lobe—in an attempt to cure the patient, and in another series *(114)*, about 45% of the patients underwent total thyroidectomy. However, in neither series did the extent of surgery influence the survival rate. The main reason to attempt resection of the neck mass is to preserve the airway. Total thyroidectomy and radical neck dissection result in an increased complication rate without conferring a clear advantage over a more conservative approach.

Airway Management. Tumor may compromise the airway by either compression, displacement, or infiltration of the malignancy. Management involves surgical decompression of the airway when there is compression or displacement, and tracheostomy with a long stomal tube when the airway is infiltrated with tumor. Many patients require tracheostomy at some time in the course of their disease, mainly to relieve airway obstruction but also as a precautionary measure before initiating external radiation therapy. External irradiation may cause tumor edema that acutely exacerbates airway obstruction. More than half the patients in one large series required tracheostomy during the course of their disease *(115)*.

MEDICAL THERAPY

External Radiotherapy. After treatment with surgery and XRT, fewer than 5% of patients with ATC survive for 5 yr, although survivors who are disease-free at 2 yr may live for longer periods *(24)*. Because conventional XRT fails to eradicate local disease, larger radiation doses given at closer intervals have been given with limited success in controlling local disease, but the toxicity is very high, resulting in severe esophagitis and dysphagia, spinal cord necrosis, and death *(116,117)*.

Chemotherapy. There is no consensus regarding the selection of chemotherapeutic agents for patients with ATC, mainly because this tumor is so resistant to chemotherapy. None provides clearly superior therapeutic efficacy, and the selection is often based as much on the side-effect profiles of the drugs as the potential efficacy. When there is a response to doxorubicin, pulmonary metastases most frequently respond to therapy, followed by bone metastases and local tumor growth; however, it may not control local disease *(24)*. Several studies *(118–120)* report that combinations of intense XRT, chemotherapy, and tumor debulking surgery marginally improve local disease recurrence and that a few patients live as long as several years after treatment. However, this therapy may be poorly tolerated and associated with severe side effects.

THYROID LYMPHOMA

Primary thyroid lymphoma is an uncommon but life-threatening disorder that often poses a major diagnostic dilemma because it is encountered so infrequently. Typically it arises in the setting of Hashimoto's thyroiditis, sometimes in patients with long-standing hypothyroidism. The neoplasm may go unrecognized for several months until the patient develops airway obstruction symptoms, and when it does become apparent that it is a malignancy, an erroneous diagnosis of ATC is sometimes made. It is important to identify the tumor as a thyroid lymphoma since its prognosis is much better than that of ATC. Nevertheless, many patients continue to die from this tumor because the diagnosis is often delayed, which is challenging because when it is diagnosed at an early stage it has an excellent prognosis.

Diagnosis

Contrary to systemic lymphomas, female preponderance is the rule for thyroid lymphoma *(29)* because it originates from active lymphoid cells in chronic lymphocytic thyroiditis, which occurs more often in women. Among 812 patients with thyroid lymphoma reported in 16 large series *(29)*, females outnumbered males by almost 3:1, and the mean age was 62.7 yr; however, the female-to-male ratio under age 60 was 1.5:1 compared with 5:1 over age 60 *(29)*. Although this is a disease of older women, about one-third of 568 patients in one review *(29)* were under age 60 yr.

CLINICAL PRESENTATION

History. A close association exists between thyroid lymphoma and Hashimoto's thyroiditis. The relative risk of thyroid lymphoma among people with Hashimoto's thyroiditis living in Sweden was 67-fold greater than expected, after an average follow-up of 8.5 yr *(121)*. Another study *(122)* found that the frequency of thyroid lymphoma among 5592 women aged 25 yr or older with chronic thyroiditis living in Japan was increased 80-fold. The interval between the diagnosis of chronic thyroiditis and thyroid lymphoma averaged 9.2 yr, but was as short as 3.5 yr in a few. Most patients have symptoms caused by a rapidly expanding goiter, which was present for a year or more in only 16% of 556 patients reported in nine large studies *(29)*. Symptoms typically exist for less than 5 mo *(29)*, contrasting sharply with the indolent course of Hashimoto's thyroiditis, and are caused by tumor pressing on and growing into vital neck organs, particularly the trachea, laryngeal nerve, esophagus, and neck muscles. The most common complaints among 281 patients reported in nine large studies *(29)* were hoarseness (21%), dysphagia, dyspnea and stridor (19%), a sensation of pressure in the neck (5%), and neck pain (5%). These important warning signs of extrathyroidal tumor extension should alert the clinician to the malignant nature of the goiter *(29)*. Stridor and hoarseness often occur together and are almost invariably a sign of laryngeal nerve paralysis. Symptoms of invasion, particularly dyspnea and dysphagia, are ominous and portend a poor outcome.

Physical Examination. On examination, there may be only an enlarged thyroid lobe or a discrete nodule or diffuse thyromegaly. The goiter is generally firm, nontender, and fixed to adjacent tissues, a sign that tumor is invading neck structures. Other signs of extrathyroidal spread include ill-defined thyroid borders with extension laterally or retrosternally. Large (>2 cm), nontender matted cervical lymph nodes are found in up to half the patients *(29)*. The chest roentgenogram may show retrosternal involvement or mediastinal widening, although lymph nodes elsewhere are seldom enlarged.

LABORATORY STUDIES

Almost all patients have clinical or histologic evidence of lymphocytic thyroiditis at the time lymphoma is diagnosed *(29)*. Antithyroglobulin and antimicrosomal antibodies were found in almost 75% of 539 patients in ten large series *(29)*, 83% of whom had histologic evidence of Hashimoto's thyroiditis. Despite these findings, few patients at the time of diagnosis have overt hypothyroidism—less than 10% of 366 patients from seven large studies *(29)*—most being euthyroid or only mildly hypothyroid with minimal TSH elevation and normal thyroid hormone levels, whereas thyrotoxicosis is very uncommon. Goiter that suddenly enlarges during long-term thyroxine therapy is an important clue to the diagnosis of lymphoma.

FNA AND OTHER TESTS

FNA should be considered in patients with Hashimoto's thyroiditis who have discrete cold thyroid nodules or diffuse or multinodular goiters with the features

Table 3
Indications for Fine-Needle Aspiration or Open
Surgical Biopsy in Patients Suspected of Having
Thyroid Lymphoma

Thyroid mass with
  • Rapid enlargement
  • Hoarseness
  • Laryngeal paralysis
  • Dysphagia
  • Stridor
  • Dyspnea
  • Pain
Hashimoto's thyroiditis
  • Hypofunctional (cold) nodule
  • Hypofunctional area on scan without nodule
  • Enlargement despite thyroid hormone therapy
  • Associated with monoclonal gammopathy

Adapted from ref. 29.

summarized in Table 3 (29). A diagnosis of lymphoma may be established by FNA cytology or by open surgical biopsy, but, regardless of the technique, good-quality smears or tissues must be obtained in sufficient quantity to perform routine studies and specific immunohistochemical stains.

Staging Tests. Although most practitioners base disease stage on surgical specimens, this is not the best approach (123). Accurate staging is important because radiation alone is often used for thyroid lymphoma, although there is little agreement regarding an optimal staging evaluation (29). Patients should have a complete blood count, blood chemistries, chest roentgenogram, and studies to investigate the extent of local disease, including regional lymph node involvement and tumor extension into neck structures and disease in the chest and abdomen. Thyroid ultrasonography may be helpful, but CT or MRI of the neck, chest, and abdomen should be done. Bone marrow examination is not necessary in every patient. One group (124) performed bone marrow examinations in most of their patients, but almost none were positive. Other studies also suggest that almost no patients with thyroid lymphoma have bone marrow involvement (29). There is lack of consensus about gastrointestinal evaluation, but at our institution, most patients have CT of the neck, chest, and abdomen.

DELAY IN DIAGNOSIS

It is important to diagnose thyroid lymphoma at an early stage. In one large study from Japan (125), the frequency of high-grade thyroid lymphomas decreased significantly after 1982, which the authors attributed to early diagnosis and therapy. Likewise, a German study found that non-Hodgkin's lymphoma with low-grade histology can undergo transformation into high-grade tumors (29). The diagnosis is usually made after a rapidly enlarging thyroid mass calls attention to the problem, but thyroid lymphoma can be discovered at an earlier stage by investigating more subtle clues in patients with Hashimoto's disease. Thyroid lymphoma should be considered when there is a discrete hypofunctional area on ^{123}I scanning of a thyroid in a patient with Hashimoto's thyroiditis, whether or not the nodule is palpable (29). Lymphoma should also be suspected when the entire thyroid gland in a patient with Hashimoto's disease or any portion of it enlarges during thyroid hormone therapy or when palpable cervical or supraclavicular lymph nodes develop.

Mortality and Recurrence Rates

Five-year survival rates with non-Hodgkin's thyroidal lymphoma was almost 60% in 368 patients reported in seven large series (29); however, survival is dependent on several variables, particularly tumor stage and grade. In one large study (126), for example, only one death occurred from lymphoma when it was limited to the thyroid (stage IE); the average survival rate was reduced to only 18 mo when there was involvement of local lymph nodes (stage IIE) or infiltration of adjacent soft tissues. Another study (127) found that 5-yr survival rates were 91% in stage IE and only 62% in stage IIE patients. Over the past several decades, 5-yr survival rates have been at least 75–100% when tumor is confined to the thyroid compared with only 35–60% when it is outside the gland (29,128,129). Histology is also prognostically important. In one large study (130) of 79 patients, 5-yr survival rates were 92% for patients with low-grade lymphomas and 79% for intermediate-grade lymphomas but only 13% for immunoblastic-type (high-grade) lymphomas.

PROGNOSTIC FACTORS

One large study (130) found that favorable prognostic factors were longer duration (>6 mo) of goiter, age less than 60 yr and goiter smaller than 10 cm. In another series (124), the important prognostic factors were tumor size and fixation, extracapsular extension, and retrosternal involvement. In a third study (131), unfavorable prognostic factors were large cell lymphoma, tumor resectability, and possibly male sex, whereas preexisting Hashimoto's thyroiditis was a favorable prognostic factor, which has also been reported by others (132). Others (128,132) find that advanced age (>65 yr), hoarseness, stridor, hepatosplenomegaly, axillary lymph nodes, vocal cord paralysis, and chest x-ray showing a superior mediastinal mass are all poor prognostic indicators.

Impact of Therapy

Treatment is not standard because large, randomized, multicenter trials for this uncommon disorder have not been done. External radiation is the treatment of choice in many centers, but controversy surrounds the optimal extent of surgery and the use of chemotherapy. Survival has improved over the past few decades, in which earlier diagnosis, better staging, and more aggressive radiation treatment has been the norm, although it is not clear which if any of these factors is responsible for the improved survival. Nonetheless, there are indications that thyroid lymphoma is being diagnosed at an earlier stage and at a lower grade now than in the past and is being more aggressively treated *(29)*. As thyroid lymphomas have become more common, adequate staging has been performed more regularly, therapy has improved, and radiation therapy has been used in nearly all cases *(29)*.

REFERENCES

1. Mazzaferri EL, Kloos RT. Current approaches to primary therapy for papillary and follicular thyroid cancer. J Clin Endocrinol Metab 2001;86:1447–1463.
2. Lin JD, Chao TC, Chen ST, Weng HF, Lin KD. Characteristics of thyroid carcinomas in aging patients. Eur J Clin Invest 2000;30:147–153.
3. Haigh PI, Ituarte PH, Wu HS, et al. Completely resected anaplastic thyroid carcinoma combined with adjuvant chemotherapy and irradiation is associated with prolonged survival . Cancer 2001;91:2335–2342.
4. Rodriguez JM, Pinero A, Ortiz S, et al. Clinical and histological differences in anaplastic thyroid carcinoma. Eur J Surg 2000;166:34–38.
5. Harada T, Ito K, Shimaoka K, Hosoda Y, Yakumaru K. Fatal thyroid carcinoma. Anaplastic transformation of adenocarcinoma. Cancer 1977;39:2588–2596.
6. Landis SH, Murray T, Bolden S, Wingo PA. Cancer statistics, 1998. CA 1998;48:6–30.
7. Kosary CL, Ries LAG, Miller BA, Hankey BF, Harras A, Edwards BK. SEER Cancer Statistic Review, 1973–1992: Tables and Graphs. NIH Pub. No. 96-2789. National Cancer Institute, Bethesda, MD, 1995.
8. Hundahl SA, Fleming ID, Fremgen AM, Menck HR. A National Cancer Data Base report on 53,856 cases of thyroid carcinoma treated in the US, 1985–1995. Cancer 1998;83:2638–2648.
9. Mazzaferri EL, Jhiang SM. Long-term impact of initial surgical and medical therapy on papillary and follicular thyroid cancer. Am J Med 1994;97:418–428.
10. Burgess JR, Duffield A, Wilkinson SJ, et al. Two families with an autosomal dominant inheritance pattern for papillary carcinoma of the thyroid. J Clin Endocrinol Metab 1997;82:345–348.
11. Stoffer SS, Van Dyke DL, Bach JV, Szpunar W, Weiss L. Familial papillary carcinoma of the thyroid. Am J Med Genet 1986;25:775–782.
12. Lupoli G, Vitale G, Caraglia M, et al. Familial papillary thyroid microcarcinoma: a new clinical entity. Lancet 1999;353:637–639.
13. Rios A, Rodriguez JM, Illana J, Torregrosa NM, Parrilla P. Familial papillary carcinoma of the thyroid: report of three families. Eur J Surg 2001;167:339–343.
14. Bell B, Mazzaferri EL. Familial adenomatous polyposis (Gardner's syndrome) and thyroid carcinoma: a case report and review of the literature. Dig Dis Sci 1993;38:185–190.
15. Cetta F, Olschwang S, Petracci M, et al. Genetic alterations in thyroid carcinoma associated with familial adenomatous polyposis: clinical implications and suggestions for early detection. World J Surg 1998;22:1231–1236.
16. Burman KD, Ringel MD, Wartofsky L. Unusual types of thyroid neoplasms. Endocrinol Metabol Clin North Am 1996;25:49–68.

17. Dahia PLM, Marsh DJ, Zheng ZM, et al. Somatic deletions and mutations in the Cowden disease gene, PTEN, in sporadic thyroid tumors. Cancer Res 1997;57:4710–4713.
18. Stratakis CA, Courcoutsakis NA, Abati A, et al. Thyroid gland abnormalities in patients with the syndrome of spotty skin pigmentation, myxomas, endocrine overactivity, and schwannomas (Carney complex). J Clin Endocrinol Metab 1997;82:2037–2043.
19. LiVolsi V, Asa SL. The demise of follicular carcinoma of the thyroid gland. Thyroid 1994;4:233–236.
20. Mazzaferri EL. Thyroid carcinoma: papillary and follicular. In: Mazzaferri EL, Samaan N, eds. Endocrine Tumors. Blackwell Scientific, Cambridge, 1993, pp. 278–333.
21. Herrera MF, Hay ID, Wu PS, et al. Hurthle cell (oxyphyilic) papillary thyroid carcinoma: a variant with more aggressive biologic behavior. World J Surg 1994;16:669–674.
22. Katoh R, Harach HR, Williams ED. Solitary, multiple, and familial oxyphil tumours of the thyroid gland. J Pathol 1998;186:292–299.
23. Ain KB. Papillary thyroid carcinoma etiology, assessment, and therapy. Endocrinol Metabol Clin North Am 1995;24:711–760.
24. Mazzaferri EL. Undifferentiated thyroid carcinoma and unusual thyroid malignancies. In: Mazzaferri EL, Samaan N, eds. Endocrine Tumors. Blackwell Scientific, Boston, 1993, pp. 378–398.
25. Mooradian AD, Allam CK, Khalil MF, Salti I, Salem PA. Anaplastic transformation of thyroid cancer: report of two cases and review of the literature. J Surg Oncol 1983;23:95–98.
26. Moore JHJr, Bacharach B, Choi HY. Anaplastic transformation of metastatic follicular carcinoma of the thyroid. J Surg Oncol 1985;29:216–221.
27. Wallin G, Backdahl M, Tallroth E, Lundell G, Auer G, Lowhagen T. Co-existent anaplastic and well differentiated thyroid carcinomas: a nuclear DNA study. Eur J Surg Oncol 1989;15:43–48.
28. Aldinger KA, Samaan NA, Ibanez ML, Hill CS Jr. Anaplastic carcinoma of the thyroid: a review of 84 cases of spindle and giant cell carcinoma of the thyroid. Cancer 1978;41:2267–2275.
29. Mazzaferri EL, Oertel YC. Primary malignant lymphoma and related lymphoproliferative disorders. In: Mazzaferri EL, Samaan N, eds. Endocrine Tumors. Blackwell Scientific, Boston, 1993, pp. 348–377.
30. Ron E, Lubin JH, Shore RE, et al. Thyroid cancer after exposure to external radiation: A pooled analysis of seven studies. Radiat Res 1995;141:259–277.
31. Hall P, Holm LE. Radiation-associated thyroid cancer—facts and fiction. Acta Oncol 1998;37:325–330.
32. Ron E, Doddy MM, Becker DV, et al. Cancer mortality following treatment for adult hyper-thyroidism. JAMA 1998;280:347–355.
33. Jacob P, Goulko G, Heidenreich WF, et al. Thyroid cancer risk to children calculated. Nature 1998;392:31–32.
34. Estimated exposures and thyroid doses received by the American people from iodine-131 in fallout following Nevada atmospheric nuclear bomb tests. A report from the National Cancer Institute. U.S. Department of Health and Human Services, National Institutes of Health, National Cancer Institute, Washington, DC 1997.
35. Committee on Exposure of the American People to I-131 from the Nevada Atomic-Bomb Test: Implications for Public Health. Institute of Medicine, National Academy of Sciences, Washington, DC, 1999.
36. Gilbert ES, Tarone R, Bouville A, Ron E. Thyroid cancer rates and ^{131}I doses from Nevada atmospheric nuclear bomb tests. J Natl Cancer Inst 1998;90:1654–1660.
37. Ries LAG, Eisner MP, Kosary CL, et al. SEER Cancer Statistics Review, 1973–1997. National Cancer Institute, Bethesda, MD, 2000.
38. Mazzaferri EL. Management of a solitary thyroid nodule. N Engl J Med 1993;328:553–559.
39. Mazzaferri EL. NCCN thyroid carcinoma practice guidelines. Oncology 1999;13(suppl 11A, NCCN Proceedings):391–442.

40. Yang GC, Liebeskind D, Messina AV. Ultrasound-guided fine-needle aspiration of the thyroid assessed by ultrafast papanicolaou stain: data from 1135 biopsies with a two- to six-year follow-up. Thyroid 2001;11:581–589.
41. Marqusee E, Benson CB, Frates MC, et al. Usefulness of ultrasonography in the management of nodular thyroid disease. Ann Intern Med 2000;133:696–700.
42. Hundahl SA, Cady B, Cunningham MP, et al. Initial results from a prospective cohort study of 5583 cases of thyroid carcinoma treated in the United States during 1996. U.S. and German Thyroid Cancer Study Group. An American College of Surgeons Commission on Cancer Patient Care Evaluation study. Cancer 2000;89:202–217.
43. Bennedbaek FN, Hegedus L. Management of the solitary thyroid nodule: results of a North American survey. J Clin Endocrinol Metab 2000;85:2493–2498.
44. Hamming JF, Goslings BM, vanSteenis GJ, Claasen H, Hermans J, Velde JH. The value of fine-needle aspiration biopsy in patients with nodular thyroid disease divided into groups of suspicion of malignant neoplasms on clinical grounds. Arch Intern Med 1990;150:113–116.
45. Bennedbaek FN, Perrild H, Hegedus L. Diagnosis and treatment of the solitary thyroid nodule. Results of a European survey. Clin Endocrinol (Oxf) 1999;50:357–363.
46. Ortiz R, Hupart KH, DeFesi CR, Surks MI. Effect of early referral to an endocrinologist on efficiency and cost of evaluation and development of treatment plan in patients with thyroid nodules. J Clin Endocrinol Metab 1998;83:3803–3807.
47. Scheumann GFW, Seeliger H, Musholt TJ, et al. Completion thyroidectomy in 131 patients with differentiated thyroid carcinoma. Eur J Surg 1996;162:677–684.
48. Kitamura Y, Shimizu K, Nagahama M, et al. Immediate causes of death in thyroid carcinoma: clinicopathological analysis of 161 fatal cases. J Clin Endocrinol Metab 1999;84:4043–4049.
49. Schneider AB, Shore Freedman E, Ryo UY, Bekerman C, Favus M, Pinsky S. Radiation-induced tumors of the head and neck following childhood irradiation. Prospective studies. Medicine (Baltimore) 1985;64:1–15.
50. Woolner LB, Beahrs OH, Black BM, McConahey WM, Keating RF Jr. Classification and prognosis of thyroid carcinoma. Am J Surg 1961;102:354–387.
51. Schlumberger MJ. Diagnostic follow-up of well-differentiated thyroid carcinoma: historical perspective and current status. J Endocrinol Invest 1999; 22(suppl to no. 11):3–7.
52. Schlumberger M, Challeton C, De Vathaire F, et al. Radioactive iodine treatment and external radiotherapy for lung and bone metastases from thyroid carcinoma. J Nucl Med 1996;37:598–605.
53. Dottorini ME, Vignati A, Mazzucchelli L, Lomuscio G, Colombo L. Differentiated thyroid carcinoma in children and adolescents: a 37-year experience in 85 patients. J Nucl Med 1997;38:669–675.
54. Harach HR, Williams ED. Childhood thyroid cancer in England and Wales. Br J Cancer 1995;72:777–783.
55. Hung W. Well-differentiated thyroid carcinomas in children and adolescents: a review. Endocrinologist 1994;4:117–126.
56. Samuel AM, Rajashekharrao B, Shah DH. Pulmonary metastases in children and adolescents with well- differentiated thyroid cancer. J Nucl Med 1998;39:1531–1536.
57. Zimmerman D, Hay ID, Gough IR, et al. Papillary thyroid carcinoma in children and adults: long-term follow-up of 1039 patients conservatively treated at one institution during three decades. Surgery 1988;104:1157–1166.
58. Schlumberger M, De Vathaire F, Travagli JP, et al. Differentiated thyroid carcinoma in childhood: long term follow-up of 72 patients. J Clin Endocrinol Metab 1987;65:1088–1094.
59. Gilliland FD, Hunt WC, Morris DM, Key CR. Prognostic factors for thyroid carcinoma—a population- based study of 15,698 cases from the surveillance, epidemiology and end results (SEER) program 1973–1991. Cancer 1997;79:564–573.

60. Samaan NA, Schultz PN, Hickey RC, Haynie TP, Johnston DA, Ordonez NG. Well-differentiated thyroid carcinoma and the results of various modalities of treatment. A retrospective review of 1599 patients. J Clin Endocrinol Metab 1992;75:714–720.

61. Brennan MD, Bergstralh EJ, van Heerden JA, McConahey WM. Follicular thyroid cancer treated at the Mayo Clinic, 1946 through 1970: initial manifestations, pathologic findings, therapy, and outcome. Mayo Clin Proc 1991;66:11–22.

62. Young RL, Mazzaferri EL, Rahe AJ, Dorfman SG. Pure follicular thyroid carcinoma: impact of therapy in 214 patients. J Nucl Med 1980;21:733–737.

63. Lin JD, Chao TC, Ho J, Weng H-F, See LC. Poor prognosis of 56 follicular thyroid carcinomas with distant metastases at the time of diagnosis. Cancer J 1998;11:190–195.

64. Akslen LA, LiVolsi VA. Prognostic significance of histologic grading compared with subclassification of papillary thyroid carcinoma. Cancer 2000;88:1902–1908.

65. Hay ID, Grant CS, Bergstralh EJ, Thompson GB, van Heerden JA. Unilateral total lobectomy: is it sufficient surgical treatment for patients with AMES low-risk papillary thyroid carcinoma? Surgery 1998;124:958–966.

66. DeGroot LJ, Kaplan EL, McCormick M, Straus FH. Natural history, treatment, and course of papillary thyroid carcinoma. J Clin Endocrinol Metab 1990;71:414–424.

67. Shaha AR, Jaffe BM. Completion thyroidectomy: a critical appraisal. Surgery 1992;112:1148–1153.

68. Sanders LE, Cady B. Differentiated thyroid cancer—reexamination of risk groups and outcome of treatment. Arch Surg 1998;133:419–424.

69. Miccoli P, Antonelli A, Spinelli C, Ferdeghini M, Fallahi P, Baschieri L. Completion total thyroidectomy in children with thyroid cancer secondary to the Chernobyl accident. Arch Surg 1998; 133:89-93.

70. Vassilopoulou-Sellin R, Klein MJ, Smith TH, et al. Pulmonary metastases in children and young adults with differentiated thyroid cancer. Cancer 1993;71:1348–1352.

71. Hay ID. Papillary thyroid carcinoma. Endocrinol Metabol Clin North Am 1990;19:545–576.

72. Mazzaferri EL. Thyroid remnant ^{131}I ablation for papillary and follicular thyroid carcinoma. Thyroid 1997;7:265–271.

73. Goldman JM, Line BR, Aamodt RL, Robbins J. Influence of triiodothyronine withdrawal time on 131-I uptake postthyroidectomy for thyroid cancer. J Clin Endocrinol Metab 1980;50:734–739.

74. Spencer CA, Takeuchi M, Kazarosyan M, et al. Serum thyroglobulin autoantibodies: prevalence, influence on serum thyroglobulin measurement, and prognostic significance in patients with differentiated thyroid carcinoma. J Clin Endocrinol Metab 1998;83:1121–1127.

75. Tsang TW, Brierley JD, Simpson WJ, Panzarella T, Gospodarowicz MK, Sutcliffe SB. The effects of surgery, radioiodine, and external radiation therapy on the clinical outcome of patients with differentiated thyroid carcinoma. Cancer 1998;82:375–388.

76. Hodgson DC, Brierley JD, Tsang RW, Panzarella T. Prescribing [131]Iodine based on neck uptake produces effective thyroid ablation and reduced hospital stay. Radiother Oncol 1998;47:325–330.

77. Taylor T, Specker B, Robbins J, et al. Outcome after treatment of high-risk papillary and non-Hurthle-cell follicular thyroid carcinoma. Ann Intern Med 1998;129:622–627.

78. Cunningham MP, Duda RB, Recant W, Chmiel JS, Sylvester JA, Fremgen A. Survival discriminants for differentiated thyroid cancer . Am J Surg 1990;160:344–347.

79. DeGroot LJ, Kaplan EL, Straus FH, Shukla MS. Does the method of management of papillary thyroid carcinoma make a difference in outcome? World J Surg 1994;18:123–130.

80. Samaan NA, Maheshwari YK, Nader S, et al. Impact of therapy for differentiated carcinoma of the thyroid: an analysis of 706 cases. J Clin Endocrinol Metab 1983;56:1131–1138.

81. Massin JP, Savoie JC, Garnier H, Guiraudon G, Leger FA, Bacourt F. Pulmonary metastases in differentiated thyroid carcinoma. Study of 58 cases with implications for the primary tumor treatment. Cancer 1984;53:982–992.

82. Pujol P, Daures JP, Nsakala N, Baldet L, Bringer J, Jaffiol C. Degree of thyrotropin suppression as a prognostic determinant in differentiated thyroid cancer. J Clin Endocrinol Metab 1996;81:4318–4323.
83. Cooper DS, Specker B, Ho M, et al. Thyrotropin suppression and disease progression in patients with differentiated thyroid cancer: results from the National Thyroid Cancer Treatment Cooperative Registry. Thyroid 1999;8:737–744.
84. Mazzaferri EL, Kloos RT. Using recombinant human TSH in the management of well-differentiated thyroid cancer: current strategies and future directions. Thyroid 2000;10:767–778.
85. Grigsby PW, Baglan K, Siegel BA. Surveillance of patients to detect recurrent thyroid carcinoma. Cancer 1999;85:945–951.
86. Haugen BR, Pacini F, Reiners C, et al. A comparison of recombinant human thyrotropin and thyroid hormone withdrawal for the detection of thyroid remnant or cancer. J Clin Endocrinol Metab 1999;84:3877–3885.
87. Robbins RJ, Tuttle RM, Sharaf RN, et al. Preparation by recombinant human thyrotropin or thyroid hormone withdrawal are comparable for the detection of residual differentiated thyroid carcinoma. J Clin Endocrinol Metab 2001;86:619–625.
88. Cailleux AF, Baudin E, Travagli JP, Ricard M, Schlumberger M. Is diagnostic iodine-131 scanning useful after total thyroid ablation for differentiated thyroid cancer? J Clin Endocrinol Metab 2000;85:175–178.
89. Sizemore GW. Medullary carcinoma of the thyroid gland. Semin Oncol 1987;14:306–314.
90. Mendelsohn G. Markers as prognostic indicators in medullary thyroid carcinoma. Am J Clin Pathol 1991;95:297–298.
91. Mulligan LM, Kwok JBJ, Healey CS, et al. Germ-line mutations of the RET proto-oncogene in multiple endocrine neoplasia type 2A. Nature 1993;363:458–460.
92. Raue F, Zink A. Clinical features of multiple endocrine neoplasia type 1 and type 2. Horm Res 1992;38(suppl 2):31–35.
93. Gagel RF, Robinson MF, Donovan DT, Alford BR. Medullary thyroid carcinoma: recent progress. J Clin Endocrinol Metab 1993;76:809–814.
94. Decker RA, Peacock ML. Update on the profile of multiple endocrine neoplasia type 2a RET mutations—practical issues and implications for genetic testing. Cancer 1997; 80:557-568.
95. Cohen R, Buchsenschutz B, Estrade P, Gardet P, Modigliani E. Causes of death in patients suffering from medullary thyroid carcinoma: report of 119 cases. Presse Med 1996;25:1819–1822.
96. Modigliani E, Cohen R, Campos JM, et al. Prognostic factors for survival and for biochemical cure in medullary thyroid carcinoma: results in 899 patients. Clin Endocrinol (Oxf) 1998;48:265–273.
97. Dottorini ME, Assi A, Sironi M, Sangalli G, Spreafico G, Colombo L. Multivariate analysis of patients with medullary thyroid carcinoma—prognostic significance and impact on treatment of clinical and pathologic variables. Cancer 1996;77:1556–1565.
98. Wells SA, Baylin SB, Leight Geal. The importance of early diagnosis in patients with hereditary medullary thyroid carcinoma. Ann Surg 1982;195:204.
99. Lips CJM, Landsvater RM, Höppener JWM, et al. Clinical screening as compared with DNA analysis in families with multiple endocrine neoplasia type 2A. N Engl J Med 1994;331:828–835.
100. Iler MA, King DR, Ginn-Pease ME, O'Dorisio TM, Sotos JF. Multiple endocrine neoplasia type 2A: a 25-year review. J Pediatr Surg 1999;34:92–96.
101. Machens A, Gimm O, Hinze R, Hoppner W, Boehm BO, Dralle H. Genotype-phenotype correlations in hereditary medullary thyroid carcinoma: oncological features and biochemical properties. J Clin Endocrinol Metab 2001;86:1104–1109.
102. Siggelkow H, Melzer A, Nolte W, Karsten K, Hoppner W, Hufner M. Presentation of a kindred with familial medullary thyroid carcinoma and Cys611Phe mutation of the RET proto-oncogene demonstrating low grade malignancy. Eur J Endocrinol 2001;144:467–473.

103. Dralle H, Gimm O, Simon D, et al. Prophylactic thyroidectomy in 75 children and adolescents with hereditary medullary thyroid carcinoma: German and Austrian experience. World J Surg 1998;22:744–751.

104. Hyer SL, Vini L, A'Hern R, Harmer C. Medullary thyroid cancer: multivariate analysis of prognostic factors influencing survival. Eur J Surg Oncol 2000;26:686–690.

105. Brierley J, Tsang R, Simpson WJ, Gospodarowicz M, Sutcliffe S, Panzarella T. Medullary thyroid cancer: analyses of survival and prognostic factors and the role of radiation therapy in local control. Thyroid 1996;6:305–310.

106. Wells SA Jr, Skinner MA. Prophylactic thyroidectomy, based on direct genetic testing, in patients at risk for the multiple endocrine neoplasia type 2 syndromes. Exp Clin Endocrinol Diabetes 1998;106:29–34.

107. Ledger GA, Khosla S, Lindor NM, Thibodeau SN, Gharib H. Genetic testing in the diagnosis and management of multiple endocrine neoplasia type II. Ann Intern Med 1995;122:118–124.

108. Skinner MA, DeBenedetti MK, Moley JF, Norton JA, Wells SA Jr. Medullary thyroid carcinoma in children with multiple endocrine neoplasia types 2A and 2B. J Pediatr Surg 1996;31:177–182.

109. O'Riordain DS, O'Brien T, Weaver AL, et al. Medullary thyroid carcinoma in multiple endocrine neoplasia types 2A and 2B. Surgery 1994;116:1017–1023.

110. Arslan N, Ilgan S, Yuksel D, et al. Comparison of In-111 octreotide and Tc-99m (V) DMSA scintigraphy in the detection of medullary thyroid tumor foci in patients with elevated levels of tumor markers after surgery 5. Clin Nucl Med 2001;26:683–688.

111. Esik O, Szavcsur P, Szakall S Jr, et al. Angiography effectively supports the diagnosis of hepatic metastases in medullary thyroid carcinoma. Cancer 2001;91:2084–2095.

112. Moley JF, DeBenedetti MK, Dilley WG, Tisell LE, Wells SA. Surgical management of patients with persistent or recurrent medullary thyroid cancer. J Intern Med 1998;243:521–526.

113. Chen HB, Roberts JR, Ball DW, et al. Effective long-term palliation of symptomatic, incurable metastatic medullary thyroid cancer by operative resection. Ann Surg 1998;227:887–893.

114. Venkatesh YS, Ordonez NG, Schultz PN, Hickey RC, Goepfert H, Samaan NA. Anaplastic carcinoma of the thyroid. A clinicopathologic study of 121 cases. Cancer 1990;66:321–330.

115. Nel CJ, van Heerden JA, Goellner JR, et al. Anaplastic carcinoma of the thyroid: a clinicopathologic study of 82 cases. Mayo Clin Proc 1985;60:51–58.

116. Mitchell G, Huddart R, Harmer C. Phase II evaluation of high dose accelerated radiotherapy for anaplastic thyroid carcinoma. Radiother Oncol 1999;50:33–38.

117. Simpson WJ. Anaplastic thyroid carcinoma: a new approach. Can J Surg 1980;23:25–27.

118. Tennvall J, Tallroth E, el Hassan A, et al. Anaplastic thyroid carcinoma. Doxorubicin, hyperfractionated radiotherapy and surgery. Acta Oncol 1990;29:1025–1028.

119. Tennvall J, Lundell G, Hallquist A, et al. Combined doxorubicin, hyperfractionated radiotherapy, and surgery in anaplastic thyroid carcinoma: report on two protocols. Cancer 1994;74:1348–1354.

120. Schlumberger M, Parmentier C, Delisle MJ, Couette JE, Droz JP, Sarrazin D. Combination therapy for anaplastic giant cell thyroid carcinoma. Cancer 1991;67:564–566.

121. Holm LE, Blomgren H, Lowenhagen T. Cancer risks in patients with chronic lymphocytic thyroiditis. N Engl J Med 1985;312:601–606.

122. Kato I, Tajima K, Suchi T. Chronic thyroiditis as a risk factor of B-cell lymphoma in the thyroid gland. Jpn J Cancer Res (Amsterdam) 1985;76:1085–1090.

123. Takashima S, Nomura N, Noguchi Y, Matsuzuka F, Inoue T. Primary thyroid lymphoma: evaluation with US, CT, and MRI. J Comput Assist Tomogr 1995;19:282–288.

124. Tupchong L, Hughes F, Harmer CL. Primary lymphoma of the thyroid: clinical features, prognostic factors, and results of treatment. Int J Radiat Oncol Biol Phys 1986;12:1813–1821.

125. Aozasa K. Hashimoto's thyroiditis as a risk factor of thyroid lymphoma. Acta Pathol Jpn 1990;40:459–468.

126. Woolner LB, McConahey WM, Beahrs OH, Black BM. Primary malignant lymphoma of the thyroid: review of forty-six cases. Am J Surg 1966;111:502–523.

127. Vigliotti A, Kong JS, Fuller LM, Velasquez WS. Thyroid lymphomas stages IE and IIE: comparative results for radiotherapy only, combination chemotherapy only, and multimodality treatment. Int J Radiat Oncol Biol Phys 1986;12:1807–1812.

128. Pedersen RK, Pedersen NT. Primary non-Hodgkin's lymphoma of the thyroid gland: a population based study. Histopathology 1996;28:25–32.

129. Sasai K, Yamabe H, Haga H, et al. Non-Hodgkin's lymphoma of the thyroid—a clinical study of twenty-two cases. Acta Oncol 1996; 35:457-462.

130. Aozasa K, Inoue A, Tajima K, Miyauchi A, Matsuzuka F, Kuma K. Malignant lymphomas of the thyroid gland. Analysis of 79 patients with emphasis on histologic prognostic factors. Cancer 1986;58:100–104.

131. Shaw JH, Dodds P. Carcinoma of the thyroid gland in Auckland, New Zealand. Surg Gynecol Obstet 1990;171:27–32.

132. Blair TJ, Evans RG, Buskirk SJ, Banks PM, Earle JD. Radiotherapeutic management of primary thyroid lymphoma. Int J Radiat Oncol Biol Phys 1985;11:365–370.

2   Hypothyroidism

Paul W. Ladenson, MD,
and Ruth M. Belin, MD

INTRODUCTION

Early diagnosis and treatment of hypothyroidism is the exception rather than the rule. Despite its high prevalence *(1–3)* and potential consequences, hypothyroidism is typically diagnosed in clinical settings at an advanced and often long-standing stage or is incidentally detected during a wide-ranging evaluation for nonspecific complaints. Even when hypothyroidism should be anticipated, such as in patients who have received neck irradiation *(4)* or amiodarone therapy *(5)*, its recognition is often delayed. Only in neonates, for whom universal thyroid function testing is mandated in most industrialized societies, is hypothyroidism identified early and treated promptly. Application of the principles of preventive medicine to hypothyroidism has occurred slowly, except in the worldwide efforts to prevent dietary iodine deficiency disorders, including endemic goiter, hypothyroidism, and cretinism *(6)*.

Preventive interventions are categorized by the stage of disease progression that they address. *Primary prevention* refers to interventions in patients without disease, in order to decrease its incidence. *Secondary prevention* aims to identify people early in a disorder's natural history. Achieved through screening and early intervention, secondary prevention attempts to avert disease morbidity,

From: *Contemporary Endocrinology: Early Diagnosis and Treatment of Endocrine Disorders*
Edited by: R. S. Bar © Humana Press Inc., Totowa, NJ

complications, and mortality. *Tertiary prevention* refers to amelioration of the course of established disease and decreasing recurrent episodes of an existing illness. The success of disease prevention may be assessed based on the benefit to treated individuals or, more often, from the perspective of cumulative benefit to an entire population. Evidence-based approaches to developing preventive practices, such as systematic literature reviews, meta-analyses, and decision and cost-effectiveness analyses, can predict whether screening is likely to achieve the desired outcome and result in more good than harm *(7)*.

PRIMARY PREVENTION OF HYPOTHYROIDISM

Primary prevention of disease focuses on risk factor identification and modification. Risk factors may stem from genetic predispositions and environmental exposures. There is a genetic predisposition to the most common cause of hypothyroidism, autoimmune thyroiditis, which occurs approximately tenfold more frequently in women than men and affects approximately one in seven female children of affected women. However, autoimmune thyroiditis appears to be a polygenic disorder *(8)* for which there can currently be only general predictions of disease risk. A number of other rare monogenic disorders causing hypothyroidism have been described. Familial combined pituitary hormone deficiencies *(9)* and isolated thyrotropin (TSH) deficiency *(10)* cause central hypothyroidism. The thyroid gland may be congenitally resistant to TSH action as the result of a mutation in the TSH receptor *(11)*, its related $G_s\alpha$ subunit *(12)*, or the TSH β-subunit *(13)*. Inherited defects in thyroid hormone biosynthesis caused by mutant thyroglobulin *(14)*, sodium-iodide symporter *(15)*, thyroid peroxidase *(16)*, and pendrin *(17)* genes can produce goiter with or without hypothyroidism. Although it is theoretically possible to detect these mutations prenatally with the goal of either preventing (primary prevention) or promptly detecting and treating (secondary prevention) congenital hypothyroidism, there is no report of this actually being done. Furthermore, the rarity of these disorders, and the ease with which hypothyroidism can be treated, makes the issue of primary prevention by genetic modification clinically inconsequential.

Several environmental influences are known to be associated with hypothyroidism, including severe dietary iodine deficiency, iodine excess, certain medications, cigarette smoke, and thyroidal irradiation. Dietary iodine deficiency is the most important of these factors epidemiologically *(18)*, affecting approximately 100 million people in underdeveloped (principally mountainous) regions around the world. The spectrum of iodine deficiency disorders includes goiter, maternal and fetal hypothyroidism, and cretinism; follicular thyroid cancer is also relatively more common in regions of mild to moderate iodine deficiency *(19)*. A full discussion of this problem and of strategies for eradication of iodine deficiency is beyond the scope of this chapter, but the topic has recently been reviewed elsewhere *(6,20)*.

Paradoxically, iodine excess is also a potential cause of hypothyroidism in two settings. First, a surfeit of iodine in the diet has been associated with higher incidences of hypothyroidism, in populations both with (21) and without autoimmune thyroiditis (22). Experimental evidence in animal models supports this relationship (23,24). Second, chronic ingestion of pharmacologic amounts of iodine in the diet or in medications can provoke hypothyroidism in individuals with underlying autoimmune thyroiditis. The most important sources of iodine in this context are dietary seaweed (25), naturopathic food supplements containing kelp, and the drug amiodarone, which is 40% iodine by weight. In North America, more than 20% of individuals treated with amiodarone develop hypothyroidism (5).

Cigarette smoke can impair thyroid function in women with iodine deficiency or autoimmune thyroiditis (26–28). One study performed in a geographic region with low dietary iodine intake suggested that in women 23% of the risk for developing autoimmune thyroiditis-related hypothyroidism could be attributed to smoking (29). Although a causal relationship between cigarette smoke and hypothyroidism has not been established, it has been postulated that increased circulating thiocyanate concentrations found in smokers may inhibit iodide transport and thyroid peroxidase-catalyzed iodide organification, precipitating hypothyroidism in patients with decreased thyroid gland reserve (30–32). Active smoking can also exacerbate established partial hypothyroidism, inhibiting both thyroid hormone secretion and peripheral thyroid hormone action (33). Consequently, smoking cessation in both populations and individual patients can contribute to both primary and secondary prevention of hypothyroidism.

Certain industrial toxins and medications cause hypothyroidism. Exposure to polybrominated biphenyls (34) and polychlorinated biphenyls (35) precipitates hypothyroidism by structural injury to the thyroid gland. Resorcinol has been reported to induce hypothyroidism in textile workers (36) and in a patient on chronic hemodialysis (37). The adrenolytic agent aminoglutethimide can impair thyroid gland function (38). The commonly used psychotropic medication lithium carbonate frequently causes hypothyroidism by inhibiting hormone release from the gland. Almost 40% of lithium-treated patients have transient TSH elevation, and approximately 10% have sustained hypothyroidism. Again, patients with underlying autoimmune thyroiditis are the most vulnerable. The immunomodulatory agent interferon-α can induce autoimmune thyroiditis and hypothyroidism, as well as hyperthyroid Graves' disease and a transiently thyrotoxic form of thyroiditis (39). Avoidance of these toxic and medicinal exposures when possible, particularly in individuals with underlying autoimmune thyroiditis, represents a form of primary prevention for hypothyroidism.

Thyroidal irradiation—either by accidental or therapeutic radioactive iodine ingestion, or by external beam radiotherapy—can cause hypothyroidism, as well as benign and malignant thyroid neoplasms. Well-defined procedures, equipment, and monitoring are important to prevent and detect accidental thyroid irradiation in the setting of research laboratories, nuclear medicine departments, and nuclear reactor facilities where workers could be exposed to radioiodine. Radioiodine has proved to be among the most dangerous radioisotopes released in nuclear power plant accidents, such as the Chernobyl nuclear power station disaster. The principal thyroid problem occurring in populations exposed as children has been thyroid cancer *(40)*, but hypothyroidism may also occur with greater frequency *(41)*. Stable iodine, as potassium iodide (KI), can effectively prevent significant thyroidal irradiation and its consequences if the compound is administered before or simultaneously with radioiodine exposure *(42)*. The potential benefits of KI, logistics of distribution, and potential side effects have been the basis for lively public debate. Similarly, thyroidal radioiodine exposure associated with the investigational use of radioimmunoglobulins to treat malignancies, such as hepatoma and Hodgkin's lymphoma *(43)*, can be prevented by administering stable iodine in advance. In patients given therapeutic 131-iodine therapy for diffuse and nodular toxic goiter, hypothyroidism is an unavoidable consequence of effective therapy in most patients *(44)*, so secondary prevention in the form of early detection is appropriate (*see* next section). External beam radiotherapy for malignancies of the head and neck commonly cause hypothyroidism, but shielding of the thyroid gland would limit the treatment field, so primary prevention is not feasible.

SECONDARY PREVENTION OF HYPOTHYROIDISM: *EARLY DIAGNOSIS AND TREATMENT*

Hypothyroidism fulfills the criteria for early detection, either through testing prompted by clinical suspicion (case finding) or by routine testing of all individuals in a defined group (screening). First, hypothyroidism is highly prevalent, particularly in clinically identifiable subsets of the population, such as older women. Second, its consequences can be clinically significant—whether one considers the morbidity of subsequent myxedema or the long-term vascular effects of associated hyperlipidemia—and these consequences can be avoided by early diagnosis and therapy. Third, clinical diagnosis alone can be inaccurate. Fourth, the diagnostic test, serum TSH measurement, can successfully identify individuals with early disease, so interventions are possible before development of adverse consequences of untreated disease. Importantly, the screening test is accurate, safe, and inexpensive. Furthermore, once hypothyroidism is diagnosed, treatment is also effective, safe, and inexpensive. For all the common causes of primary hyperthyroidism, measurement of a serum TSH can establish or exclude the diagnosis in a straightforward manner. For central hypothyroidism caused by hypothalamic or pituitary disorders, a serum free thyroxine measurement (FT4) is required.

Table 1
Indications to Test for Hypothyroidism

Symptoms and Signs

Fatigue	Muscle weakness	Bradycardia
Dry skin	Muscle cramps	Diastolic hypertension
Impaired memory	Deep tendon reflex delay	Hoarseness
Slowed mentation	Cold intolerance	Periorbital edema
Depression	Constipation	Weight gain

Risk factors for thyroid failure
  Autoimmune thyroiditis
    Established serologic or tissue diagnosis
    Diffuse goiter
    Family history of autoimmune thyroid disease
    Previous Graves' disease or painless (postpartum) thyroiditis
    Personal or family history of associated autoimmune disorders (e.g., vitiligo,
      pernicious anemia, adrenal insufficiency, diabetes mellitus)
    Interferon-α therapy
  Previous thyroid injury
    Surgery
    Radioactive iodine
    External radiotherapy
  Postpartum status
  Drug impairing thyroid function
    Lithium carbonate
    Amiodarone
    Aminoglutethimide
  Hypothalamic or pituitary disease, known or suspected
    Other elements of hypopituitarism
    Manifestations of a sellar mass (headache, decreased temporal vision, or diplopia).
    Disorders known to cause hypothalamic or pituitary dysfunction (sarcoidosis or
      metastatic cancer).

Routine laboratory test abnormalities
  Hypercholesterolemia
  Anemia
  Hyponatremia
  Hyperprolactinemia
  ↑Creatine phosphokinase

Suspicion that a patient has hypothyroidism can be based on the presence of clinical findings, recognition of risk factors for thyroid gland failure, or abnormalities in routinely measured laboratory parameters (Table 1). Case finding is particularly important in populations at high risk of developing hypothyroidism,

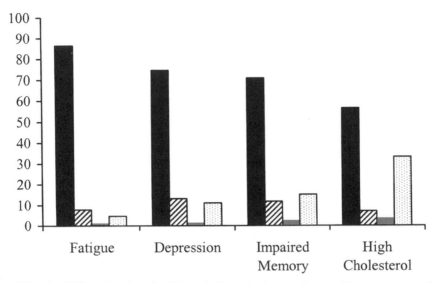

Fig. 1. TSH testing by physicians in hypothetical patients with symptoms and hypercholesterolemia potentially attributable to hypothyroidism. (Adapted from ref. *48*.)

e.g., patients who have been treated with lithium carbonate, amiodarone, or thyroid irradiation. Various strategies have been described for systematic follow-up of patients at risk of developing hypothyroidism after radioiodine therapy *(45–47)*.

The extent to which practicing physicians actually consider the diagnosis of hypothyroidism in patients with nonspecific clinical and laboratory findings is unknown. However, a recently published survey of 1721 primary care physicians revealed the frequency with which TSH testing was employed in the differential diagnosis of hypothetical patients who had potential manifestations of hypothyroidism—either one of three nonspecific symptoms or hypercholesterolemia *(48)* (Fig. 1). Seventy-five to 87% of physicians requested a serum TSH measurement, among other investigations, at the first visit in symptomatic patients, but only 56% of physicians ordered a TSH at the first visit in the hypercholesterolemic patient. Familiarity with managed care guidelines regarding the evaluation of hypercholesterolemic patients for secondary causes of hyperlipidemia was associated with a significantly higher rate of TSH testing.

The argument for population screening for hypothyroidism is particularly persuasive in neonates, since untreated thyroid hormone deficiency can lead to irreversible abnormalities in neuropsychological development. The rationale and procedures for neonatal thyroid function screening have been reviewed elsewhere *(49)*. Guidelines for hypothyroidism screening in adults have been articulated by several professional societies *(50)* (Table 2). The cost-effectiveness of TSH screening every 5 years has been shown to be as favorable as, or even more favorable than, screening for hypertension, breast cancer, and hypercholesterolemia *(51)*.

TERTIARY PREVENTION OF HYPOTHYROIDISM: *AVOIDING COMPLICATIONS*

Potential complications of recognized hypothyroidism and its treatment are preventable with sustained thyroxine therapy and appropriate clinical and laboratory monitoring. Myxedema coma is a life-threatening syndrome of multisystem organ failure resulting from prolonged profound thyroid hormone deficiency, usually with superimposed sepsis, drug intoxication, or an ischemic vascular event *(52)*. Anecdotally, the hypothyroid patient who is elderly or has a history of previous noncompliance, other systemic illness, alcohol abuse, social isolation, and economic deprivation is at greatest risk. A second potential complication in hypothyroid patients who are suboptimally treated is persistence of risk factors for atherosclerosis. In this setting, the serum low-density lipoprotien cholesterol *(53)* concentration may remain elevated. In one small trial of patients with treated hypothyroidism and ischemic heart disease undergoing follow-up coronary catheterization after angioplasty, the patients with inadequately treated hypothyroidism (i.e., persistently elevated serum TSH concentrations) had a significantly higher rate of progression of their coronary arterial lesions than did patients on an optimal thyroxine replacement dose *(54)*.

For patients with treated hypothyroidism, tertiary prevention includes avoiding complications of thyroid hormone therapy. The first of these is iatrogenic thyrotoxicosis, which in one large population survey was found to occur in more than one-fifth of thyroid hormone-treated patients *(2)*. Appropriate dose selection and adjustment with TSH monitoring can avoid this problem *(55)*. Even the appropriate restoration of euthyroidism with thyroxine can also be associated with two unusual complications that should be anticipated and (when they are probable) prevented. First, ischemic heart disease can be exacerbated by thyroid hormone's positive chronotropic and inotropic actions, which have been reported to cause angina, myocardial infarction, dysrthythmia, and death *(56)*. Consequently, in patients with known coronary artery disease, prominent risk factors for it, or age older than 65 years, treatment should be initiated with a low dose of thyroxine, e.g., 0.025 mg/d. Second, institution of thyroid hormone replacement alone can provoke adrenal insufficiency in patients with associated borderline adrenal cortical function caused by autoimmune adrenalitis in patients with

Table 2
Clinical Practice Guidelines for Thyroid Function Testing and Screening

Guideline	Methods used to analyze evidence	Organization, year	Summary of relevant recommendations
American Thyroid Association guidelines for the detection of thyroid dysfunction (58)	Narrative literature review; Expert opinion[a]	American Thyroid Association, 2000	Screening with serum thyrotropin (TSH) every 5 yr for women and men over age 35 yr; Screening for individuals with symptoms and risk factors; Addition of serum free thyroxine (FT4) when pituitary or hypothalamic disease suspected
Consensus statement for good practice and audit measures in the management of hypo-thyroidism and hyper-thyroidism (59)	Narrative literature review; Expert opinion[c]	Royal College of Physicians of London Society for Endocrinology, 1996	General testing of population unjustified; Screening for congenital hypothyroidism; Screening patients after thyroid surgery, radioactive iodine treatment, or longstanding lithium treatment; low threshold for screening patients on amiodarone; Consideration of screening patients with type I diabetes during first-trimester pregnancy by measuring antithyroid antibody; Biochemical confirmation of hypothyroidism with serum TSH and total thyroxine (T4) or FT4

Laboratory medicine practice guidelines for the diagnosis and monitoring of thyroid disease testing (60,61)	Narrative literature review Expert opinion[c]	American Association of Clinical Chemists American Association of Clinical Endocrinologists American Thyroid Association National Academy of Clinical Biochemistry, 1990 (update in progress)	Serum TSH for evaluating patients with stable thyroid status; FT4 in patients during first 2–3 mo treatment of thyroid dysfunction Prepregnancy or first-trimester pregnancy screening with serum TSH In patients receiving amiodarone, baseline TSH, thyroid peroxidase antibody, FT4, and FT3; biannual screening of TSH, FT4, and FT3 Assessment of thyroid status (using FT4 or T4 and TSH) in hospitalized patients, when clinical suspicion high
Newborn screening for congenital hypo-thyroidism: recommended guidelines (62)	Narrative literature review Expert opinion[c]	American Academy of Pediatrics, 1993	Screening within first week of life either with filter paper blood spot primary T4 and backup TSH; or primary TSH with backup T4; or combined primary TSH and T4 Cord serum measurements in offspring of mothers with thyroid abnormalities Confirmatory serum measurements, serial serum T4 and TSH, as well as consideration of thyroid scan in infants with abnormalities Confirmation after age 3 yr with discontinuation of levothyroxine for 30 d, followed by serum TSH, T4

(continued)

Table 2 (*continued*)

Guideline	Methods used to analyze evidence	Organization, year	Summary of relevant recommendations
Periodic Health Examinations: Summary of AAFP Policy Recommendations and Age Charts (63)	Systematic literature review performed by U.S. Preventive Services Task Force Expert opinion[c]	American Academy of Family Physicians, 1996, 2001	Screening patients over age 60 yr recommended
Screening for congenital hypothyroidism (64)	Systematic literature review[b]	Canadian Task Force on Preventive Health Care, 1994, 1998	Good evidence to support screening on all newborns during first week of life using routine TSH followed by T4 if necessary
Screening for congenital hypothyroidism (65)	Systematic literature review[b]	U.S. Preventive Services Task Force, 1996	Good evidence to support screening on all newborns, including those born at home, optimally between d 2 and 6 Choice of screening test determined by state requirements
Screening for thyroid disease (66)	Systematic literature review Meta-analysis of observational trials[b]	American College of Physicians–American Society of Internal Medicine, 1997	Screening women older than 50 yr with a sensitive TSH; FT4 when TSH is undetectable or ≥ 10 mU/L Poor evidence to support screening women younger than age 50 and men Careful follow-up of patients with mild hypothyroidism
Screening for thyroid disease (67)	Systematic literature review[b]	U.S. Preventive Services Task Force, 1996	Fair evidence to support exclusion of routine screening of thyroid disease in asymptomatic adults in periodic health examination

Topic	Method	Organization, Year	Recommendation
Screening for thyroid disorders and thyroid cancer in asymptomatic adults (68)	Systematic literature review adapted from U.S. Preventive Services Task Force[b]	Canadian Task Force on Preventive Health Care, 1994, 1999	Despite insufficient evidence, recommend low threshold for screening with serum TSH in high-risk patients, including elderly, postpartum women, and persons with Down's syndrome. Poor evidence to support screening of asymptomatic adults. High level of clinical suspicion should be maintained in perimenopausal and postmenopausal women
Subclinical hypothyroidism during pregnancy (69)	Narrative literature review Expert opinion[c]	American Association of Clinical Endocrinologists, 1999	Routine screening with serum TSH reasonable early in pregnancy. Screening with TSH recommended in women considering pregnancy. Screening with serum TSH recommended in pregnant women with: goiter, antithyroid antibodies, family history of thyroid disease, autoimmune endocrine disease, symptoms suggestive of hypothyroidism, history of levothyroxine treatment

[a]Self-funded.
[b]Governmental funding.
[c]Not specified.

autoimmune thyroiditis (*see* next paragraph) and in patients with hypopituitarism. Therefore, in patients with clinical features suggesting primary adrenal insufficiency (e.g., weight loss, hyperpigmentation, nausea, or vomiting) or pituitary disease (e.g., visual field deficits, diplopia, or hypogonadism), the possibility of hypoadrenalism should be excluded by adrenocorticotropic hormone stimulation testing.

Although autoimmune thyroiditis is not a complication of hypothyroidism *per se*, patients affected with it are also at risk of developing a relatively small set of associated autoimmune disorders. The polyglandular autoimmune syndrome type II includes hypothyroidism, primary adrenal insufficiency, and type I diabetes *(57)*. Less commonly, hypothyroidism may occur in the autoimmune polyendocrinopathy-candidiasis-ectodermal dystrophy syndrome (or polyglandular autoimmune syndrome type I). Autoimmune thyroid disorders are associated with increased risk of developing pernicious anemia and gastric achlorhydria caused by intrinsic factor and parietal cell autoimmunity. Patients with autoimmune thyroiditis should be monitored for vitamin B12 deficiency with periodic complete blood counts and, whenever the disorder is seriously suspected, serum vitamin B12 measurement. Vitiligo, leukotrichia (prematurely gray hair), and alopecia areata have also been associated with autoimmune thyroiditis; although these disorders are often distressing, their prevention is not currently possible.

In conclusion, hypothyroidism occurs commonly, generates morbidity and mortality, and may be prevented at all stages of disease progression. Once hypothyroidism has been identified and treated with thyroxine, special attention to optimal dose management, complications of therapy, and the potential development of associated diseases can improve the clinical course and quality of life for affected individuals.

REFERENCES

1. Hollowell JG, Staehling NW, Flanders WD, et al. Serum TSH, T(4), and thyroid antibodies in the United States population (1988 to 1994): National Health and Nutrition Examination Survey (NHANES III). J Clin Endocrinol Metab 2002;87:489–499.
2. Canaris GJ, Manowitz NR, Mayor G, Ridgway EC. The Colorado thyroid disease prevalence study. Arch Intern Med 2000;160:526–534.
3. Vanderpump MPJ, Tunbridge WMG. The epidemiology of thyroid diseases. In: Braverman LE, Utiger RD, eds. Werner & Ingbar's The Thyroid: A Fundamental and Clinical Text, 8th ed. Lippincott Williams & Wilkins, Philadelphia, 2000, pp. 467–473.
4. Hancock SL, Cox RS, McDougall IR. Thyroid diseases after treatment of Hodgkin's disease. N Engl J Med 1991;325:599–605.
5. Martino E, Safran M, Aghini-Lombardi F, et al. Environmental iodine intake and thyroid dysfunction during chronic amiodarone therapy. Ann Intern Med 1984;101:28–34.
6. Delange F, de Benoist B, Pretell E, Dunn JT. Iodine deficiency in the world: where do we stand at the turn of the century? Thyroid 2001;11:437–447.
7. Powe NR, Danese M, Ladenson PW. Decision analysis in endocrinology and metabolism. J Clin Endocrinol Metab 1997;26:89–112.

8. Barbesino G, Chiovato L. The genetics of Hashimoto's disease. Endocrinol Metab Clin North Am 2000;29:357–374.
9. Rosenbloom AL, Almonte AS, Brown MR, Fisher DA, Baumbach L, Parks JS. Clinical and biochemical phenotype of familial anterior hypopituitarism from mutation of the PROP1 gene. J Clin Endocrinol Metab 1999;84:50–57.
10. Hayashizaki Y, Hiraoka Y, Tatsumi K, et al. Deoxyribonucleic acid analyses of five families with familial inherited thyroid stimulating hormone deficiency. J Clin Endocrinol Metab 1990;71:792–796.
11. Yen PM. Thyrotropin receptor mutations in thyroid diseases. Rev Endocr Metab Disord 2000;1:123–129.
12. Spiegel AM. Hormone resistance caused by mutations in G proteins and G protein-coupled receptors. J Pediatr Endocrinol Metab 1999;12(suppl 1):303–309.
13. Pohlenz J, Dumitrescu A, Aumann U, et al. Congenital secondary hypothyroidism caused by exon skipping due to a homozygous donor splice site mutation in the TSHbeta-subunit gene. J Clin Endocrinol Metab 2002;87:336–339.
14. Targovnik HM, Frechtel GD, Mendive FM, et al. Evidence for the segregation of three different mutated alleles of the thyroglobulin gene in a Brazilian family with congenital goiter and hypothyroidism. Thyroid 1998;8:291–297.
15. Pohlenz J, Refetoff S. Mutations in the sodium/iodide symporter (NIS) gene as a cause for iodide transport defects and congenital hypothyroidism. Biochimie 1999;81:469–476.
16. Pannain S, Weiss RE, Jackson CE, et al. Two different mutations in the thyroid peroxidase gene of a large inbred Amish kindred: power and limits of homozygosity mapping. J Clin Endocrinol Metab 1999;84:1061–1071.
17. Kopp P. Pendred's syndrome: identification of the genetic defect a century after its recognition. Thyroid 1999;9:65–69.
18. Delange F. The disorders induced by iodine deficiency. Thyroid. 1994;4:107–128.
19. Feldt-Rasmussen U. Iodine and cancer. Thyroid 2001;11:483–486.
20. Wolff J. Physiology and pharmacology of iodized oil in goiter prophylaxis. Medicine (Baltimore) 2001;80:20–36.
21. Laurberg P, Pedersen KM, Hreidarsson A, Sigfusson N, Iversen E, Knudsen PR. Iodine intake and the pattern of thyroid disorders: a comparative epidemiological study of thyroid abnormalities in the elderly in Iceland and in Jutland, Denmark. J Clin Endocrinol Mctab 1998;83:765–769.
22. Konno N, Makita H, Yuri K, Iizuka N, Kawasaki K. Association between dietary iodine intake and prevalence of subclinical hypothyroidism in the coastal regions of Japan. J Clin Endocrinol Metab 1994 78:393–397.
23. Allen EM, Braverman LE. The effect of iodine on lymphocytic thyroiditis in the thymectomized buffalo rat. Endocrinology 1990;127:1613–1616.
24. Rose NR, Rasooly L, Saboori AM, Burek CL. Linking iodine with autoimmune thyroiditis. Environ Health Perspect 1999;107(suppl. 5):749–752.
25. Tajiri J, Higashi K, Morita M, Umeda T, Sato T. Studies of hypothyroidism in patients with high iodine intake. J Clin Endocrinol Metab 1986;63:412–417.
26. Fukata S, Kuma K, Sugawara M. Relationship between cigarette smoking and hypothyroidism in patients with Hashimoto's thyroiditis. J Endocrinol Invest 1996;19:607–612.
27. Nystrom E, Bengtsson C, Lapidus L, et al. Smoking—a risk factor for hypothyroidism. J Endocrinol Invest 1993;16:129–131.
28. Muller B, Zulewski H, Huber P, et al. Impaired action of thyroid hormone associated with smoking in women with hypothyroidism. N Engl J Med 1995;333:964–969.
29. Vestergaard P, Rejnmark L, Weeke J, et al. Smoking as a risk factor for Graves' disease, toxic nodular goiter, and autoimmune hypothyroidism. Thyroid 2002;12:69–75.
30. Fukata S, Kuma K, Sugawara M. Relationship between cigarette smoking and hypothyroidism in patients with Hashimoto's thyroiditis. J Endocrinol Invest 1996;19:607–612.

31. Colzani R, Fang SL, Alex S, et al. The effect of nicotine on thyroid function in rats. Metabolism 1998;47:154–157.
32. Utiger RD. Effects of smoking on thyroid. Eur J Endocrinol 1998;138:368–369.
33. Muller B, Zulewski H, Huber P, et al. Impaired action of thyroid hormone associated with smoking in women with hypothyroidism. N Engl J Med 1995;333:964–969.
34. Bahn AK, Mills JL, Synder PJ, et al. Hypothyroidism in workers exposed to polybrominated biphenyls. N Engl J Med 1980;302:31–33.
35. Byrne JJ, Carbone JP, Hanson EA. Hypothyroidism and abnormalities in the kinetics of thyroid hormone metabolism in rats treated chronically with polychlorinated biphenyl and polybrominated biphenyl. Endocrinology 1987;121:520–527.
36. Roberts FP, Wright AL, O'Hagan SA. Hypothyroidism in textile workers. J Soc Occup Med 1990;40:153–156.
37. Katin MJ, Teehan BP, Sigler MH, Schleifer CR, Gilgere GS. Resorcinol-induced hypothyroidism in a patient on chronic hemodialysis. Ann Intern Med 1977;86:447–449.
38. Dowsett M, Mehta A, Cantwell BM, Harris AL. Low-dose aminoglutethimide in postmenopausal breast cancer: effects on adrenal and thyroid hormone secretion. Eur J Cancer 1991;27:846–849.
39. Koh LK, Greenspan FS, Yeo PP. Interferon-alpha induced thyroid dysfunction: three clinical presentations and a review of the literature. Thyroid 1997;7:891–896.
40. Robbins J, Schneider AB. Thyroid cancer following exposure to radioactive iodine. Rev Endocr Metab Disord 2000;1:197–203.
41. Goldsmith JR, Grossman CM, Morton WE, et al. Juvenile hypothyroidism among two populations exposed to radioiodine. Environ Health Perspect 1999;107:303–308.
42. Becker DV, Braverman LE, Dunn JT, et al. The use of iodine as a thyroidal blocking agent in the event of a reactor accident. Report of the Environmental Hazards Committee of the American Thyroid Association. JAMA 1984;252:659–661.
43. Order SE, Sleeper AM, Stillwagon GB, Klein JL, Leichner PK. Current status of radioimmunoglobulins in the treatment of human malignancy. Oncology (Huntingt) 1989;3:115–120
44. Allahabadia A, Daykin J, Sheppard MC, Gough SC, Franklyn JA. Radioiodine treatment of hyperthyroidism—prognostic factors for outcome. J Clin Endocrinol Metab 2001;86:3611–3617.
45. Jones SJ, Hedley AJ, Curtis B, et al. Do we need thyroid follow-up registers? A cost-effective study. Lancet 1982;1:1229–1233.
46. Harrison LC, Buckley JD, Martin FI. Use of a computer-based postal questionnaire for the detection of hypothyroidism following radioiodine therapy for thyrotoxicosis. Aust N Z J Med 1977;7:27–32.
47. Falkenberg M, Nilsson OR, Rosenqvist U. Value of thyroid follow-up registers. Scand J Prim Health Care 1987;5:181–185.
48. Meyer CM, Ladenson PW, Scharfstein JA, Danese MD, Powe NR. Evaluation of common problems in primary care: effect of physician, practice and financial considerations. J Manag Care 2000;6:457–472.
49. LaFranchi S. Congenital hypothyroidism: etiologies, diagnosis, and management. Thyroid 1999;9:735–740.
50. Belin RM, Ladenson PW, Robinson KA, Powe NR. Development and use of evidence-based clinical practice guidelines for thyroid disease. Endocrinol Metab Clin North Am 2002;31:795–817.
51. Danese MD, Powe NR, Sawin CT, Ladenson PW. Screening for mild thyroid failure at the periodic health examination: a decision and cost-effectiveness analysis. JAMA 1996;276:285–292.
52. Nicoloff JT, LoPresti JS. Myxedema coma. A form of decompensated hypothyroidism. Endocrinol Metab Clin North Am 1993;22:279–290.

53. Danese MD, Ladenson PW, Meinert CL, Powe, NR. Effect of thyroxine therapy on serum lipoproteins in patients with mild thyroid failure: a quantitative review of the literature. J Clin Endocrinol Metab 2000;85:2993–3001.
54. Perk M, O'Neill BJ. The effect of thyroid hormone therapy on angiographic coronary artery disease progression. Can J Cardiol 1997;13:273–276.
55. Ladenson, PW. Problems in the management of hypothyroidism. In: Braverman LE, ed. Diseases of the Thyroid, 2nd ed. Humana, Totowa, NJ, 2002, pp. 161–176.
56. Klein I, Ojamaa K. Thyroid hormone and the cardiovascular system. N Engl J Med 2001;344:501–509.
57. Trence DL, Morley JE, Handwerger BS. Polyglandular autoimmune syndromes. Am J Med 1984;77:107–116.
58. Ladenson PW, Singer PA, Levy EG, et al. American Thyroid Association guidelines for detection of thyroid dysfunction. Arch Intern Med 2000;160:1573–1575. (http://www.thyroid.org/publications/guidelines.html).
59. Vanderpump, MP, Ahlquist, JA, Franklyn, JA, et al. Consensus statement for good practice and audit measures in the management of hypothyroidism and hyperthyroidism. BMJ 1996;313:539–544. (http://bmj.com/cgi/content/full/313/7056/539).
60. Spencer CA. National Academy of Clinical Biochemistry laboratory medicine practice guidelines for the diagnosis and monitoring of thyroid disease testing. The American Thyroid Association. (Last updated 9-12-2001. http://www.thyroid.org/resources/professional/nacb_comment.rtf).
61. Surks MI, Chopra IJ, Mariash CN, et al. American Thyroid Association guidelines for use of laboratory tests in thyroid disorders. JAMA 1990;263:1529–1532.
62. American Academy of Pediatrics. Newborn screening for congenital hypothyroidism: recommended guidelines. Pediatrics 1993;91:1203–1209.
63. Commission on Clinical Policies and Research, Working Group on Periodic Health Examinations, AAFP Board of Directors: Periodic Health Examinations: Summary of AAFP Policy Recommendations & Age Charts. American Academy of Family Physicians. (Last updated 2001. http://www.aafp.org/exam/intro.html).
64. Beaulieu MD. Screening for congenital hypothyroidism. Canadian Task Force on Preventive Health Care. (Last updated 1994. http://www.ctfphc.org/).
65. U.S. Preventive Services Task Force: Screening for congenital hypothyroidism. In Guide to Clinical Preventive Services, 2nd ed. Williams & Wilkins, Baltimore, 1996, pp 503–507. (http://hstat.nlm.nih.gov/ftrs/directBrowse.pl?collect=cps&dbName=cps&href=CH45).
66. Helfand M, Redfern C. Screening for thyroid disease: an update. Ann Intern Med 1998;129:141–158. (http://www.acponline.org/journals/annals/15jul98/ppthyroid2.htm).
67. U.S. Preventive Services Task Force: Screening for thyroid disease. In: Guide to Clinical Preventive Services, 2nd ed. Williams & Wilkins, Baltimore, 1996, pp 209–218. (http://hstat.nlm.nih.gov/ftrs/directBrowse.pl?collect=cps&dbName=cps&href=CH20).
68. Beaulieu MD. Screening for thyroid disorders and thyroid cancer in asymptomatic adults. Canadian Task Force on Preventive Health Care. (Last updated 1994. http://www.ctfphc.org/).
69. Gharib H, Cobin RH, Dickey RA. Subclinical hypothyroidism during pregnancy: position statement from the American Association of Clinical Endocrinologists. Endocr Pract 1999;5:367–368. (http://www.aace.com/clin.guidelines/pregnancy.pdf).

3 Hyperthyroidism

Elizabeth N. Pearce, MD, and Lewis E. Braverman, MD

CONTENTS

INTRODUCTION
WHO TO SCREEN
SCREENING METHODS
DIFFERENTIAL DIAGNOSIS
EARLY SIGNS AND SYMPTOMS
EFFECTS OF THYROTOXICOSIS
TREATMENT OF OVERT HYPERTHYROIDISM
TREATMENT OF SUBCLINICAL THYROTOXICOSIS
REFERENCES

INTRODUCTION

The introduction of increasingly sensitive serum thyroid-stimulating hormone (TSH) assays over the past decade has led to the ability to detect thyrotoxicosis at an early stage, before the development of overt disease. TSH screening is now widely advocated for some groups of asymptomatic patients. The clinical consequences of subclinical thyrotoxicosis are becoming better understood, but the best method for the workup and treatment of subclinical disease remains controversial.

The generic term thyrotoxicosis refers to the clinical syndrome in which serum total and free triiodothyronine (T3) or free thyroxine (T4) concentrations or both are elevated and the peripheral tissues are hypermetabolic, irrespective of the source of the excess hormones. Hyperthyroidism is one cause of thyrotoxicosis and is defined as increased endogenous thyroid hormone synthesis and release. Another cause of thyrotoxicosis is excess outpouring of hormone from a damaged thyroid in the absence of excess production, including the various causes of thyroiditis. A third cause is excess thyroid hormone ingestion. Subclinical thyrotoxicosis is defined as the presence of a low serum TSH level with normal total and free T3 and T4 concentrations.

From: *Contemporary Endocrinology: Early Diagnosis and Treatment of Endocrine Disorders*
Edited by: R. S. Bar © Humana Press Inc., Totowa, NJ

Overt thyrotoxicosis is relatively common in the general population. However, it has been difficult to quantify the prevalence of subclinical disease. The observed prevalence of subclinical thyrotoxicosis varies regionally depending on dietary iodine intake *(1)* and the prevalence of thyroid autoantibodies; nonthyroidal illness, especially in institutionalized or elderly patients, may be difficult to differentiate from subclinical disease, and the sensitivity of TSH assays used in various studies has differed *(2)*. Some studies have excluded patients on L-thyroxine (L-T4) therapy, a major cause of subclinical thyrotoxicosis, whereas others have not. The Whickham survey, a large English cross-sectional study begun in the 1970s, found that overt thyrotoxicosis was present in 2% of adult women (and was ten times more common than in men) *(3)*. In the 20-yr follow-up of the Whickham survey, 2–3% of the cohort had a suppressed TSH without overt symptoms *(4)*. One U.S. study found suppressed TSH values in 2.5% of the population over age 55 *(5)*. Data from the original Framingham Heart Study cohort evaluated 2575 ambulatory subjects over age 60 and found suppressed serum TSH values in 3.9% (half of whom were ingesting exogenous thyroid hormone) and overt thyrotoxicosis in only 0.2% *(15)*. More recently, a Colorado prevalence study found overt thyrotoxicosis in 0.1% and subclinical disease in 2.1% of adults overall, but found some degree of thyrotoxicosis in 21% of those taking thyroid medication *(6)*. Finally, the third National Health and Nutrition Examination Survey in the United States (1988–1994) found overt thyrotoxicosis in 0.5% and subclinical disease in 0.8% of the U.S. population ages 12 and older *(7)*. Of interest is the fact that both autoimmune thyroid disease and mean serum TSH values were lower in African Americans than in Caucasians.

WHO TO SCREEN

It is clear that individuals who present with signs and symptoms of thyrotoxicosis should have thyroid function tests carried out. However, there has been an ongoing debate about the role of screening in asymptomatic patients. In 1990, American Thyroid Association guidelines recommended against screening of asymptomatic patients, as it was unclear whether early diagnosis conferred any benefit *(8)*. As recently as 1996, the U.S. Preventive Services Task Force recommended against TSH screening for asymptomatic adults *(9)*. In 1998 the American College of Physicians issued guidelines recommending routine TSH screening for all women over age 50 *(10)*. More recently, given the high prevalence of thyroid dysfunction in the general population, and the potentially serious consequences of undetected disease, the American Thyroid Association has advocated the screening of all adults aged 35 yr or over with serum TSH measurements every 5 yr *(11)*. This approach has been found to be cost-effective, particularly in women, although only because of the detection of overt and subclinical hypothyroidism, which is more prevalent than thyrotoxicosis *(12)*. We believe that this recommendation is somewhat arbitrary but that serum TSH testing should certainly be carried out in women over age 55 yr on a regular basis.

More frequent screening is indicated in patients with known risk factors such as the presence of a goiter, a history of type 1 diabetes mellitus, previous thyroid surgery or radiation, pernicious anemia, premature gray hair, vitiligo, or any previous history or family history of thyroid disease. Additionally, in any patient with an unexplained laboratory abnormality such as hypercholesterolemia, hyponatremia, anemia, hypercalcemia, or creatine kinase elevation serum TSH levels should be determined (11). Patients with new-onset atrial fibrillation should also be tested, since approximately 15% will be thyrotoxic (13,14). Patients should be evaluated for thyroid dysfunction before starting therapy with iodine-containing medications and then periodically while taking those medications.

SCREENING METHODS

The serum TSH should be the first thyroid function test obtained in patients suspected of thyroid dysfunction or in the screening of older patients or those at risk for thyroid disease. A serum TSH level below the lower limits of detectability in any given assay raises the suspicion of thyrotoxicosis. A patient with a TSH value below the normal range but still detectable is probably not thyrotoxic, and the test should be repeated in a few months.

Further studies are warranted in patients whose serum TSH is undetectable and who are not receiving thyroid hormone therapy (Fig. 1). A careful physical exam, especially of the thyroid, should be carried out in all patients, since the presence of a goiter would make the diagnosis of thyroid dysfunction more likely. We usually obtain thyroperoxidase (TPO) and thyroglobulin (Tg) antibodies and some measure of thyroid hormone levels, primarily a serum T4, free T4 (or index), and total T3 (or free T3). If either or both of the thyroid antibodies are positive, autoimmune thyroid disease is present. If either of the circulating free thyroid hormones is elevated, then the patient almost certainly has some form of overt thyrotoxicosis. If circulating thyroid hormone levels are normal, suggesting subclinical disease, a serum TSH should be repeated in a few months, since a suppressed TSH may be a transient finding. For example, in the Framingham Heart Study, 88% of those who had subclinical thyrotoxicosis at baseline had serum TSH values more than 0.1 on repeat testing 4 yr later (15). Additionally, subclinical disease must be differentiated from other causes of low serum TSH values including nonthyroidal illness, first-trimester pregnancy, pituitary or hypothalamic insufficiency, and the use of medications including glucocorticoids, dopamine, aspirin, furosemide, and fenclofenac, which suppress TSH release (16). Finally, a serum Tg might prove to be of interest. If the serum Tg is in the upper normal range or elevated, this would suggest that the thyroid may indeed be hyperfunctioning and secreting Tg. On the other hand, if the serum Tg

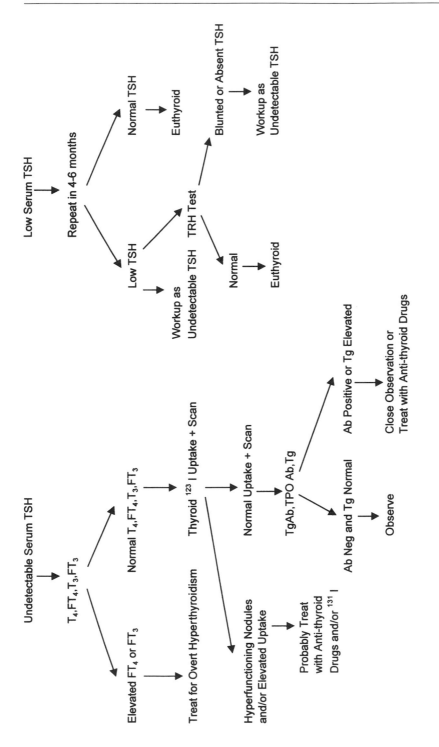

Fig. 1. Laboratory evaluation for suspected endogenous hyperthyroidism. Tg, thyroglobulin; TPO, thyroperopidase; TRH, thyrotropin-releasing hormone; TSH, thyroid-stimulating hormone.

Table 1
Thyrotoxicosis Associated with an Elevated Thyroid RAIU (Hyperthyroidism)

Type	Etiology
Circulating thyroid stimulators	
Graves' disease	Circulating TSH receptor antibody
Inappropriate TSH hypersecretion	TSH secreting pituitary tumor ($\uparrow$ α-subunit)
	Pituitary resistance to thyroid hormone
Trophoblastic tumor	
Choriocarcinoma	Circulating asialo HCG
Hyperemesis gravidarum	
Autonomous thyroid function	
Solitary hyperfunctioning adenoma	Autonomous function owing to a
Multinodular goiter	somatic point mutation of the TSH receptor (TSHR) in some cells, causing constitutive activation
Non-autoimmune autosomal dominant hyperthyroidism	Germline point mutation of the TSHR, causing constitutive activation
Familial gestational hyperthyroidism	Mutant TSHR hypersensitive to HCG
Lithium	Variable

HCG, human chorionic gonadotropin; TSH, thyroid-stimulating hormone.

is in the low-normal range, endogenous thyroid hyperfunction is less likely; if the serum Tg is suppressed, then thyrotoxicosis factitia should be ruled out.

Once overt or subclinical thyrotoxicosis has been identified, the radioiodine uptake (RAIU) and scan may be used to help determine the etiology (Tables 1 and 2). The thyroid RAIU is elevated in Graves' disease. It may be normal or only mildly elevated in patients with a toxic multinodular goiter. It will be low in thyrotoxicosis owing to exogenous L-T4 administration, or from the thyrotoxic phase of thyroiditis, but the serum Tg will be low in the former and elevated in the latter. A scan may be helpful in differentiating between Graves' disease (diffuse uptake) and toxic multinodular goiter (one or more focal areas of uptake) (17). In some cases, measurement of TSH receptor-stimulating antibodies can be helpful in confirming a diagnosis of Graves' disease. These antibodies are detectable in over 90% of adults with newly diagnosed Graves' disease (18).

DIFFERENTIAL DIAGNOSIS

In iodine-sufficient regions such as the United States, overt hyperthyroidism is most commonly caused by Graves' disease. The first and only abnormality in early Graves' disease may be a suppressed serum TSH. Multinodular or

Table 2
Thyrotoxicosis Associated with a Low Thyroid RAIU

Type	Etiology
Inflammatory disease	Release of stored hormone
Silent lymphocytic thyroiditis	
Subacute painful thyroiditis	
Drug-induced (amiodarone, lithium,	
interferon-α, interleukin-2	
High-dose x-ray therapy	
Surgical manipulation	
Infarction of thyroid adenoma	Release of stored hormone
Thyrotoxicosis factitia	Excess thyroid hormone in
	medication or food
Metastatic thyroid cancer	Foci of functional autonomy
Iodine-induced (hyperthyroidism)	Iodine excess plus goiter
Struma ovarii (hyperthyroidism)	Ovarian teratoma

RAIU, radioiodine uptake.

uninodular toxic goiter is another major cause of hyperthyroidism, especially in areas of marginal iodine intake. The natural history of multinodular goiter (Plummer's disease) appears to be the gradual development of autonomy, leading first to subclinical and then to overt hyperthyroidism *(19)*. The prevalence of thyroid nodularity generally increases with age, especially in women—in one English postmortem study, 23% of women over age 60 had nodular glands *(20)*. A German postmortem study (in an area of moderate iodine deficiency) found nodules in 88% of elderly women *(21)*.

Thyrotoxicosis is frequently iatrogenic, the result of overzealous thyroid hormone replacement therapy for hypothyroidism or of TSH-suppressive therapy for thyroid cancer. In older patients with autonomous nodules, hyperthyroidism may be precipitated by an exogenous iodine load owing to radiocontrast agents and other iodine-containing medications, including all forms of kelp. In particular, amiodarone is an important cause of thyrotoxicosis. Amiodarone-induced thyrotoxicosis can be the result of excess iodine-induced thyroid hormone synthesis in an abnormal thyroid gland (Type I) or of amiodarone-related destructive thyroiditis (Type II) *(22)*.

Thyrotoxicosis may occur secondary to thyroiditis—in this case it is caused not by increased thyroid hormone production but by the release of excess hormone from a damaged gland. Very rarely, hyperthyroidism may be caused by excess TSH secretion from a pituitary adenoma, by metastatic thyroid carcinoma, or by pituitary resistance to thyroid hormone *(23)*.

The causes of subclinical hyperthyroidism are similar to those that cause overt thyrotoxicosis *(24)*.

EARLY SIGNS AND SYMPTOMS

The clinical presentation of overt thyrotoxicosis can be subtle and nonspecific. Some patients may complain of classic symptoms such as nervousness, sweating, fatigue, heat intolerance, weakness, tremor, hyperactivity, changes in weight or appetite, insomnia, exertional dyspnea, hyperdefecation, or palpitations. Oligomenorrhea occurs in about one in four women with thyrotoxicosis *(25)*. Thyrotoxic patients, especially among the elderly, may have higher rates of depression than their euthyroid counterparts *(26)*. Although subclinical thyrotoxicosis is usually assumed to be asymptomatic, some studies suggest it may be possible to elicit subtle physical and psychiatric symptoms in these patients *(27)*.

Physical findings in thyrotoxicosis may include hyperactivity, tachycardia or atrial fibrillation, systolic hypertension, warm, moist, smooth skin, stare and eyelid retraction, tremor, hyperreflexia, and muscle weakness *(28)*. Goiter is not invariably present: one study found that 37% of thyrotoxic patients over age 60 did not have thyroid enlargement *(29)*. In Graves' disease, ophthalmologic findings may include exopthalmos, extraocular muscle dysfunction, periorbital edema, conjunctival chemosis and injection, and exposure keratitis *(30)*. Pretibial myxedema is rarely seen in patients with Graves' disease and only when eye disease is also present.

After the fifth decade of life, there is a gradual decrease in the number of classic presenting signs and symptoms of thyrotoxicosis *(31–33)*. Even overt thyrotoxicosis may go undiagnosed in older patients in the absence of routine TSH screening. Rather than appearing hyperactive as younger patients do, older individuals with thyrotoxicosis may seem placid or depressed, i.e., the "apathetic hyperthyroidism" described by Lahey in 1931 *(34)*. Although older patients with hyperthyroidism are less likely than younger ones to have a resting tachycardia, they are more likely to have atrial arrhythmia *(35)*. Weight loss in younger patients is usually associated with increased appetite, whereas in older patients it may instead be associated with anorexia *(36)*.

EFFECTS OF THYROTOXICOSIS

Bone Effects

Postmenopausal women are at high risk for losing bone density. Up to 3% of bone mass is commonly lost within each of the first 5 yr after menopause *(37)*. It is estimated that 30% of Caucasian women in the United States have osteoporosis *(38)*. Concomitant thyrotoxicosis, whether subclinical or overt, has been shown to exacerbate this risk for postmenopausal osteoporosis. In thyrotoxicosis there is an increase in both osteoblast and osteoclast activity. This results in increased bone turnover, as measured by increased urine, and serum *N*-telopeptide, and serum osteocalcin, with a net increase in bone resorption *(39,40)*. In overtly thyrotoxic patients, the increased bone resorption may occasionally lead to hypercalcemia *(41)* and more commonly to decreased bone density *(42)*. Cortical bone is affected more severely than trabecular bone *(43)*.

Multiple studies of the effects of subclinical thyrotoxicosis on bone have provided conflicting results since the first study by Ross et al. *(44)* demonstrating reduced bone density in patients receiving TSH-suppressive doses of L-T4. Grant et al. *(45)* found no significant differences in forearm bone mineral density among postmenopausal women on long-term TSH-suppressive doses of L-T4, those on replacement L-T4 doses, and euthyroid controls. However, in a large study of postmenopausal women, Schneider et al. *(46)* found significantly lower bone density at multiple skeletal sites in women taking more than 200 µg of L-T4 daily versus those taking smaller doses of thyroid hormone. Studies by Lehmke et al. *(47)* and Kung et al. *(48)* found lower bone densities in postmenopausal women with subclinical thyrotoxicosis secondary to TSH-suppressive doses of L-T4. Campbell et al. *(49)* showed increased markers of bone turnover in hypothyroid postmenopausal women treated with TSH-suppressive versus replacement doses of L-T4. L-T4 therapy does not seem to have a deleterious effect on bone density, however, when given in replacement, rather than TSH-suppressive, doses *(50)*. In fact, in a 2-yr prospective study, Guo et al. *(51)* were able to show that bone density increased and markers of bone turnover decreased after postmenopausal women were switched from suppressive to replacement doses of L-T4. Endogenous subclinical hyperthyroidism seems to confer the same risks as TSH-suppressive L-T4 doses. Mudde et al. *(52)* found that women with subclinical hyperthyroidism owing to untreated multinodular goiter had significantly lower bone densities at the forearm than age- and menopausal status-matched euthyroid controls *(52)*.

Although overt hyperthyroidism is known to be associated with increased fracture risk, data are less clear for subclinical hyperthyroidism despite the known reductions in bone density and increase in markers of bone turnover. In a Scottish study, primarily of postmenopausal women, no differences in the rate of fractures requiring hospitalization were seen over an average 8.6 yr of follow-up between hypothyroid patients treated with replacement doses of L-T4 versus those treated with TSH-suppressive doses *(53)*. A recent large prospective study found that postmenopausal women over age 65 with serum TSH levels of 0.1 mIU/L or less at baseline had increased risk for both vertebral and hip fractures over a mean follow-up period of 3.7 yr. T3 and T4 were not measured in this study, so it is not clear how many of these women had overt versus subclinical thyrotoxicosis. The authors did note that thyroid hormone use was not associated with increased fracture risk if the serum TSH values were normal *(54)*.

In men and premenopausal women, the effects of subclinical hyperthyroidism on bone are of uncertain significance. Marcocci et al. *(55)* reported that there was no evidence of decreased bone mineral density in men receiving TSH-suppressive doses of L-T4. Lecomte et al. *(56)* found a significant increase in serum osteocalcin between premenopausal women on suppressive L-T4 therapy and euthyroid controls. Foldes et al. *(57)* found that bone density of the lumbar spine, femoral neck, and midshaft radius was not significantly decreased in premeno-pausal women with endogenous subclinical hyperthyroidism. Although Harvey et al. *(40)* documented increased urinary markers of bone turnover in postmeno-pausal women on suppressive doses of L-T4, they did not find any increase in bone turnover in premenopausal women on similar L-T4 doses. Similarly, Gurlek and Gedik *(58)* did not find any increase in bone turnover, or decrease in bone density, in a sample of premenopausal women with endogenous subclinical hyperthyroidism compared with euthyroid controls, although an older study by Paul et al. *(59)* reported a small but significant decrease in hip but not spine bone mineral density in TSH-suppressed premenopausal women.

There are some discrepancies in the literature on the effects of TSH-suppres-sive doses of L-T4 on bone in pre- compared with postmenopausal women, but two large meta-analyses reached similar conclusions: that TSH-suppressive doses of L-T4 decrease bone mineral density in postmenopausal but not in pre-menopausal women *(60,61)*.

Postmenopausal or perimenopausal women with subclinical thyrotoxicosis may be particularly good candidates for estrogen or bisphosphonate therapy, which can prevent the thyroid-associated bone loss. Rosen et al. *(62)* reported that cyclic intravenous pamidronate increased bone density in patients receiving TSH-suppressive doses of L-T4. Women taking both estrogen replacement therapy and L-T4 have been shown to have significantly higher bone densities than those taking L-T4 alone *(46)*. Lecomte et al. *(56)* showed no difference in bone turnover or bone mineral density between postmenopausal women on TSH-suppressive doses of L-T4 and estrogen replacement therapy compared with euthyroid controls.

Cardiac Effects

Overt thyrotoxicosis, especially when associated with tachycardia or atrial arrhythymias, has long been known to aggravate underlying cardiac disease, worsening angina secondary to increased myocardial oxygen demand. Thyro-toxicosis leads to increased cardiac contractility at rest, although there may be impaired ventricular function with exertion. Tachycardia decreases diastolic coronary perfusion time *(63)*. All these factors can contribute to the development of cardiomyopathy and congestive heart failure. Significant cardiac dysfunction may also result from subclinical thyrotoxicosis. A recent review summarizes the effects of thyroid hormones on the cardiovascular system *(64)*.

Biondi et al. *(65)* examined cardiac function and exercise tolerance in a group of ten subjects, all of whom had been treated with TSH-suppressive doses of L-T4 for at least 5 yr, and all of whom complained of exertional dyspnea. They showed impaired resting left-ventricular diastolic filling, increased exertional left-ventricular ejection fraction, and significantly reduced exercise capacity in the TSH-suppressed group compared with controls. Notably, these findings all improved after 4 mo of β-blocker therapy. Another study by the same group noted significantly higher average heart rates, a higher prevalence of atrial premature beats, and left-ventricular hypertrophy on echocardiography in patients on long-term TSH-suppressive L-T4 therapy compared with controls (66). However, when Shapiro et al. (67) looked at a group of 17 asymptomatic patients on TSH-suppressive L-T4 therapy, they found no difference between these subjects and controls in mean heart rate, prevalence of atrial premature contractions, or mean ejection fraction. Left-ventricular mass index was significantly increased in the L-T-4-treated group, although it was still within normal limits (67).

Tenerz et al. (68) studied 40 patients with subclinical thyrotoxicosis compared with a control group and found that atrial fibrillation was present in 28% of the subclinical group compared with 10% of the controls. Data from the Framingham Heart Study demonstrated that, over 10 yr of follow-up in patients over age 60, the cumulative incidence of atrial fibrillation was 28% in those with low serum TSH values (>0.1) at baseline, compared with 11% of patients with normal TSH levels. Only 2 of the 13 patients with suppressed TSH values in this study who developed atrial fibrillation also developed overt hyperthyroidism during the follow-up period; the rest were subclinically thyrotoxic (69). This finding has important clinical implications, as thyrotoxicosis-associated atrial fibrillation may be complicated by thromboembolism in up to 15% of patients (13).

TREATMENT OF OVERT HYPERTHYROIDISM

Patients with overt hyperthyroidism from Graves' disease or from toxic multinodular goiter should clearly be treated. One therapeutic option for patients with Graves' disease is medical management with methimazole (MMI) or propylthiouracil (PTU), both of which decrease thyroid hormone synthesis. Therapy with one of these drugs will induce long-term remission of Graves' disease in about half of all patients, although those patients with large goiters are less likely to remain euthyroid (70). Since remission of the hyperthyroidism caused by toxic multinodular goiter almost never occurs, therapy with MMI or PTU is only given prior to definitive therapy, as described below. Side effects of both of these medications include rash or urticaria. More seriously, agranulocytosis occurs in approximately 0.3% of patients (71). Patients starting on these medications should be cautioned to discontinue them and call their physician if they develop fever, rash, jaundice, arthralgia, or sore throat.

More definitive therapy with radioactive iodine may also be elected, especially in older patients. After radioactive iodine treatment, patients may become transiently more thyrotoxic owing to damage to the gland and release of stored hormone. Pretreatment with antithyroid medications may help protect older patients or others at risk for cardiac complications by decreasing thyroid hormone stores *(71)*, although this concept has recently been challenged *(72,73)*. Most patients will become euthyroid within weeks after receiving a single large dose of radioiodine; the remaining 10–20% of patients require retreatment 6 mo to a year later. Within a year of treatment, up to 90% of patients will become hypothyroid; the other 10% become hypothyroid at a rate of 2–3% per year *(70)*.

Surgery is another option for treatment of younger patients with hyperthyroidism. It is especially useful for patients with very large goiters and/or compressive symptoms who often require multiple doses of ^{131}I. Subtotal or near-total thyroidectomy is the procedure of choice. The most common adverse effects of thyroidectomy are injury to the parathyroids, resulting in hypocalcemia, and injury to the recurrent laryngeal nerve. Patients should be treated with antithyroid drugs to restore euthyroidism preoperatively. Additionally, they should receive iodine for 7–10 d before surgery to decrease thyroid blood flow. When a patient with a large goiter is noncompliant with medical therapy and thyroidectomy is planned, euthyroidism can be achieved in 5–7 d by a regimen similar to that employed in some patients with thyroid storm. Large doses of PTU or MMI decrease hormone synthesis. One milligram of dexamethasone twice a day decreases peripheral conversion of T4 to T3 by inhibiting the outer ring 5'-deiodinase. The iodine-rich contrast agent iopanoic acid (0.5 g twice a day) decreases T4 to T3 generation, release of hormone from the gland, and thyroid blood flow. A β-blocker decreases the catecholamine effects of thyrotoxicosis. All these medications are given, under careful supervision, at home or preferably in the hospital *(74)*.

β-Blockers can be used as adjunctive treatment to slow the heart rate and improve symptoms of anxiety, tremor, palpitations, heat intolerance, and tremor. β-blockade should be used as primary therapy only in patients with transient thyrotoxicosis secondary to thyroiditis and a low thyroid RAIU *(71)*.

Once patients become biochemically euthyroid, symptoms of hyperthyroidism should resolve within a few weeks. Patients with atrial fibrillation in the setting of hyperthyroidism will often spontaneously convert to sinus rhythm once the hyperthyroidism has been corrected, generally within 4 mo of normalization of serum T3 and T4 concentrations *(75)*.

TREATMENT OF SUBCLINICAL THYROTOXICOSIS

Whereas overt thyrotoxicosis clearly requires therapy, the question of whether early, subclinical hyperthyroidism should be treated remains controversial *(76,77)*. To date, large, long-term randomized trials examining this question have not been carried out. Clinical manifestations of subclinical hyperthyroidism, if present, can be managed without antithyroid therapies: osteoporosis can be treated with estrogen replacement and bisphosphonates and tachycardia with β-blockers. However, once a persistently suppressed TSH level has been documented, the goal of specific therapy is to normalize the serum TSH using small doses of MMI or PTU. Definitive therapy with ^{131}I may be carried out, especially in patients with goiter, although large doses may be required in the setting of a normal 24-h RAIU. The thyroid ^{131}I uptake may be enhanced by the prior administration of recombinant human TSH *(78,79)*. Early therapy may be especially beneficial for patients with multinodular goiter, given an expected progression to overt hyperthyroidism *(80)*. Treatment with antithyroid drugs has been shown to have a beneficial effect on osteoporosis in two small studies *(81,82)*. Additionally, treatment of subclinical hyperthyroidism does seem to decrease the risk for atrial fibrillation *(77)*. Some authors *(16,35)* advocate aggressive treatment for subclinical hyperthyroidism, whereas others suggest a policy of watchful waiting, deferring treatment until the hyperthyroidism becomes overt *(76,83)*. Samuels *(2)* suggests that good candidates for treatment include elderly patients with unexplained weight loss, women with osteopenia, and those with additional known risk factors for atrial fibrillation. Regardless of whether one opts to treat patients with subclinical hyperthyroidism, the diagnosis mandates close follow-up to prevent the deleterious effects of overt thyrotoxicosis.

If the serum TSH is low during therapy for hypothyroidism (in nonthyroid cancer patients), the dose of L-T4 should be decreased every 3–4 mo until the serum TSH normalizes.

REFERENCES

1. Laurberg P, Bulow Pedersen I, Knudsen N, Ovesen L, Andersen S. Environmental iodine intake affects the type of nonmalignant thyroid disease. Thyroid 2001;11:457–469.
2. Samuels MH. Subclinical thyroid disease in the elderly. Thyroid 1998;8:803–813.
3. Tunbridge WMG, Evered DC, Hall R, et al. The spectrum of thyroid disease in a community: The Whickham Survey. Clin Endocrinol 1977;7:481–493.
4. Vanderpump PJ, Tunbridge WMG. The epidemiology of thyroid diseases. In: Braverman LE, Utiger RD, eds. Werner and Ingbar's The Thyroid, 8th ed. JB Lippincott, Philadelphia, 2000, pp. 467–473.
5. Bagchi N, Brown TR, Parish RF. Thyroid dysfunction in adults over age 55 years: a study in an urban US community. Arch Intern Med 1990;150:785–787.
6. Canaris GJ, Manowitz NR, Mayor G, Ridgway EC. The Colorado Thyroid Disease Prevalence Study. Arch Intern Med 2000;160:526–534.
7. Hollowell JG, Staehling NW, Hannon WH, et al. Serum thyrotropin, thyroxine, and thyroid antibodies in the United States population (1988 to 1994): National Health and Nutrition Examination Survey (NHANES III). J Clin Endocrinol Metab, 2002;87:489–499.
8. Surks MI, Chopra IJ, Mariash CN, et al. American Thyroid Association guidelines for use of laboratory tests in thyroid disorders. JAMA 1990;263:1529–1532.
9. US Preventive Services Task Force. Guide to Clinical Preventive Services, 2nd ed. Williams & Wilkins, Baltimore, 1996.
10. Helfand M, Redfern CC. Screening for thyroid disease: an update. Ann Intern Med 1998;129:144–158.

11. Ladenson PW, Singer PA, Ain KB, et al. American Thyroid Association guidelines for detection of thyroid dysfunction. Arch Intern Med 2000;160:1573–1575.
12. Danese MD, Powe NR, Sawin CT, Ladenson PW. Screening for mild thyroid failure at the periodic health examination: a decision and cost-effectiveness analysis. JAMA 1996;276:285–292.
13. Ladenson PW. Thyrotoxicosis and the heart: something old and something new. J Clin Endocrinol Metab 1993;77:332–333.
14. Sulimani RA. Diagnostic algorithm for atrial fibrillation caused by occult hyperthyroidism. Geriatrics 1989;44:61–64.
15. Sawin CT, Geller A, Kaplan MM, Bacharach P, Wilson PWF, Hershman JM. Low serum thyrotropin (thyroid-stimulating hormone) in older persons without hyperthyroidism. Arch Intern Med 1991;151:165–168.
16. Surks MI, Ocampo E. Subclinical thyroid disease. Am J Med 1996;100:217–223.
17. McDougall IR, Cavalieri RR. In vivo radionuclide tests and imaging. In: Braverman LE, Utiger RD, eds. Werner and Ingbar's The Thyroid, 8th ed. JB Lippincott, Philadelphia, 2000, pp. 355–375.
18. Marcocci C, Chiovato L. Thyroid-directed antibodies. In: Braverman LE, Utiger RD, eds. Werner and Ingbar's The Thyroid, 8th ed. JB Lippincott, Philadelphia, 2000, pp. 414–431.
19. Berghout A, Wiersinga WM, Smits NJ, Touber JL. Interrelationships between age, thyroid volume, thyroid nodularity, and thyroid function in patients with sporadic nontoxic goiter. Am J Med 1990;89:602–608.
20. Denham MJ, Wills EJ. A clinico-pathological survey of thyroid glands in old age. Gerontology 1980;26:160–166.
21. Pullen R, Hintze G. Size and structure of the thyroid in old age. J Am Geriatr Soc 1997;5:1539.
22. Martino E, Bartalena L, Bogazzi F, Braverman LE. The effects of amiodarone on the thyroid. Endocr Rev 2001;22:240–254.
23. Mokshagundam S, Barzel US. Thyroid disease in the elderly. J Am Geriatr Soc 1993;41:1361–1369.
24. Charkes ND. The many causes of subclinical hyperthyroidism. Thyroid 1996;6:391–396.
25. Krassas GE, Pontikides N, Kaltsas T, et al. Menstrual disturbances in thyrotoxicosis. Clin Endocrinol 1994;40:641–644.
26. Whybrow PC, Bauer M. Behavioral and psychiatric aspects of thyrotoxicosis. In: Braverman LE, Utiger RD, eds. Werner and Ingbar's The Thyroid, 8th ed. JB Lippincott, Philadelphia, 2000, pp. 673–678.
27. Schlote-Sautter B, Schmidt R, Kaumeier S, Teuber J, Vardarli I, Usaldel KH. Subclinical hyperthyroidism: do physical and mental symptoms exist that justify treatment? In: Reinwein D, Scriba PC, eds. The Various Types of Hyperthyroidism. Urban & Schwartzenberg, Munich, 1990, 319–322.
28. Braverman LE, Utiger RD. Introduction to thyrotoxicosis. In: Braverman LE, Utiger RD, eds. Werner and Ingbar's The Thyroid, 8th ed. JB Lippincott, Philadelphia, 2000, pp. 515–517.
29. Davis PJ, Davis FB. Hyperthyroidism in patients over the age of 60 years: clinical features in 85 patients. Medicine 1974;53:161–181.
30. Bahn RS, Heufelder AE. Mechanisms of disease: pathogenesis of Graves' ophthalmopathy. N Engl J Med 1993;329:1468–1475.
31. Marnini P, Piantanida E, Venco A. Hyperthyroidism in the elderly: difference in the clinical findings compared with younger patients. J Endocrinol Invest 1999;22 (suppl to no. 10):44.
32. Nordyke RA, Gilbert FI, Harada AS. Graves' disease: influence of age on clinical findings. Arch Intern Med 1988;148:626–631.
33. Trivalle C, Doucet J, Chassagne P, et al. Differences in the signs and symptoms of hyperthyroidism in older and younger patients. J Am Geriatr Soc 1996;44:50–53.
34. Lahey FH. Nonactivated (apathetic) type of hyperthyroidism. N Engl J Med 1931;204:747–748.
35. Jayme JJ, Ladenson PW. Subclinical thyroid dysfunction in the elderly. Trends Endocrinol Metab 1994;5:79–86.

36. Sirota DK. Thyroid function and dysfunction in the elderly: a brief review. Mt Sinai J Med 1980;47:126–131.
37. Riggs BL, Melton LJ. Involutional osteoporosis. N Engl J Med 1986;314:1676–1686.
38. Wasnich RD. Epidemiology of osteoporosis. In: Primer on the Metabolic Bone Diseases and Disorders of Mineral Metabolism, 4th ed. Lippincott, Philadelphia, 1999, pp. 257–259.
39. Baran DT, Braverman LE. Editorial: thyroid hormones and bone mass. J Clin Endocrinol Metab 1991;72:1182-1183.
40. Harvey RD, McHardy KC, Reid IW, et al. Measurement of bone collagen degradation in hyperthyroidism and during thyroxine replacement therapy using pyridium cross-links as specific urinary markers. J Clin Endocrinol Metab 1991;72:1189–1194.
41. Burman KD, Monchik JM, Earll JM, Wartofsky L. Ionized and total serum calcium and parathyroid hormone in hyperthyroidism. Ann Intern Med 1976;84:668–671.
42. Lee MS, Kim SY, Lee MC, et al. Negative correlation between the change in bone mineral density and serum osteocalcin in patients with hyperthyroidism. J Clin Endocrinol Metab 1990;70:766–770.
43. Ross DS. Hyperthyroidism, thyroid hormone therapy and bone. Thyroid 1994;4:319–326.
44. Ross DS, Neer RM, Ridgway RC, Daniels GH. Subclinical hyperthyroidism and reduced bone density as a possible result of prolonged suppression of the pituitary-thyroid axis with L-thyroxine. Am J Med 1987;82:1167–1170.
45. Grant DJ, McMurdo MET, Mole PA, Paterson CR, Davies RR. Suppressed TSH levels secondary to thyroxine replacement therapy are not associated with osteoporosis. Clin Endocrinol 1993;39:529–533.
46. Schneider DL, Barrett-Connor EL, Morton DJ. Thyroid hormone use and bone mineral density in elderly women: effects of estrogen. JAMA 1994;271:1245–1249.
47. Lehmke J, Bogner U, Felsenberg D, Peters H, Schleusener H. determination of bone mineral density by quantitative computed tomography and single photon absorptiometry in subclinical hyperthyroidism: a risk of early osteopaenia in post-menopausal women. Clin Endocrinol 1992;36:511–517.
48. Kung AWC, Lorentz T, Tam SCF. Thyroxine suppressive therapy decreases bone mineral density in post-menopausal women. Clin Endocrinol 1993;39:535–540.
49. Campbell J, Day P, Diamond T. Fine adjustments in thyroxine replacement and its effect on bone metabolism. Thyroid 1996;6:75–78.
50. Hanna FWF, Pettit RJ, Ammari F, Evans WD, Sandeman D, Lazarus JH. Effect of replacement doses of thyroxine on bone mineral density. Clin Endocrinol 1998;48:229–234.
51. Gou CY, Weetman AP, Eastell R. Longitudinal changes of bone mineral density and bone turnover in postmenopausal women on thyroxine. Clin Endocrinol 1997;46:301–307.
52. Mudde AH, Reijnders FJL, Kruseman CAN. Peripheral bone density in women with untreated multinodular goiter. Clin Endocrinol 1992;37:35–39.
53. Leese GP, Jung RT, Guthrie C, Waugh N, Browning MCK. Morbidity in patients on L-thyroxine: a comparison of those with a normal TSH to those with a suppressed TSH. Clin Endocrinol 1992;37:500-503.
54. Bauer DC, Ettinger B, Nevitt MC, Stone KL. Risk for fracture in women with low serum levels of thyroid-stimulating hormone. Ann Intern Med 2001;134:561–568.
55. Marcocci C, Golia F, Vignali E, Pinchera A. Skeletal integrity in men chronically treated with suppressive doses of L-thyroxine. J Bone Miner Res 1997;12:72–77.
56. Lecomte P, Lecureuil N, Osorio-Salazar C, Lecureuil M, Valat C. Effects of suppressive doses of levothyroxine treatment on sex-hormone-binding globulin and bone metabolism. Thyroid 1995;5:19–23.
57. Foldes J, Tarjan G, Szathmari M, Varga F, Kresznal I, Horvath C. Bone mineral density in patients with endogenous subclinical hyperthyroidism: is this thyroid status a risk factor for osteoporosis? Clin Endocrinol 1993;39:521–527.

58. Gurlek A, Gedik O. Effect of endogenous subclinical hyperthyroidism on bone metabolism and bone mineral density in premenopausal women. Thyroid 1999;9:539–543.
59. Paul TL, Kerrigan J, Kelly AM, Braverman LE, Baran DT. Long-term l-thyroxine therapy is associated with decreased hip bone density in pre-menopausal women. JAMA 1988;259:3137–3141.
60. Uzzan B, Campos J, Cucherat M, Nony P, Boissel JP, Perret GY. Effects on bone mass of long term treatment with thyroid hormones: a meta-analysis. J Clin Endocrinol Metab 1996;81:4278–4289.
61. Faber J, Galloe AM. Changes in bone mass during prolonged subclinical hyperthyroidism due to L-thyroxine treatment: a meta-analysis. Eur J Endocrinol 1994;130:350–356.
62. Rosen HN, Moses AC, Garber J, et al. Randomized trial of pamidronate in patients with thyroid cancer: bone density is not reduced by suppressive doses of thyroxine, but is increased by cyclic intravenous pamidronate. J Clin Endocrinol Metab 1998;83:2324–2330.
63. Kahaly GJ, Nieswandt J, Mohr-Kahaly S. Cardiac risks of hyperthyroidism in the elderly. Thyroid 1998;8:1165–1169.
64. Klein I, Ojamaa K. Thyroid hormone and the cardiovascular system. N Engl J Med 2001;344:501–509.
65. Biondi B, Fazio S, Cuocolo A, et al. Impaired cardiac reserve and exercise capacity in patients receiving long-term thyrotropin-suppressive therapy with thyroxine. J Clin Endocrinol Metab 1996;81:4224–4228.
66. Biondi B, Fazio S, Carella C, et al. Cardiac effects of long term thyrotropin-suppressive therapy with thyroxine. J Clin Endocrinol Metab 1993;77:334–338.
67. Shapiro LE, Sievert R, Ong L, et al. Minimal cardiac effects in asymptomatic athyreotic patients chronically treated with thyrotropin-suppressive doses of L-thyroxine. J Clin Endocrinol Metab 1997;82:2592–2595.
68. Tenerz A, Forberg R, Jansson R. Is a more active attitude warranted in patients with subclinical thyrotoxicosis? J Intern Med 1990;228:229–233.
69. Sawin CT, Geller A, Wolf PA, et al. Low serum thyrotropin concentrations as a risk factor for atrial fibrillation in older persons. N Engl J Med 1994;331:1249–1252.
70. Cooper DS. Treatment of thyrotoxicosis. In: Braverman LE, Utiger RD, eds. Werner and Ingbar's The Thyroid, 8th ed. JB Lippincott, Philadelphia, 2000, pp. 691–715.
71. Singer PA, Cooper DS, Levy EG, et al. Treatment guidelines for patients with hyperthyroidism and hypothyroidism. JAMA 1995;273:808–812.
72. Andrade VA, Gross JL, Maia AL. Effect of methimazole pretreatment on serum thyroid hormone levels after radioactive treatment in Graves' hyperthyroidism. J Clin Endocrinol Metab 1999;84:4012–4016.
73. Burch HB, Solomon BL, Wartofsky L, et al. Discontinuing antithyroid drug therapy before ablation with radioactive iodine in Graves' disease. Ann Intern Med 1994;121:553–559.
74. Baeza A, Aguayo J, Barria M, Pineda G. Rapid preoperative preparation in hyperthyroidism. Clin Endocrinol 1991;35:439–442.
75. Nakazawa HK, Sakurai K, Hamada N. Management of atrial fibrillation in the post-thyrotoxic state. Am J Med 1982;72:903–906.
76. Koutras DA. Subclinical hyperthyroidism.Thyroid 1999;9:311–315.
77. Ross DS. Subclinical thyrotoxicosis. In: Braverman LE, Utiger RD, eds. Werner and Ingbar's The Thyroid, 8th ed. JB Lippincott, Philadelphia, 2000, pp. 1007–1012.
78. Huysmans DA, Nieuwlatt WA, Erdtsieck RJ, et al. Administration of a single low dose of recombinant human thyrotropin significantly enhances thyroid radioiodide uptake in nontoxic nodular goiter. J Clin Endocrinol Metab 2000;85:3592–3596.
79. Torres MS, Ramirez L, Simkin PH, Braverman LE, Emerson CH. Effect of various doses of recombinant human thyrotropin on the thyroid radioactive iodine uptake and serum levels of thyroid hormones and thyroglobulin in normal subjects. J Clin Endocrinol Metab 2001;86:1660–1664.

80. Toft AD. Clinical practice: subclinical hyperthyroidism. N Engl J Med 2001;345:512–516.
81. Faber J, Jensen IW, Petersen L, Nygaard B, Hegedus L, Siersbaek-Nielsen K. Normalization of serum thyrotropin by means of radioiodine treatment in subclinical hyperthyroidism: effect on bone loss in postmenopausal women. Clin Endocrinol 1998;48:285–290.
82. Mudde AH, Houben AJHM, Kruseman CAN. Bone metabolism during anti-thyroid drug treatment of endogenous subclinical hyperthyroidism. Clin Endocrinol 1994;41:421–424.
83. Utiger RD. Subclinical hyperthyroidism—just a low serum thyrotropin concentration, or something more? N Engl J Med 1994;331:1302–1303.

4   Type 1 Diabetes

Yogish C. Kudva, MB BS, Rita Basu, MD, and Robert A. Rizza, MD

CONTENTS

INTRODUCTION

Diabetes is a complex metabolic disorder diagnosed on the basis of hyperglycemia. Diagnostic criteria for the disorder are periodically revised *(1)*. Diabetes may be classified mainly into types 1 and 2 based on the etiology and severity of insulin deficiency *(1)*. Most patients with type 1 diabetes show evidence of immune-mediated damage to the insulin-secreting β-cells. Diabetes is characterized by considerable morbidity and mortality. About 50% of patients with type 2 diabetes are not aware of having the disorder. Many patients are diagnosed with diabetes when being evaluated for a complication of diabetes. In contrast, patients with type 1 diabetes are dependent on insulin and need to be prescribed a complex insulin program consisting of rapidly absorbable insulin with each meal and long-acting insulin between meals and during the night. The incidence of type 1 diabetes has risen worldwide. The disorder is occurring earlier and is increasing

From: *Contemporary Endocrinology: Early Diagnosis and Treatment of Endocrine Disorders*
Edited by: R. S. Bar © Humana Press Inc., Totowa, NJ

even in regions with low prevalence *(2)*. It is projected that the greatest increase in the prevalence of type 1 diabetes will occur in regions that currently have a low incidence *(3)*. It is estimated that the incidence of type 1 diabetes in Finland will exceed 50/100,000 by the year 2010 *(3)*. The Diabetes Control and Complications Trial proved that improved glycemic control decreases the incidence and progression of retinopathy and neuropathy *(4)*. However, achieving long-term satisfactory glycemic control in people with type 1 diabetes is often difficult in clinical practice. Therefore, diagnosis of type 1 diabetes at an early stage and preservation of insulin secretion are important public health issues. This chapter addresses the following questions that are pertinent to the diagnosis and treatment of early type 1 diabetes.

1. What is type 1 diabetes?
2. What is the natural history of type 1 diabetes?
3. What is early type 1 diabetes?
4. Which are the autoantigens present in type 1 diabetes?
5. What is the natural history of autoantibodies in type 1 diabetes?
6. Which metabolic test is used to evaluate insulin secretory reserve?
7. Can treatment prevent the loss of β-cell function in individuals with early type 1 diabetes?
8. What factors should be considered in future trials?

What is Type 1 Diabetes?

Most patients with type 1 diabetes eventually need insulin for survival *(1)*. At the time of diagnosis, 85–90% of patients show antibodies to certain antigens *(1)*. Traditionally, type 1 diabetes has been considered a disorder of childhood, with a peak incidence between age 10 and 14 yr *(2)*. Recent studies indicate that it may occur at any age *(5,6)*. Five to 30% of what has previously been considered to be type 2 diabetes may be immune mediated *(5,6)*. That type 1 diabetes is immune mediated is supported by several findings:

1. Type 1 diabetes in humans is similar to immune-mediated diabetes in certain rodent models. Immune-mediated diabetes in rodents may be transferred by adoptive transfer (i.e., infusion of T-cells from a diabetic donor into a nondiabetic recipient animal that does not reject these cells, lacks T-cells, and does not naturally develop diabetes) *(7)*.
2. Insulitis is evident in patients who died soon after diagnosis of type 1 diabetes and in individuals whose pancreas has been biopsied at the time of diagnosis *(8,9)*.
3. Autoantibodies are present at the time of diagnosis in most individuals *(10)*.
4. Linkage to certain HLA haplotypes is common in people who develop type 1 diabetes *(11)*.
5. People with type 1 diabetes commonly develop other immune-mediated disorders such as autoimmune thyroid disease.
6. Early treatment with certain immunomodulatory medications has been shown to delay the progress of type 1 diabetes *(12)*.

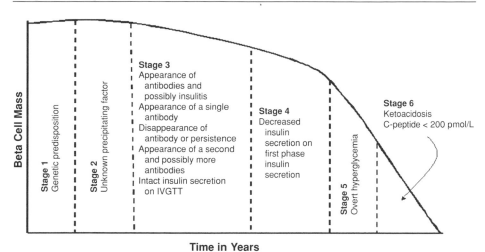

Time in Years

Fig. 1. Natural history of type 1 diabetes. IVGTT, intravenous glucose tolerance test.

Natural History

Eisenbarth *(13)* proposed a model hypothesizing that the natural history of immune-mediated type 1 diabetes can be divided into six stages (Fig. 1). The first stage represents a genetic susceptibility to autoimmune destruction of islets, and the second stage entails exposure to a triggering event. Stage 2 is hypothetical, since specific triggering events have rarely been identified. Overt immunologic changes such as peripheral T-cell responses to autoantigens and/or the presence of certain autoantibodies constitute stage 3. Insulin release in response to an intravenous glucose tolerance test (IVGTT) injection is normal in stages 2 and 3. Stage 4 is characterized by decreased insulin release during IVGTT in the presence of a normal fasting glucose. Stage 5 is characterized by overt diabetes diagnosed incidentally or because of symptomatic hyperglycemia (symptoms of polyuria, polydipsia, and weight loss). Although markedly decreased, endogenous insulin secretion (measured as basal or an increase in C-peptide concentration following stimulation) is generally present when type 1 diabetes is clinically diagnosed. Insulin secretion is severely impaired or totally absent in stage 6, resulting in the development of diabetic ketoacidosis if insulin is not given. Insulin secretion may temporarily improve in stage 6 following treatment with insulin (commonly referred to as the *honeymoon phase*). However, with current forms of treatment, progression to severe insulin deficiency almost invariably occurs once stage 6 has been reached.

At the time of diagnosis, most patients do not have a family history of type 2 diabetes. Such patients are generally diagnosed in stage 5 or 6. In contrast, patients with a family history of type 1 diabetes may be diagnosed earlier since

Table 1
Classification of Prediabetes

Stage	Characteristic
1	Presence of one autoantibody with normal insulin secretion on intravenous glucose tolerance testing
2	Presence of two autoantibodies with normal insulin secretion on intravenous glucose tolerance testing
3	Presence of two or more autoantibodies with impaired insulin secretion on intravenous glucose tolerance testing

Adapted from ref. *15*.

screening programs for autoimmune markers are more feasible in such individuals. At the time of diagnosis, most patients with type 2 diabetes have autoantibodies to one or more proteins such as insulin, glutamic acid decarboxylase (GAD), and the insulinoma-associated tyrosine phosphatase-like molecule IA-2 *(2)*.

Early Type 1 Diabetes

Prior to the identification of autoantigens in type 1 diabetes, patients with type 1 diabetes were diagnosed with symptomatic hyperglycemia or ketoacidosis. Patients may sometimes be diagnosed in stage 4 when an elevated fasting glucose is found during a routine medical evaluation . Autoantibodies enable identification of people in stage 3 of the disorder. Patients in stage 4 almost always develop diabetes within 5 yr after identification *(14)*. Patients in stage 3 may or may not progress to clinical diabetes. The presence of more than one antibody and high titers is associated with a higher risk of progression. Kimpimaki et al. have suggested that stages 3 and 4 be referred to as "prediabetes" and have proposed the classification system described in Table 1 *(15)*.

Autoantigens Present in Type 1 Diabetes

The islet cell antibody test has been used as an index of autoimmunity for over 2 decades *(21)*. This test measures the degree of binding to islets compared with acini; it is commonly performed using a frozen section of human pancreas. The test is hard to standardize and is subject to considerable variability. Nevertheless, a positive islet cell antibody has been shown to increase the probability of developing type 1 diabetes and has been extensively used to identify volunteers for enrollment in intervention studies. Newer tests include measurement of antibodies to insulin, GAD, and insulinoma-associated cDNA(IA-2) (Table 2). These tests are more sensitive, specific, and reproducible than measurement of islet-cell antibodies (ICA). These tests are now available for three antigens. A small percentage of islet cell antibodies do not interact with any of these major antigens, confirming the heterogeneity of the disorder and the need to identify more antigens. A

Table 2
Candidate Autoantigens in Type 1 Diabetes Mellitus in Humans

Antigen	Comments	Relevance in diabetes diagnosis
GAD (16)	Neuroendocrine protein	Anti-GAD antibodies present both in early-onset type 1 diabetes with rapid progression to insulin deficiency and in late-onset diabetes with slowly progressive course
Insulin (10)	Only antigen identified so far that is β-cell-specific	Antiinsulin antibodies present in patients who develop diabetes early in life (<5 yr)
IA-2 (17)	Neuroendocrine protein Integral membrane protein that is a putative protein tyrosine phosphatase	Anti-IA-2 antibodies commonly present in patients whose diabetes is rapidly progressive and develops after 5 yr of age
Phogrin (18)	Putative protein tyrosine phosphatase present in membrane of secretory vesicles	Phogrin antibodies commonly present in patients whose diabetes is rapidly progressive and develops after 5 yr of age
GM-1 islet ganglioside (19)	Antibodies reported by some authors	Further work necessary to describe natural history of this antibody
Heat shock protein 60 (Hsp60) (20)	Peripheral T-cell responses described in some studies	Further work necessary to describe natural history of this antibody

GAD, glutamic acid decarboxylase; IA-2, insulinoma-associated cDNA 2A antibodies

Table 3
Autoantibodies in New-Onset Type 1 Diabetes
in Relation to Age of Onset of Disorder

No. of patients	Age at onset (yr)	IA-2A [no. (%)]	Phogrin [no. (%)]	GAD antibodies [no. (%)]
8	0–5	6(75)	4(50)	2(25)
192	5–40	106 (55.2)	72 (37.5)	129 (67.2)
123	<20	86 (69.9)	60 (48.8)	84 (68.3)
46	21–30	19 (41.3)	11 (23.9)	28 (60.9)
31	31–40	7 (22.6)	5 (16.1)	19 (61.3)

GAD, glutamic acid decarboxylase; IA-2A, insulinoma-assocated cDNA 2A antibodies.
Adapted from ref. 22.

fourth autoantigen, called phogrin or IA-2B, has been recently described (18). Although other islet antigens have been proposed, their ability to predict the development of type 1 diabetes remains an area of active investigation.

A large, multicenter study has documented the presence of GAD, IA-2A, and IA-2B (phogrin) antibodies in 65.5, 56, and 38%, respectively, of patients with new-onset type 1 diabetes (22). In the same study, whereas GAD antibodies were present in 2.8% of 785 type 2 diabetes patients of variable duration, only 0.1% showed IA-2A or phogrin antibodies. The same study also noted a relationship between age and the presence of distinct antibody patterns (Table 3). Patients with age of onset less than 20 yr show primarily IA-2 and GAD antibodies. GAD antibodies are present with similar prevalence in older patients. However, IA-2 antibodies decrease with increasing age. The role of autoantibodies in the pathogenesis of type 1 diabetes remains to be determined, and immune interventions initiated once the autoantibodies are present have met with limited success as yet. On the other hand, tests for autoantibodies may help to determine whether or not newly diagnosed or suboptimally controlled diabetes may benefit from a complex insulin program including both preprandial rapidly absorbed insulin and intraprandial basal insulin coverage.

People with DR3/DR4 alleles appear to be genetically predisposed to the development of type 1 diabetes. In addition, approximately 90% of patients with type 1 diabetes have DR3/DR4 alleles (23). However, testing for these alleles is of little value since they are relatively common, and most people with these alleles do not develop the disorder. Of interest, type 1 diabetes appears to be the only autoimmune disorder for which a "protective" HLA haplotype (i.e., HLA DQB1*0602) has been identified (23).

Natural History of Autoantibodies

Population-based studies of children reveal that transplacental antibodies disappear by 6–9 mo of age *(2)*. Children first show antibodies at 9 mo to 3 yr, the most frequent antibody being against insulin followed by antibodies to GAD. These children develop multiple antibodies before progressing to type 1 diabetes (Table 4) *(15, 24–26)*. The best predictor of progression remains a combination of autoantibodies and impaired insulin secretion *(14)*.

Reproducible, sensitive, and specific assays are necessary to predict accurately who will develop type 1 diabetes. A recent workshop has taken a significant step toward standardizing these assays *(27)*. This workshop has shown that measurement of anti-GAD and IA-2 antibodies appears to be more reliable than measurement of antiinsulin antibodies *(27)*. To date, data also suggest that the radioimmunoassays are more reliable than enzyme-linked immunosorbent assay *(2)*.

Metabolic Testing for Evaluation of Insulin Secretory Reserve

The IVGTT has traditionally been used to evaluate insulin secretory reserve in prospective studies of type 1 diabetes. Lack of first-phase insulin response (i.e., the sum of the insulin concentrations observed during the first 10 min after intravenous glucose injection) indicates substantial β-cell destruction and strongly suggests that the disease process is progressing.

An IVGTT is performed after an overnight fast. A glucose load of 0.5g/kg total body weight (maximum dose, 35 g) is administered, usually as a 25% dextrose solution in a square wave pattern over 3 min. Blood is sampled prior to the glucose infusion and at 1, 3, 5, 7, and 10 min after the glucose infusion is complete. The sum of the plasma insulin values at 1 and 3 min post infusion, referred to as first-phase insulin release (FPIR), is calculated by adding the insulin concentrations present at 1 and 3 min. This value is used to stratify risk for progression to type 1 diabetes. A value less than the 10th percentile (i.e., <60 µU/mL if age 3–7 yr, or <100 µU/mL if age ≥ 8 yr) on two separate IVGTTs (Diabetes Prevention Trial-1 protocol) indicates moderate risk. However, a value that falls to less than the 1st percentile (i.e., <50 µU/mL at age ≥ 8 yr) on two separate IVGTTs indicates high risk. Indeed, more than 50% of these individuals will progress to type 1 diabetes within 5 yr, and more than 90% will do so within 10 yr *(27,28)*. The probability of progression is greater if islet cell antibodies are also present. In contrast, individuals with an FPIR value of between 50 and 100 µU/mL have a 48% risk for 5 yr, and those with an FPIR greater than 100 µU/mL have a 17% risk for developing type 1 diabetes in the same time period *(29)*.

Among other independent risk factors, the loss of FPIR is most strongly associated with rapid progression to type 1 diabetes *(14)*. Annual measurement of the FPIR provides the most reliable means of predicting the time of onset of overt type 1 diabetes *(30)*. Not only does a markedly decreased FPIR have a high

Table 4
Studies of Natural History of Type 1 Diabetes in Offspring Followed from Birth and Early in Life

Study	No. of patients enrolled	Follow-up Period	No.	One auto-antibody (%)	Two or more antibodies (%)	Diabetes (%)	Comments
BABYDIAB (24)	1353	All followed for 0.9 yr	114 at 5 yr	11	3.5	1.8	Insulin auto-antibodies were the first to appear in almost all patients.
DAISY (25)	NA	NA	NA	41 at 4 yr	NA	NA	NA
Australian study (26)	357	Mean 3.1 yr	NA	5	2.8	1.1	Insulin antibodies first to appear in 64% of high-risk patients
Childhood Diabetes in Finland Study Group (15)	180	4 yr	180 at 4 yr after study commencement	18.3	9	8.3	Study enrolled patients up to 6 yr of age and followed them to 10 yr

positive predictive value, but a normal FPIR also has a high negative predictive value. Furthermore, in the absence of high levels of islet and insulin autoantibodies, individuals with an FPIR of more than the 10th percentile rarely progress to diabetes within 3 yr of follow up *(31–33)*.

Thus, a significantly reduced FPIR, as obtained from a standardized IVGTT, and the presence of high titers of insulin and islet cell autoantibodies are strong predictors of progression to overt type 1 diabetes *(31–33)*.

Treatment to Prevent Loss of β-Cell Function in Early Type 1 Diabetes

A complex insulin program consisting of preprandial injection of a rapidly absorbed form of insulin combined with a means of maintaining constant intraprandial basal levels is the treatment of choice in type 1 diabetes. Since islet dysfunction generally progressively worsens over several years, clinical trials have sought to preserve or restore insulin secretion in predisposed individuals who have evidence of islet autoimmunity. Interventions have included injections of long-acting insulin, immunomodulatory therapy such as cyclosporine A (CsA), and putative β-cell protective agents such as nicotinamide.

To date, clinical trials have been initiated at different stages in the evolution of type 1 diabetes and therefore have had differing endpoints (Tables 5 and 6, Fig. 2).

The ideal stage for intervention is a matter of active debate. Opposing points of view have been recently published *(34)*. First-degree relatives with two or more antibodies have a 70% risk of diabetes over 5 yr. However, 30% of the subjects will not develop diabetes. Therefore, the risk of the intervention must be small and of limited severity.

Trial to Reduce IDDM in the Genetically at Risk (TRIGR)

This study is enrolling infants born in families with at least one first-degree relative with type 1 diabetes. After exclusive breast feeding, infants are randomized into one of two groups at weaning. The control group is given a regular formula with 20% casein hydrolysate, added and the intervention group is given a casein hydrolysate formula. The endpoint is the presence of antibodies associated with type 1 diabetes in the first 2 yr of life. Preliminary data suggests that hydrolyzed formulas significantly decrease the formation of autoantibodies *(34)*.

Cyclosporine A

Since type 1 diabetes is T-cell-mediated, agents that selectively affect T-cells may alter the natural history of the disorder. With the advent of CsA in the 1980s, this agent was used at multiple centers *(12,34–36)*. Outcome and long-term follow-up data for these patients have now been published (Table 7). CsA slows the rate of loss of β-cells but does not alter the destruction of all insulin-secreting cells. Although one group has documented the absence of long-term side effects

Table 5
Stages in the Evolution of Type 1 Diabetes at Which Intervention May Be Tested

Intervention stage	Endpoint
At birth	Islet cell antibodies during early years of life
After islet cell antibodies have been established but with intact insulin secretion on IVGTT	Decreased insulin secretion during IVGTT
Islet cell antibodies > 20 JDF units and decreased insulin secretion on IVGTT	C-peptide secretion
At onset of clinical type 1 diabetes.	C-peptide secretion

IVGTT, intravenous glucose tolerance test; JDF, Juvenile Diabetes Foundation

Table 6
Pros and Cons of Trials to Prevent Type 1 Diabetes Mellitus

Pros
   Lessens public health burden
   Accurate identification of high-risk individuals
   Safe intervention, which may be worthwhile even if it decreases incidence by only
      10–15%
Cons
   Ability to identify high-risk individuals at best 70% over 5 yr
   Etiology unknown
   Pathogenesis of disorder unknown

Data from ref. *34*.

in subjects treated with CsA, Parving et al. have reported that treatment with CsA results in a small but statistically significant decrease in glomerular filtration rate (GFR) on long-term follow-up *(35,36)*. Treatment of individuals who had reached stage 4 of type 1 diabetes slowed but did not prevent the loss of β-cell function. However, concern about potential short- and long-term side effects has led to the consensus that intervention with CsA is not appropriate for people with new-onset type 1 diabetes *(37)*.

Nicotinamide

Nicotinamide may theoretically preserve β-cell function by increasing the resistance of β-cells to apoptosis, increasing β-cell regeneration, and altering immune cell function. Therefore, this agent has been used in several trials (Table 8). The Deutsche nicotinamide Intervention Study (DENIS) showed that Nicotinamide did not prevent progression to phase 5 when used in patients at phase 3 *(38)*. Patients in this study were younger than 5 yr, and β-cell destruction may be more rapid in such patients. The European Nicotinamide Intervention Trial

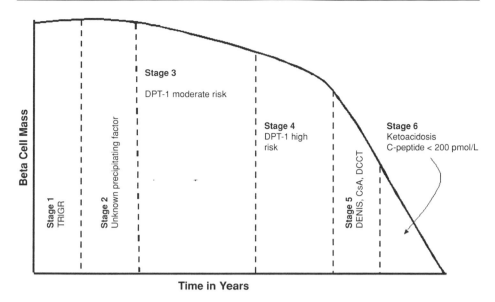

Fig. 2. Trials carried out at different stages in the pathogenesis of type 1 diabetes. CsA, cyclosporine; DCCT, Diabetes Control and Complications Trial; DPT, Diabetes Prevention Trial; DENIS, Deutsche Nicotinamide Intervention Study; TRIGR, Trial to Reduce IDDM in the Genetically at Risk.

(ENDIT) has enrolled more than 550 patients who are in phase 3 *(34)*. Patients have been randomized to either nicotinamide or placebo and will be followed for 5 yr. The endpoint is a decrease in C-peptide secretion. The study will be unblinded in 2002. A metaanalysis of smaller, previously published trials of nicotinamide suggested beneficial effects at 1 yr on C-peptide secretion but no clinical difference over the long run when used in new-onset type 1 diabetes *(39)*.

Insulin

To date, insulin is the only β-cell specific autoantigen described in type 1 diabetes. Both the whole molecule and a peptide that is metabolically inactive have been demonstrated to alter autoimmunity in NOD mice. A pilot study reported that endogenous insulin secretion was preserved when first-degree relatives in stage 4 of type 1 diabetes were treated with annual intravenous insulin infusion and twice-daily long-acting human insulin *(40)*. Based on this pilot trial, the Diabetes Prevention Trial (DPT-1) was designed with primary and secondary prevention cohorts *(41)*. The secondary prevention cohort enrolled first-degree relatives with islet cell antibodies more than 20 JDF units (Juvenile Diabetes Foundation units), HLA type that was not DQB1* 0602, and decreased first-phase insulin secretion. Results presented in abstract form in 2001 indicated no

Table 7
Trials Using Cyclosporine as Intervention in Type 1 Diabetes

Study	No. of patients	Intervention stage	Endpoint	Results	Long-term follow-up/ adverse effects
DeFilippo et al. (35)	130	5	C-peptide secretion	130 patients were followed for at least 6 yr 83 patients had received CsA, and 47 were treated with placebo. C-peptide in patients treated with CsA was detectable for 3.2 yr in the placebo group compared with 5.8 yr in the CsA group	By 6 yr after initiation of the trials, C-peptide secretion was not different between the two groups.
Canadian-European Randomized Control Trial Group (12) Parving et al. (36)	188	5	C-peptide secretion	33.5% in the CsA group vs 21% in the placebo group showed remission	Long-term follow-up of kidney function showed a decrease in GFR of 6.3 ± 6.0 compared with an increase of 7 ± 4.5 in the placebo group
Carel et al. (37)	15	4	C-peptide secretion	All nine untreated patients developed diabetes within 12 mo. Two of six nondiabetics after 47 mo when treated with CsA. One developed diabetes in the first year and three from 1 to 4 yr after treatment	Reservations about long-term toxicity and enrollment of patients in trials of safer therapy have rendered CsA therapy obsolete

CsA, cyclosporine A; GFR, glomerular filtration rate.

Table 8
Nicotinamide Intervention Trials in Type 1 Diabetes

Study	Intervention stage	No. of subjects	Age (yr)	Endpoint	Comments
DENIS (38)	Stage 3	25 in the nicotinamide group and 30 in the placebo group	3–5	Phase 5 disease; patients followed for 3 yr	Nicotinamide did not prevent overt diabetes Progression is probably more rapid in such patients
ENDIT (34)	Phase 3	>550	<20	C-peptide secretion	Double-blind placebo-controlled Results to be reported in 2003 Interim analysis in 1998 showed dose used (1.2 g/d) to be safe
Pozzilli et al. (39) Metaanalysis of ten studies of which five were placebo-controlled	Phase 5	211 in the nicotinamide group and 178 in the placebo-controlled group	10–23	C-peptide secretion	Nicotinamide-treated patients showed significantly preserved C-peptide secretion at 1 yr

DENIS, Deutsche Nicotinamide Intervention Study; ENDIT, European Nicotinamide Intervention Trial

Table 9
Trials Evaluating Insulin to Preserve β-Cell Function in Type 1 Diabetes

Study	Stage at enrollment	Intervention	No. of subjects	Endpoint	Results
DPT-1 (42)					
Intermediate risk	3	Oral insulin	490	Insulin secretion on IVGTT	Recruitment continuing
High risk	4	IV insulin once-yearly and twice-daily Human Ultra-lente® injections	326	C-peptide secretion	Intervention not successful
DCCT (44)	5	Intensive diabetes management	303	Stimulated C-peptide >200 pmol/L	Intensive therapy preserved C-peptide response (risk reduction 57%)
Chaillous et al. (45)	5	Oral insulin 2.5 or 7.5 mg daily compared with placebo	131	C-peptide secretion	Intervention not successful

DCCT, Diabetes Control and Complications Trial; DPT, Diabetes Prevention Trial; IVGTT, intravenous glucose tolerance test.

benefit from this approach *(42)*. A trial of oral insulin versus placebo is ongoing. *See* Table 9 for trial results.

Intensive insulin treatment at diagnosis of type 1 diabetes for 2 wk has been shown to increase stimulated plasma C-peptide concentrations 1 yr after treatment *(43)*. A substudy of the Diabetes Control and Complications Trial (DCCT) enrolled 303 patients who had C-peptide concentrations of more than 200 pmol/L after glucagon stimulation. Individuals randomized to intensive insulin therapy had slightly but significantly greater C-peptide concentrations over a mean of 6.5 yr than did individuals randomized to what then was standard (i.e., associated with suboptimal glycemic control) insulin therapy *(44)*. On the other hand, auto-antibody-positive type 1 diabetes patients aged 7–40 yr treated within 2 wk of diagnosis with intensive subcutaneous insulin plus either placebo, oral insulin 2.5 mg daily, or oral insulin 7.5 mg daily showed no difference in the rate of loss of β-cell function *(45)*.

Anti-CD3 Antibodies

Modified anti-CD3 antibodies have been shown to induce remission in NOD mice *(46)*. These antibodies are directed against the T-cell receptor but do not activate T-cells in vivo. A trial in humans enrolled patients within 6 wk of diagnosis of clinical type 1 diabetes at a single center to receive intervention with a modified anti-CD3 antibody or placebo *(47)*. Patients were randomized in a 2:1 ratio (antibody/placebo) with escalating doses for 4 d and full dose for 10 more d. HbA1$_c$ at 6 mo was better in the intervention group (6.2 vs 7.7, $p > 0.02$). Stimulated C-peptide concentrations increased in the intervention group. Side effects included eczematoid rash, lymphopenia, and fever but were managed with symptomatic treatment. Serum cytokine measurements showed a possible change in T-cell subset function in the antibody-treated group. A multicenter trial involving eight centers with the same design is currently being conducted.

DiaPep277™

Some investigators have identified Hsp60 as a self-antigen in type 1 diabetes *(20)*. A 24-amino-acid sequence of this protein (p277) induces remission of diabetes in the NOD mouse, a model of spontaneous type 1 diabetes *(48)*. Raz et al. *(49)*, in a recently reported clinical trial, randomized 35 patients with type 1 diabetes to intervention with DiaPep277™ or placebo at entry and at 1 and 6 mo and showed preservation of glucagon-secreted C-peptide secretion in the intervention group 10 mo after enrollment.

FACTORS TO BE CONSIDERED IN FUTURE TRIALS

The past several years have revealed several important features about prediabetes and early type 1 diabetes. Patients who are DQB1*0602 have a lower incidence of type 1 diabetes compared with the general population. Younger patients progress more rapidly to type 1 diabetes. The presence of more than one autoantibody increases the risk of progression to overt diabetes. All potential therapies need to be carefully evaluated in animal models. The potential therapies need to be carefully studied in pilot studies prior to the design of a multicenter trial. Multicenter trials need to be adequately powered to answer the hypotheses of intervention. Previous clinical trials attempting to preserve β-cell function have met with limited success, and several trials of novel therapies are ongoing. The design of future trials will probably benefit from new information regarding the pathogenesis of autoimmune β-cell destruction.

ACKNOWLEDGMENTS

Yogish C. Kudva is supported by the Mayo Foundation. Dr. Rita Basu is supported by an American Diabetes Association Mentorship award. Dr. R.A. Rizza is supported by National Institutes of Health grant DK29953. We thank Dr. A. Basu for critical review of the manuscript, and we gratefully acknowledge Michelle Papaconstandinou for her secretarial support.

REFERENCES

1. Report of the Expert Committee on the Diagnosis and Classification of Diabetes Mellitus. Diabetes Care 1997;20:1183–1197.
2. Atkinson MA, Eisenbarth GS. Type 1 diabetes: new perspectives on disease pathogenesis and treatment. Lancet 2001;358:221–229.
3. Onkamo P, Väänänen S, Karvonen M, Tuomilehto J. Worldwide increase in incidence of type 1 diabetes—the analysis of the data on published incidence trends. Diabetologia 1999;42:1395–1403.
4. The Diabetes Control and Complications Trial Research Group. The effect of intensive treatment of diabetes on the development and progression of long-term complications in insulin-dependent diabetes mellitus. N Engl J Med 1993;329:977–986.
5. Zimmet PZ, Tuomi T, Mackay R, et al. Latent autoimmune diabetes mellitus in adults (LADA): the role of antibodies to glutamic acid decarboxylase in diagnosis and prediction of insulin dependency. Diabet Med 1994;11:299–303.
6. Turner R, Stratton I, Horton V, et al. UKPDS 25: autoantibodies to islet-cell cytoplasm and glutamic acid decarboxylase for prediction of insulin requirement in type 2 diabetes. UK Prospective Diabetes Study Group. Lancet 1997;350:1288–1293.
7. Brown GR, Silva MD, Thompson PA, Beutler B. Lymphoid hyperplasia, CD45RB[high] to CD45RB[low] T-cell imbalance, and suppression of type 1 diabetes mellitus: results from TNF blockade in NOD{{fi}}NOD-*scid* adoptive T-cell transfer. Diabetologia 1998;41:1502–1510.
8. Foulis AK, Liddle CN, Farquharson MA, Richmond JA, Weir RS. The histopathology of the pancreas in type 1 (insulin-dependent) diabetes mellitus: a 25-year review of deaths in patients under 20 years of age in the United Kingdom. Diabetologia 1986;29:267–274.
9. Pipeleers D. Ling Z. Pancreatic beta cells in insulin-dependent diabetes. Diabetes Metab Rev 1992;8:209–227.
10. Palmer JP, Asplin CM, Clemons P, et al. Insulin antibodies in insulin-dependent diabetics before insulin treatment. Science 1983;222:1337–1339.
11. Nerup J, Platz P, Andersen OO, et al. HL-A antigens and diabetes mellitus. Lancet 1974;2:864–866.

12. Cyclosporin-induced remission of IDDM after early intervention. Association of 1 year of cyclosporin treatment with enhanced insulin secretion. The Canadian-European Randomized Control Trial Group. Diabetes 1988;37:1574–1582.
13. Eisenbarth GS. Type I diabetes mellitus. A chronic autoimmune disease. N Engl J Med 1986;314:1360–1368.
14. Verge CF, Gianani R, Kawasaki E, et al. Prediction of type 1 diabetes in first-degree relatives using a combination of insulin, GAD, and ICA512bdc/IA-2 autoantibodies. Diabetes 1996;45:926–933.
15. Kimpimaki T, Kulmala P, Savola K, et al. Disease-associated autoantibodies as surrogate markers of type 1 diabetes in young children at increased genetic risk. Childhood Diabetes in Finland Study Group. J Clin Endocrinol Metab 2000;85:1126–1132.
16. Baekkeskov S, Aanstoot HJ, Christgau S, Reetz A, Solimena M, Cascalho M. Identification of the 64K autoantigen in insulin-dependent diabetes as the GABA-synthesizing enzyme glutamic acid decarboxylase. Nature 1990;347:151–156.
17. Lan MS, Wassefall C, Maclaren NK, Notkins AL. IA-2, a transmembrane protein of the tyrosine phosphatase family, is a major autoantigen in insulin-dependent diabetes mellitus. Proc Natl Acad Sci USA 1992;93:6367–6370.
18. Payton MA, Hawkes CJ, Christie MR. Relationship of the 37,000- and 40,000-M(r) tryptic fragments of islet antigens in insulin-dependent diabetes to the protein tyrosine phosphatase-like molecule IA-2 (ICA512). J Clin Invest 1995;96:1506–1511.
19. Dotta F, Gianani R, Previti M, et al. Autoimmunity to the GM2-1 islet ganglioside before and at the onset of type I diabetes. Diabetes 1996;45:1193–1196.
20. Abulafia-Lapid R, Elias D, Raz I, Keren-Zur Y, Atlan H, Cohen IR. T-cell responses of type I diabetes patients and healthy individuals to human hsp60 and its peptides. J Autoimmun 1999;12:121–129.
21. Botazzo GF, Florin-Christensen A, Doniach D. Islet-cell antibodies in diabetes mellitus with autoimmune polyendocrine deficiencies. Lancet 1974;2:1279–1283.
22. Seissler J, de Sonnaville JJ, Morgenthaler NG, et al. Immunological heterogeneity in type I diabetes: presence of distinct autoantibody patterns in patients with acute onset and slowly progressive disease. Diabetologia 1998;41:891–897.
23. Greenbaum CJ, Schatz DA, Cuthbertson, D, Zeidler A, Eisenbarth GS, Krischer JP. Islet cell antibody-positive relatives with human leukocyte antigen DQA1*0102, DQB1*0602: identification by the Diabetes Prevention Trial-Type 1. J Clin Endocrinol Metab 2000;85:1255–1260.
24. Ziegler AG, Hummel M, Schenker M, Bonifacio E. Autoantibody appearance and risk for development of childhood diabetes in offspring of parents with type 1 diabetes: the 2-year analysis of the German BABYDIAB Study. Diabetes 1999;48:460–468.
25. Rewers M, Eisenbarth GS, Elsey C, et al. Target population for prevention trials of β-cell autoimmunity in early childhood. Diabetologia 1998;41(suppl 1):A86.
26. Colman PG, Steele C, Couper JJ, Beresford SJ, Powell T, Kewming K. Islet autoimmunity in infants with a type I diabetic relative is common but is frequently restricted to one autoantibody. Diabetologia 2000;43:203–209.
27. Verge CF, Stenger D, Bonifacio E, et al. Combined use of autoantibodies (IA-2 autoantibody, GAD autoantibody, insulin autoantibody, cytoplasmic islet cell antibodies) in type 1 diabetes: Combinatorial Islet Autoantibody Workshop. Diabetes 1998;47:1857–1866.
28. Beer SF, Heaton DA, Alberti KG, Pyke DA, Leslie RD. Impaired glucose tolerance precedes but does not predict insulin-dependent diabetes mellitus: a study of identical twins. Diabetologia 1990;33:497–502.
29. Bingley PJ, Colman P, Eisenbarth GS. Standardization of IVGTT to predict IDDM. Diabetes Care 1992;15:1313–1316.
30. Bingley PJ. Interactions of age, islet cell antibodies, insulin autoantibodies, and first phase insulin response in predicting risk of progression to IDDM in ICA+ relatives: the ICARUS data set. Islet Cell Antibody Register Users Study. Diabetes 1996;45:1720–1728.

31. Bleich D, Jackson RA, Soeldner JS, Eisenbarth GS. Analysis of metabolic progression to type 1 diabetes in ICA+ relatives of patients with type 1 diabetes. Diabetes Care 1990;13:111–118.
32. Eisenbarth GS, Gianani R, Yu L, et al. Dual parameter model for prediction of type 1 diabetes mellitus. Proc Assoc Am Physicians 1998;110:126–135.
33. Diabetes Prevention Trial-Type 1 Study Protocol. Revised: October 2000.
34. Rosenbloom AL, Schatz DA, Krischer JP, et al. Prevention and treatment of diabetes in children. J Clin Endocrinol Metab 2000;85:494–522.
35. De Filippo G, Carel JC, Boitard C, Bougneres PF. Long-term results of early cyclosporine therapy in juvenile IDDM. Diabetes 1996;45:101–104.
36. Parving HH, Tarnow L, Nielsen FS, et al. Cyclosporine nephrotoxicity in type 1 diabetic patients. A 7-year follow-up study. Diabetes Care 1999;22:478–483
37. Carel JC, Boitard C, Eisenbarth G, Bach JF, Bougneres PF. Cyclosporine delays but does not prevent clinical onset in glucose intolerant pre-type 1 diabetic children. J Autoimmun 1996;9:739–745.
38. Lampeter EF, Klinghammer A, Scherbaum WA, et al. The Deutsche Nicotinamide Intervention Study: an attempt to prevent type 1 diabetes. DENIS Group. Diabetes 1998;47:980–984.
39. Pozzilli P, Browne PD, Kolb H, The Nicotinamide Trialists. Correct analysis of nicotinamide in patients with recent onset insulin dependent diabetes. Diabetes Care 1996;19:1356–1363.
40. Keller RJ, Eisenbarth GS, Jackson RA. Insulin prophylaxis in individuals at high risk of type I diabetes. Lancet 1993;341:927–928.
41. DPT-1 Study Group. The Diabetes Prevention Trial (DPT-1): Implementation of screening and staging of relatives. Transplant Proc 1995;27:3377.
42. Skyler J. Results of the DPT-1. Diabetes 2001;50(suppl 2):35.
43. Shah SC, Malone JI, Simpson NE. A randomized trial of intensive insulin therapy in newly diagnosed insulin-dependent diabetes mellitus. N Engl J Med 1989;320:550–554.
44. The Diabetes Control and Complications Trial Research Group. Effect of intensive therapy on residual beta-cell function in patients with type 1 diabetes in the diabetes control and complications trial. A randomized, controlled trial. Ann Intern Med 1998;128:517–523.
45. Chaillous L, Lefevre H, Thivolet C, Boitard C. Lahlou N, Atlan-Gepner C. Oral insulin administration and residual beta-cell function in recent-onset type 1 diabetes: a multicentre randomised controlled trial. Diabete Insuline Orale group. Lancet 2000;356:545–549.
46. Chatenoud L, Primo J, Bach JF. CD3 antibody-induced dominant self tolerance in overtly diabetic NOD mice. J Immunol 1997;158:2947–2954.
47. Herald KC, Hagopian W, Auger J, et al. Treatment with Anti-CD3 monoclonal antibody (mAb) hOKT3γl(Ala-Ala) improves glycemic control during the first year of type 1 diabetes mellitus. Diabetes 2001;50(suppl 2):A34.
48. Elias D, Cohen IR. Peptide therapy for diabetes in NOD mice. Lancet 1994;343:704–706.
49. Itamar R, Elias D, Avron A, Tamir M, Metzger M, Cohen I. β-cell function in new-onset type 1 diabetes and immunomodulation with a heat-shock protein peptide (DiaPep277): a randomized, double-blind, phase II trial. Lancet 2001;358:1749–1753.

5 Type 2 Diabetes

Preethi Srikanthan, MD, *Jeffrey E. Pessin,* PhD,
and Robert S. Bar, MD

CONTENTS

INTRODUCTION

Impaired glucose tolerance (IGT), a precursor to type 2 diabetes, has received important attention in the past year. Two large clinical trials have suggested that individuals with IGT can be prevented, or at least delayed, from progressing to type 2 diabetes and its complications *(1–3)*. The data from these trials are important in regard to the well-publicized national and worldwide epidemics of type 2 diabetes. To discuss early diagnosis and early treatment of type 2 diabetes means discussing IGT—who to screen and how to approach the therapy of IGT *(4)*. This chapter primarily discusses IGT, its recognition, how and who to screen, and its treatment. Finally, we suggest measures for pre-IGT recognition of the at-risk population, and we also suggest preventive therapy even *before* IGT develops *(5–7)*.

In the United States IGT is currently estimated to be present in 6–7% of individuals in the 20–44-yr-old age group and progressively increases to ≥20% in those over 70 yr of age. With length of life further extending, the tendency to gain weight

From: *Contemporary Endocrinology: Early Diagnosis and Treatment of Endocrine Disorders*
Edited by: R. S. Bar © Humana Press Inc., Totowa, NJ

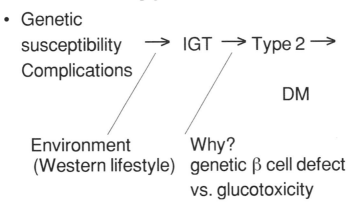

Stages in Development of
Type 2 Diabetes

- Genetic
  susceptibility → IGT → Type 2 →
  Complications

  DM

  Environment   Why?
  (Western lifestyle) genetic β cell defect
                       vs. glucotoxicity

Fig. 1. Pathogenesis of type 2 diabetes mellitus (DM). IGT, impaired glucose tolerance.

increasing, and the level of physical activity decreasing, the prevalence of IGT in all age groups will markedly increase in the next 20 yr *(8)*. The screening and formal definition of IGT are still controversial in the United States *(9,10)*. Based on the criteria of the expert panel of the American Diabetes Association (ADA) in 1997, impaired fasting glucose was defined by a fasting blood sugar of 110–125 mg% and IGT by a serum glucose 2 h after ingesting glucola (75 g) of 140–199 mg%. The ADA panel also discouraged routine use of the more difficult oral glucose tolerance test. However, the World Health Organization (WHO) now defines IGT as a fasting blood glucose of less than 126 mg% and a serum glucose drawn 2 h after ingesting 75 g of glucola of 140–200 mg%. The WHO standards identified approx 30% more subjects with abnormal glucose concentration than the 1997 ADA criteria *(11–13)*. Therefore, we believe that the fasting glucose and 2-h post glucola blood sugar is the test of choice for the diagnosis of IGT *(14–16)*.

The course of events in the progression to type 2 diabetes, with IGT being a precursor, is shown in Fig. 1 *(17)*. IGT is seen here as the beginning process in the development of diabetes (Fig. 2) *(18–23)*. This concept is further reinforced by IGT having the same risk factors as those for type 2 diabetes (Table 1) *(24,25)*. The increased cardiovascular disease associated with IGT *per se* and the findings of microvascular disease in some newly diagnosed type 2 patients suggest that even the microvascular complications of diabetes may have been initiated several years prior to the formal diagnosis of diabetes. Thus the recognition of IGT and its treatment take on added importance.

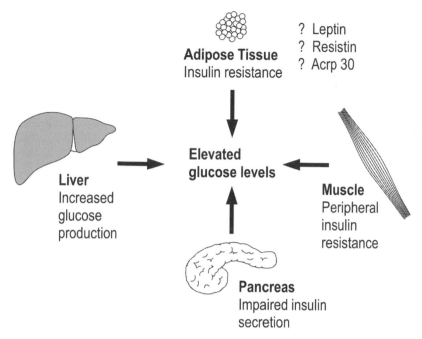

Fig. 2. Mechanisms of hyperglycemia in type 2 diabetes.

Table 1
Risk Factors for Impaired Glucose Tolerance and Type 2 Diabetes

Family history of diabetes
Older age
Obesity
Gestational diabetes
Polycystic ovarian syndrome (PCOS)
Increased waist/hip ratio
Having had a baby weighing more than 9 pounds
Sedentary lifestyle
Hispanic/Native American/Asian-American/African-American/Pacific Island descent
Hypertension or dyslipidemia

Risk factors for IGT are also the same risk factors for type 2 diabetes (Table 1). These include family history of diabetes, older age, obesity, gestational diabetes, polycystic ovarian syndrome (PCOS), increased waist/hip ratio, having had a baby weighing more than 9 pounds, sedentary lifestyle, Hispanic/Native American/Asian-American/African-American/Pacific Island descent, hypertension, or dyslipidemia *(26–34)*. The precipitating factor (s) causing someone to go from normal glucose tolerance to IGT are not precisely known. Several factors though, are clearly associated with this progression, including genetic (racial) factors, obesity, diet, and lack of physical exercise *(35–49)*. Likewise, the specific factors that cause IGT to progress to type 2 diabetes are also unknown *(50)*, but they probably include the same factors associated with the initial development of IGT. The importance of overweight/obesity cannot be stressed enough *(51)*. In our society, obesity and its accompanying complications are increasing at a frightening pace. A recent report covering the period 1980–1998 *(52)* assessed the percent of children who were overweight and demonstrated a steady increase in the United States from 1980 through 1998, with the greatest increase seen in African Americans and Hispanics, minorities with a particular susceptibility to develop type 2 diabetes. By 1998, "overweight" increased to 21.5% among African Americans, 21.8% among Hispanic Americans, and 12.3% among non-Hispanic whites. In addition, overweight children were heavier in 1998 compared with overweight children in 1980. These findings in children have been accompanied by a substantial increase in type 2 diabetes in the pediatric population *(53)*. This would have been a major surprise 25–30 yr ago, but it is not today. The increase in type 2 diabetes in our pediatric population is now requiring pediatricians to become familiar with its diagnosis and treatment.

The same trend toward overweight or obesity in the pediatric population is also being observed in the adult population *(54)*. According to the Behavior Risk Factor Study, the prevalence of overweight in adults has risen by 50% in the period 1991–1999. Of further concern are statistics just released from the Centers for Disease Control and Prevention (CDC) estimating the incidence of an entity associated with adult obesity, cardiovascular disease, and frequently IGT or type 2 diabetes—the dysmetabolic or metabolic syndrome *(55)*. In this study the dysmetabolic syndrome was defined according to the ATP111 criteria by the presence of at least three of the following criteria: (1) abdominal obesity with waist circumference more than 102 cm in men and 88 cm in women; (2) serum triglycerides 150 mg% or more; (3) high-density lipoprotein (HDL) less than 40 mg% in men and 50 mg% in women; (4) blood pressure 130/85 mmHg or more; and (5) fasting blood glucose 100 mg% or higher. In this study of 8814 men and women, the overall prevalence of the metabolic syndrome was 22%, ranging from a low of 6.7% in those 20–29 yr old and progressively increasing to a maximum of 43.5% in those older than 60 yr. These disheartening figures will probably worsen in the next 20 yr.

CELLULAR RESPONSE TO INSULIN

In both IGT and type 2 diabetes, defect (s) exist in insulin action and/or insulin secretion from the pancreatic β-cell *(21,55–60)*. Although the specific cellular and molecular defects have not yet been defined, the evolving delineation of the complex molecular events in insulin signaling and insulin synthesis/secretion has given increasing information on the polygenic diseases that manifest as IGT and type 2 diabetes. The cellular effects of insulin have been generally agreed on for type 2 diabetes (Fig. 2). Specifically, all patients with type 2 diabetes have two defects: impaired insulin release by the pancreatic β-cell and resistance to the cellular response to insulin, or insulin resistance. All treatments for type 2 diabetes are directed at improving one of these two defects. In many patients with type 2 diabetes, there are decreases in insulin secretion over time, such that initial treatment of hyperglycemia can be successfully managed by diet/exercise or use of a single oral hypoglycemic agent. Over time, patients often need the addition of a second agent, then a third, and finally exogenous insulin injections. For IGT the defects are not as clearly defined. Some authors feel that insulin resistance is the initiating event for IGT, others feel that insulin secretion is the primary culprit, and still others argue that both defects, as in type 2 diabetes, must be present for IGT to occur. Is it really important to determine which of these possibilities is the true initiating event? The answer is probably *yes*. Knowledge of the initiating process would give us a lead in developing precise screening tests for early diagnosis of IGT and perhaps guide our early therapy of IGT.

Knowledge of the cellular effects of insulin has greatly expanded in the last 10 yr (Fig. 3). The three primary peripheral target tissues of insulin action are the liver, skeletal muscle, and adipose tissue (Fig. 2). In the liver, insulin functions to suppress gluconeogenesis, lipogenesis, and amino acid and glucose release, whereas glycogen and protein synthesis are enhanced. Similarly, insulin increases glucose and amino acid uptake into both striated muscle and adipose tissue. All these biologic responses result from the binding of insulin to the cell surface insulin receptor that is highly expressed in these tissues (Fig. 3).

At the cellular/molecular level, the insulin receptor is a plasma membrane disulfide-linked heterotetrameric protein, consisting of two extracellular α-subunits and two transmembrane β-subunits (Fig. 3). The α-subunits contain the high-affinity insulin binding sites; upon ligand occupancy, they transmit a transmembrane signal through the plasma membrane activating the intracellular tyrosine kinase domain of the β-subunits (61–63). Following receptor autophosphorylation, the β-subunit tyrosine kinase domain becomes catalytically active toward exogenous substrates and tyrosine-phosphorylates a number of intracellular proteins (64–68). Mutations in the insulin receptor that impair its processing, cell surface exposure, insulin binding or activation of its tyrosine kinase domain result in severe forms of insulin resistance (69–71). However, insulin receptor mutations are quite rare and do not account for a significant number of insulin-resistant patients.

Once activated, the insulin receptor can tyrosine-phosphorylate a number of proximal substrates involved in several distinct intracellular signaling pathways. In general, these can be grouped into signals activating the MAP kinase, the

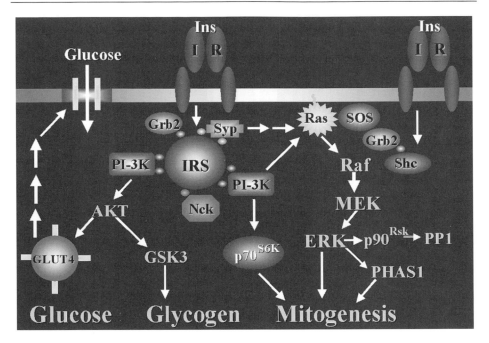

Fig. 3. Cellular signaling for insulin action. ERK, extracellular signal-regulated kinase; GSK3, glycogen synthase kinase 3; Ins, insulin; IR, insulin receptor; MEK, mitogen activated extracellular signal-regulated kinase kinase; PI-3K, phosphatidylinositol 3-kinase, PP1, protein phosphatase 1; IRS, insulin receptor substrate; Rsk, p90 ribosomal S6 kinase; SOS, son-of-sevenless; Syp, protein tyrosine phosphatase 2.

phosphatidylinositol 3-kinase (PI 3-kinase), and the CAP/Cbl pathways (72–74). The MAP kinase pathway is thought to be primarily responsible for the control of growth and development, whereas the PI 3-kinase pathway is involved in growth, antiapoptosis, and metabolic signaling including enhancement of glucose uptake and utilization. Similarly, the recently described CAP/Cbl pathway is thought to be involved in enhanced insulin stimulation of glucose uptake and to function cooperatively with the PI 3-kinase pathway in this response.

It is generally accepted that the ability of insulin to enhance glucose uptake is owing to the presence of a specific facilitative glucose transporter protein isoform, GLUT4, in striated muscle and adipose tissue. In these tissues, GLUT4 is sequestered away from the cell surface membrane and stored in specialized intracellular membrane compartments. However, following insulin stimulation, this protein undergoes a massive redistribution to the cell surface, thereby increasing the number of glucose transporter proteins and increasing glucose uptake. Several lines of evidence have established that the PI 3-kinase pathway is essential, but not necessarily sufficient, for this biologic response. Although several models of insulin resistance have been correlated with reduction in the insulin action of the

PI 3-kinase pathway, downstream targets of PI 3-kinase are unaffected, bringing into question the relevance of small changes in PI 3-kinase activity as a mechanism for insulin resistance *(75)*.

The study of another insulin receptor downstream target termed the insulin receptor substrate (IRS) has generated much interest. Currently, there are four known isoforms, IRS1, -2, -3, and -4, which function as proximal substrates of the insulin receptor. The tyrosine phosphorylation of these proteins generates recognition sites for several additional effector proteins including the PI 3-kinase. Mice deficient in IRS1 display peripheral tissue insulin resistance and growth retardation but do not become diabetic, owing to pancreatic β-cell compensation *(76,77)*. In contrast, IRS2-deficient mice have impaired β-cell insulin secretion and display a clear diabetic phenotype *(78)*. Although extensive investigation has not revealed any systematic gene defect in IRS structure or expression, recent data have suggested a novel mechanism inactivating IRS function. In many systems, serine/threonine phosphorylation is known to impair the ability of tyrosine kinases to tyrosine-phosphorylate their substrates. Several lines of evidence have demonstrated that serine/threonine phosphorylation of IRS markedly impairs insulin-stimulated tyrosine phosphorylation and inhibits insulin action *(79)*. Since insulin resistance is a highly heterogenous disease with both genetic and environmental components, is it possible that IRS proteins underlie a single signaling defect that can account for this phenotype? Probably not.

One important clue has emerged from the study of the inflammatory/cytokine signaling pathway. It is well known that many factors that activate the inflammatory pathway also induce insulin resistance and serine/threonine phosphorylation of IRS. More compelling are studies showing that inhibition of the inflammatory kinase pathway (IκB kinase) enhances insulin sensitivity, whereas activation of this pathway induces insulin resistance *(80,81)*. In hindsight, these recent findings are consistent with numerous anecdotal reports on the ability of high-dose aspirin to reduce hyperglycemia in diabetic patients. In addition to being a cyclooxygenase (COX) inhibitor, high-dose salicylates also apparently function to inhibit IκB kinase. Thus, the development of specific inhibitors of the inflammatory pathway may eventually provide a powerful new clinical tool in the management of peripheral tissue insulin sensitivity.

In addition to striated muscle, liver, and adipocytes, the fourth major organ intimately controlling glucose metabolism is the pancreas (Fig. 2). The β-cells of the pancreatic islets of Langerhans store insulin in dense-core granules that are released in response to various fuel secretagogues such as fatty acids, arginine, and glucose. It is clear that elevated circulating glucose levels are sensed (glucose sensor) by a low-K_m glucose transporter isoform, GLUT2, which couples to glucokinase. This allows glucose to enter the glycolytic pathway to generate ATP in a manner directly proportional to the physiologic range of circulating glucose. This change in β-cell energy status (ATP/ADP ratio) provides a critical metabolic signal, which closes an ATP-sensitive potassium channel/sulfonyl-urea receptor complex, resulting in membrane depolarization. In turn, membrane depolarization opens a voltage-sensitive calcium channel, thereby increasing intracellular calcium levels. The increase in intracellular calcium then provides a trigger for the fusion of insulin-containing granules and the subsequent increase in circulating insulin levels.

This complex regulation of insulin secretion underscores the extremely tight control of this process and provides multiple potential targets that can be dysregulated in states of insulin resistance and diabetes. One potential clue has arisen from the observation that peripheral tissue insulin resistance is not sufficient to induce diabetes. There must also be an additional insulin secretion defect. Furthermore, the same types of states that induce peripheral tissue insulin resistance have a high propensity to impair insulin secretion. Is it therefore possible that defects in insulin receptor signaling also directly affect pancreatic β-cell insulin release? Although it has been very difficult to demonstrate directly a specific insulin receptor signaling role in isolated β-cells, insulin receptor knockout mice display altered glucose-sensitive insulin secretion properties and develop type 2 diabetes (82). Thus, one exciting possibility is that the initial development of peripheral tissue insulin resistance eventually leads to pancreatic β-cell insulin resistance and thus triggers the full-blown diabetic phenotype.

TYPE 2 DIABETES AND IGT

Type 2 diabetes in the United States is increasing at an alarming rate; it is predicted that as many as 10% of the country's population will have diabetes by the year 2025 (83). Individuals with type 2 diabetes pass through a stage of IGT prior to diabetes onset (Fig. 1) (84,85). Depending on the criteria used for the diagnosis of IGT, 30–40 million Americans now have IGT, with 20% or more of the elderly being affected (86). This compares with the 16 million individuals who now have type 2 diabetes. As the average lifespan of Americans continues to increase, the frequency of progression of IGT to type 2 diabetes will also probably increase. IGT has two major associated problems: increased cardiovascular disease and the progression to type 2 diabetes. The risk of cardiovascular disease with IGT is not as great as that seen in overt type 2 diabetes, but it is clearly greater than in age-matched controls (87). Progression to type 2 diabetes increases if individuals with IGT decrease their physical activity and/or increase their weight (88). The rate of progression to diabetes in the United States ranges from 30 to 60% within 10 yr after the diagnosis of IGT. Rates of progression to diabetes in different countries are extremely variable. Whether this is caused by different genetic backgrounds or different lifestyles is not entirely clear.

Central components of the successful treatment of IGT have been diet (89–91) and exercise, which are appropriately termed lifestyle changes (92,93). Several

Table 2
Recent Studies in Lifestyle Management in Impaired Glucose Tolerance (IGT)

	No. of patients	Study period	Reduction in progression of DM with exercise or dietary intervention
Da Qing Study (93)	577	6 yr	21% reduction in DM
Malmo Study (49)	181	6 yr	50% normalization of IGT in 5 yr
Tuomilehto et al. (3)	522	4 yr	57% reduction in rate of progression of IGT to DM
Wing et al. (94)	154	2 yr	No significant result at 3 yr
DPP (1,2,143,144)	3234	3 yr	58% reduction in DM2 with lifestyle changes

DM, daibetes mellitus; DPP, Diabetes Prevention Program; IGT, impaired glucose tolerance.

different diets have been used successfully in IGT, usually combined with some form of exercise. The recommended exercises have mostly been some form of light aerobic exercise or resistance training. The various diets have several characteristics in common, including decreased calories for weight reduction, decreased fat (<30% of total calories), decreased saturated fat (<10% of diet), and increased fiber (15 g/d). The combined exercise and diet were intended to result in weight loss, of 5% or more, but this goal was rarely achieved in any study. Even so, patients in many of these studies showed improvement in IGT and decreased progression to type 2 diabetes.

Successful large-scale, long-term studies of lifestyle changes in IGT have been reported since 1991 (Table 2), with the most recently published study in February 2002, the DPP (Table 2). Against this background of effective therapy of IGT, it is important to realize that other studies of IGT treatment with lifestyle changes have not demonstrated sustained long-term improvement. An example of such negative findings is the well-designed study of IGT by Wing et al. published in 1998 (94). These authors showed positive results after the first year of the study that were not sustained at the end of 3 yr. However, the published literature, in total, does show a positive effect of lifestyle changes on slowing the progression of IGT to type 2 diabetes.

Recent Large-Scale Trials in IGT

Two important studies on IGT and lifestyle changes were recently completed, the NIH-sponsored DPP (143,144) and the Finnish Cooperative Diabetes Trial (Table 2) (1–3). These are of particular importance because they both included a large population (the Finnish study 552 and the DPP 3234 IGT patients) and also provide insight into the time, the effort, and the multidisciplinary team needed to impact on IGT effectively (3,143,144). The NIH DPP, a study of 3234 individuals with IGT aged 25–85 yr, compared treatment with diet/exercise or with metformin (850 mg twice daily) in the prevention of the progression of IGT to type 2 diabetes. The results of this trial were sufficiently positive to stop the study in August, 2001, well before its scheduled completion in 2002.

The DPP was a major clinical trial including 27 centers of individuals with IGT and body mass index (BMI) greater than 25. IGT was diagnosed on the basis of an oral glucose tolerance test. Forty-five percent of the 3234 participants were from the minority groups that are disproportionately affected with type 2 diabetes, including African Americans, Native Americans, Hispanic Americans, Asian Americans and Pacific Islanders. At 3-yr follow-up, there was a 29% progression to type 2 diabetes in the placebo group and a 58% *reduction* in expected progression to type 2 diabetes in those in the intensive lifestyle intervention group. Metformin was also effective, causing a 31% reduction in the expected diabetes rate. Thus, the risk of developing diabetes was decreased in both study groups, with rates in the modified lifestyle changes group being substantially better than in those treated with metformin *(95,96)*. Although labeled "intensive lifestyle intervention," diet and exercise were not pushed to extreme levels. This patient group maintained an average of 30 min of exercise daily, usually consisting of walking for 30 min a day or other moderate exercise, and a weight loss program aimed toward a 7% reduction in the initial body weight. All ages benefited, with the greatest prevention rate in individuals older than 65 yr (71%). Although similar positive results were previously found in other reports (Table 2), the DPP was distinguished by the magnitude of the IGT population studied, the diversity of the ethnic groups, and the age range (25–85 yr) of the participants.

The authors of the DPP highlight several areas they considered key elements in successfully implementing their lifestlye changes *(143,144)*. These include: clearly defined goals of 7% weight loss and 150 min exercise per wk, individual case managers or "lifestyle coaches," frequent contact, intensive interventions, 16–24-session core curriculum, extra classes, consistent motivation, feedback support, restart opportunities, monthly visits, and telephone calls. The weight loss was most important to decrease the risk of diabetes, with each kilogram loss equaling a 13% decrease in risk of diabetes. Exercise without weight loss was not associated with an increase in diabetes, but exercise was especially relevant for maintaining weight loss. The latter is especially relevant since it has been shown that exercise programs can be maintained for greater the 10 yr *(145)*.

In the recently published Finnish study on IGT *(3)*, five goals were set by the trial investigators: (1) a decrease in body weight of 5% of initial weight or more; (2) fat component in diet 30% or less of total ingested kcal; (3) saturated fat less than 10% of the diet; (4) increased fiber to 15 g or more per kcal; and (5) moderate exercise of 30 min or more daily. At 1-yr, there was an inverse relationship between goals met and the proportion of individuals who progressed to type 2 diabetes. Most impressively, this inverse relationship was observed at each of the 5 yr of the multicenter trial. Quarterly visits were made with the individuals who formed the intervention group of the study, frequent contacts were maintained throughout the trial, and repeated education sessions were held related to the importance of the lifestyle modifications. The Finnish trial, a five-center study, enrolled 552 participants (vs 3234 in the DPP NIH trial). The average age was 55-yr and the average BMI was 31. The intervention group received seven dietary counseling sessions in yr 1 and every 3 mo thereafter. Dietary advice was individualized and focused on weight loss, decrease in fat (especially saturated fat) (97), and total calories consumed. The individualized exercise program concentrated more on muscle strengthening, with weight lifting and resistance training, and placed somewhat less emphasis on aerobic exercising (vs 30 min of daily walking or light aerobics in the DPP). Free health club memberships were given at two of the five centers. Individuals in the control group were given yearly advice about diet and exercise regimens.

The greatest decrease in weight loss was seen at the end of yr 1 (−4.2 kg vs −0.8 kg in controls). However, the difference in prevention of progression to type 2 diabetes was statistically significant at yr 1–5, with the final rate in the intervention group being a 57% reduction in expected progression to diabetes. It is of interest that in the DPP there was a similar 58% decrease at 3 yr in progression to diabetes, even though there was a slight difference in the type of exercise performed in each study (94,95).

IMPORTANT ILLUSTRATIVE STUDIES

To illustrate further the importance of diet and exercise, at least four other studies have contributed to our thinking on slowing the progression of IGT to frank diabetes. In the first, published in 1984, ten urbanized Australian aborigines with type 2 diabetes returned to their traditional hunter-gatherer lifestyle for 7 wk (98). During this time they gathered all their food, which necessitated a marked increase in physical exercise. In the 7 wk period, they consumed a diet low in calories (average of 1200 kcal/person/d) and low in fat (98,99). After only 7 wk, all participants lost weight at an average of 8 kg/person. Fasting blood glucose either decreased or normalized, fasting insulin level decreased, and glucose-stimulated insulin release markedly improved.

In a second study, the Pima Indians who settled in Arizona were compared with the Pimas who settled in Mexico (100). The Mexican Pimas had less obesity, expended more energy, and had a strikingly lower incidence of IGT and type 2 diabetes (101,102). This report emphasized that individuals of the same genetic background can have markedly different rates of IGT and type 2 diabetes depending on their diet and exercise pattern (103).

A third study showed the effect of weight loss in very obese individuals on the progression of IGT to type 2 diabetes (104). The effect of weight loss by gastric bypass surgery on the progression of IGT to frank type 2 diabetes was assessed in a population of severely obese individuals with IGT. After surgery, subsequent weight loss was accompanied by improvement or, commonly, "cure" of

IGT, even though patients remained substantially obese at the time of major improvement/cure of IGT.

Finally, in a fourth report published in September, 2001 *(30)*, a large number (84,941) of nurses was followed from 1980 to 1996. During the 16-yr of follow-up, 3300 new cases of type 2 diabetes were found. Being overweight or obese was the single most important predictor of developing type 2 diabetes. Lack of exercise and a "poor diet" were also found in those who developed type 2 diabetes.

These last four studies strikingly illustrate the important treatment concepts: (1) diet and exercise can rapidly slow the progression of IGT to diabetes and can also improve glycemic control in those with type 2 diabetes; (2) losing weight, well short of ideal body weight, can also cause IGT to improve or return to normal; and (3) the best predictor of development of IGT and type 2 diabetes is being overweight or obese, which is further compounded by lack of exercise *(105)*.

SPECIFIC RISK FACTORS FOR IGT:
POLYCYSTIC OVARIAN SYNDROME AND SYNDROME X

Two of the risk factors for IGT, polycystic ovarian syndrome (PCOS) and the dysmetabolic or metabolic syndrome, or syndrome X, are now being seen with increasing frequency by the family practitioner, the internist, and the endocrinologist (Table 1). Chapter 9 (The Polycystic Ovarian Syndrome) and 7 (Obesity) explore these topics in detail. The following discussion covers these two syndromes briefly, with an emphasis on their relationship to IGT.

Polycystic Ovarian Syndrome

PCOS is a common disorder of premenstrual women characterized by hyperandrogenism, chronic anovulation, menstrual irregularity, hyperinsulinemia, and often (for which it is a major cause) infertility (106,107). Prevalence estimates range from 5 to 10% of menstruating females. It was first reported in 1980 that women with PCOS had hyperinsulinemia, suggesting the presence of insulin resistance *(108–110)*. Subsequently, many women with PCOS were found to have subtle acanthosis nigricans, a skin darkening often associated with insulin resistance. Women with chronic anovulation and hyperandrogenemia *(111,112)* without secondary causes were found to have glucose intolerance and elevated insulin levels *(55)*. That PCOS is associated with insulin resistance and hyperglycemia following an oral glucose tolerance test (OGTT) was first demonstrated by Dunaif in 1987 *(109)*. Forty percent of PCOS patients who are also obese have IGT or frank type 2 diabetes, and this remains consistent despite ethnic or geographic variation. Most of these PCOS patients are diagnosed in their third and fourth decades of life. PCOS-related insulin resistance accounts for 20–40% of IGT and type 2 diabetes in reproductive age women *(113)*. The percentage of occurrence of IGT or diabetes is further increased by the presence of obesity or a family history of type 2 diabetes. Screening patients with PCOS, especially in the presence of other risk factors for IGT (Table 1), should clearly be done. Again, screening should include fasting glucose with the diagnosis of IGT confirmed by 2-h glucose after ingestion of 75 g glucola.

Treatment of PCOS, especially if fertility is desired, should probably consist of metformin (113–117) and possibly lifestyle changes in diet and exercise (118). Drugs that improve insulin sensitivity, such as metformin and the glitizones (rosiglitizone and pioglitazone), are thought to reverse not only the metabolic features of PCOS but also the excess ovarian steroidogenesis and gonadotropin stimulation (119). Treatment with metformin or a thiazolidinedione can often normalize menses and can result in conception in a previously infertile woman. Metformin inhibits glycogenolysis, decreasing hepatic glucose output and also improving peripheral insulin sensitivity. Metformin was first used for PCOS in 1994 by Velazquez et al. (120). Their study in 26 women with PCOS used metformin at 1500 mg/d for 8 wk. Not only did the women have significant improvement in hyperglycemia, but there was a 52% drop in testosterone levels and several spontaneous pregnancies. Subsequently, at least eight publications have shown the positive effects of metformin in decreasing androgen levels, improving metabolic profiles, and increasing fertility in PCOS (121).

Dysmetabolic (Metabolic) Syndrome (Syndrome X)

The original definition of syndrome X, by Reaven (20), emphasized insulin resistance. The dysmetabolic syndrome consists of insulin resistance in association with dyslipidemia, obesity (particularly with excess visceral fat), hypertension, and often IGT or type 2 diabetes. This constellation of abnormalities is associated with an accelerated onset of atherosclerosis (18,122). Patients with syndrome X have a 20–40% incidence of type 2 diabetes and probably an even greater association with IGT (123).

The obesity in the abdomen tends to be deep or visceral adiposity, which is associated with accelerated atherosclerosis and coronary artery disease (104). The presence of visceral fat in this syndrome is an example of the fact that not all forms of obesity are functionally the same and that different forms can pose different health risks. Patients with fat distributed in subcutaneous regions around the gluteofemoral areas and upper abdomen are at much less risk for complications such as hypertension, lipid abnormalities, and insulin resistance than those with visceral fat (124,125). The idea that adipose tissue releases important metabolites has been fueled by recent findings showing that fat may not be just a storage compartment but rather an active source for production of proteins central to obesity, insulin resistance, and lipid disorders. Adipose tissue has been demonstrated to produce leptin (126), resistin (127,128), and Acrp 30/AdipoQ (129–132), which have been proposed to mediate obesity, insulin resistance, and hepatic insulin sensitivity, respectively (132–134) (Fig. 2).

Visceral adipose tissue is drained by the portal venous system and has a direct connection with the liver. Free fatty acids are quickly mobilized from these depots, compared with other peripheral fat stores. The lipolytic activity in visceral adipocytes is higher than in other fat depots, whereas, at the same time, the antilipolytic effect of insulin is more in the subcutaneous than the visceral fat. The concentration of free fatty acids in the portal system is thus elevated. This apparently results in stimulation of gluconeogenesis, resulting in hyperglycemia and increased triglyceride synthesis with associated dyslipidemia. Visceral obesity is also associated with increased levels of plasminogen activator inhibitor-1 (PAI-1) *(135–140)*. PAI-1 lessens the fibrinolytic activity of tissue plasminogen by complexing with it. Low levels of plasminogen activator compared with PAI-1 are a risk factor for cardiovascular disease. PAI-1 is atherogenic, and its levels increase with hyperinsulinemia. The potential role of PAI-1 in atherosclerosis associated with obesity, atherosclerosis, and cardiovascular disease of diabetics needs to be further explored.

Detection of patients with syndrome X (the dysmetabolic syndrome) is important because of the markedly increased cardiovascular disease associated with the syndrome *(141,142)*. It also must be recognized that treatment of this complex syndrome is difficult for both the patient and the health care team. Both must understand the components of the syndrome, medications needed, treatment goals, and lifestyle changes in diet and exercise required if the cardiovascular risks are to be lessened. Treatment should target a blood pressure of 130/80 or less, low-density lipoprotein (LDL) cholesterol of 100 or less, prevention of diabetes, and, if diabetes is present, maintenance of hemoglobin A_1c at 7% or less, discontinuation of smoking, and aspirin prophylaxis. To care for patients with this complex syndrome, effectively, the health care team should ideally include a well-informed patient (which is extremely critical), a physician, an exercise therapist, a nutritional consultant, and a psychologist.

MULTIDISCIPLINARY TREATMENT TEAMS

In an attempt to stem the rising tide of type 2 diabetes, multidisciplinary teams have been formed in a few areas of the country. One such program has been ongoing at the University of Iowa since 1999. Led by a physical therapist/exercise therapist (Rhonda Barr), the team is composed of a psychologist, a certified diabetes nurse educator, a nutritionist, and a diabetologist. All persons on the team had a strong interest in disease prevention and IGT in particular. All had read extensively about IGT and clearly were aware of the difficulties in establishing such a team (Table 3). The team, called REACH (Reaching Euglycemia and Comprehensive Health), designed an 8-wk program that incorporated requisite lifestyle changes for healthier daily living patterns in individuals with IGT (Table 4). These included dietary counseling with group and individual dietary

Table 3
Incentives and Disincentives for Forming a REACH-Type Program

Incentives
Diet and exercise do work to decrease or slow progression of IGT to diabetes
Diet and exercise are also helpful for hypertension, dyslipidemia, and cardiovascular
    disease, each of which commonly accompanies diabetes
Even small improvements in diet and/or exercise clearly help
Disincentives
Compliance is difficult
Increased time commitment of staff
Little, if any, reimbursement through health insurance and other third-party carriers
Need of a committed, multidisciplinary team

IGT, impaired glucose tolerance; REACH, Reaching Euglycemia and Comprehensive Health.

Table 4
REACH General Schedule

| 5:30–6:30 | Education topics, goal-setting and support |
| 6:30–7:30 | Group exercise and exercise instruction |

Week	Tuesday	Thursday
1	Program overview	Labeling your challenges
	Developing a support system	Portion sizes
2	Ask the expert: IGT and DM— what are they?	Ask the expert: monitoring health risks
3	Ask the expert: current diet fads	Realistic goal setting and time management
4	Individualized goal setting	Foot and shoe clinic
5	Exercise for health	Ask the expert: dyslipidemia
6	Cardiovascular health: mark your progress	Dining out with ease
7	Decision making and self-esteem	Cooking demonstration: meals in a hurry
8	Stress management: relaxation and reinforcing activities	REACH for health: round table

DM, diabetes mellitus; IGT, impaired glucose tolerance; REACH, Reaching Euglycemia and Comprehensive Health.

change advice, concepts of lifestyle changes, home blood glucose monitoring, and an understanding of IGT and diabetes. Each session of the 8-wk program emphasized individualized exercise training, with 1 h of each session devoted to personalized exercise. The 8-wk classes began in May, 2000. Twelve groups have already completed an 8-wk program. Each group had four to six individuals with IGT and their significant others. The first three groups were intentionally kept small to maximize individual attention and allow the addition of relevant changes or added components that were suggested by REACH team members or IGT participants in completed programs. Data were collected at baseline and at the completion of the 8-wk program. All patients, except two with newly found diabetes through our screening, had IGT by OGTT criteria.

Results of the 8-wk program indicate that even short-term adherence to the program can result in improvement of several objective parameters. For example, participants showed a triglyceride decrease of 61 mg/dL, an LDL cholesterol decrease of 51 mg/dL, an HDL cholesterol increase of 9 mg/dL, a weight loss of 21 pounds, a decrease in systolic blood pressure of 36 mmHg, a decrease in submaximal heart rate of 39 beats per minute, and a decrease in waist circumference of 11.8 cm. These examples represent the maximal positive response after the completion of the 8-wk program. However, it should be noted that most participants had changes that moved in the desired direction. Whether these changes will continue in a positive direction will be determined by follow-up studies in the next year.

For programs such as REACH to be successful in decreasing type 2 diabetes requires several major changes in our health care system. At a minimum, these include testing of trial programs to determine the optimal composition of the multidisciplinary team best suited for such a program, the most effective programs (including those designed for different cultures afflicted with type 2 diabetes) (Table 1), and a redirection of third-party carriers to pay for these prevention programs. The cost of such changes in our health care system for prevention of diabetes must be measured against the present expense for diabetes care, which is now $60 billion a year, not including days lost from work or the personal impact that diabetes has on daily living. At the rate that type 2 diabetes is increasing in the United States, a conservative cost of diabetes in 25 yr has been estimated to be $200 billion a year.

FINAL THOUGHTS

It should be clear that the authors do not consider IGT and type 2 diabetes as two separate illnesses, but rather as two stages in the course of the same disease. By the time one develops IGT, the disease process has already begun. This chapter was primarily aimed at IGT and its treatment. If IGT already indicates the presence of disease, then when should we be intervening? It is our strong opinion that individuals at high risk for IGT/type 2 diabetes (Table 1) should be identified early and be treated at that time, before disease is manifested. Treatment should include specific lifestyle changes with assessment of maintenance of such changes in diet and exercise. The "cynic," or perhaps the "realist," would argue that you cannot get people, including children, to do things that they often do not like to do. Such lifestyle changes may have only small immediate returns and, they would say, people will probably not maintain such changes with the aim of *possibly* preventing disease that could develop in 15–20 yr. They will argue that you are talking about 60–100 million people now, spanning the spectrum of children to the elderly, and that you would need a massive education process directed at children in schools, teachers, parents, the elderly, and several minorities, all of different cultures. Finally, they would sum up by saying that we do not know who would direct such a massive program, who would administer its many branches, and who would pay for such an expensive endeavor.

All these issues are certainly valid. However, it is critical to be aware of the alternative: to remain on the present path, which is leading to a striking increase in type 2 diabetes in our pediatric population and a likely doubling of persons with type 2 diabetes in the next 30 yr. The first step in dealing with such a major health problem is to recognize the existence of the problem. The next step would be the development of a program to begin to address this situation. Such a program would probably need funding from the National Institutes of Health, the American Diabetes Association, the Juvenile Diabetes Foundation, the U.S. government, organizations sponsoring health care research, and private health care organizations. Developing such a program will not be easy and certainly will be very expensive. Without this intervention, the cost will be measured in human suffering from the ravages of type 2 diabetes. The recently published Finnish study *(3)* and the DPP *(143,145)* show that there is real hope of preventing this epidemic from continuing. It is now the task of physicians, behavior therapists, and other allied medical personnel to make this happen.

REFERENCES

1. The Diabetes Prevention Program. Design and methods for a clinical trial in the prevention of type 2 diabetes. Diabetes Care 1999;22:623–634.
2. The Diabetes Prevention Program: baseline characteristics of the randomized cohort. The Diabetes Prevention Program Research Group. Diabetes Care 2000;23:1619–1629.
3. Tuomilehto J, Lindstrom J, Eriksson JG, et al. Prevention of type 2 diabetes mellitus by changes in lifestyle among subjects with impaired glucose tolerance. N Engl J Med 2001;344:1343–1350.
4. Narayan KM, Bowman BA, Engelgau ME. Prevention of type 2 diabetes. BMJ 2001;323:63–64.
5. Perry RC, Baron AD. Impaired glucose tolerance. Why is it not a disease? Diabetes Care 1999;22:883–885.
6. Alberti KG. The clinical implications of impaired glucose tolerance. Diabet Med 1996;13:927–937.
7. Matsumoto K, Miyake S, Yano M, et al. Glucose tolerance, insulin secretion, and insulin sensitivity in nonobese and obese Japanese subjects. Diabetes Care 1997;20:1562–1568.
8. Heine RJ, Mooy JM. Impaired glucose tolerance and unidentified diabetes. Postgrad Med J 1996;72:67–71.
9. Johnson KC, Graney MJ, Applegate WB, Kitabchi AE, Runyan JW, Shorr RI. Prevalence of undiagnosed non-insulin-dependent diabetes mellitus and impaired glucose tolerance in a cohort of older persons with hypertension. J Am Geriatr Soc 1997;45:695–700.
10. Uusitupa M, Louheranta A, Lindstrom J, et al. The Finnish Diabetes Prevention Study. Br J Nutr 2000;83 Suppl 1:S137–S142.

11. Harris TJ, Cook DG, Wicks PD, Cappuccio FP. Impact of the new American Diabetes Association and World Health Organisation diagnostic criteria for diabetes on subjects from three ethnic groups living in the UK. Nutr Metab Cardiovasc Dis 2000;10:305–309.
12. Matsuda M, DeFronzo RA. Insulin sensitivity indices obtained from oral glucose tolerance testing: comparison with the euglycemic insulin clamp. Diabetes Care 1999;22:1462–1470.
13. Metcalf PA, Scragg RK. Comparison of WHO and ADA criteria for diagnosis of glucose status in adults. Diabetes Res Clin Pract 2000;49:169–180.
14. Bolli G, Compagnucci P, Cartechini MG, et al. HbA1 in subjects with abnormal glucose tolerance but normal fasting plasma glucose. Diabetes 1980;29:272–277.
15. Breda E, Cavaghan MK, Toffolo G, Polonsky KS, Cobelli C. Oral glucose tolerance test minimal model indexes of beta-cell function and insulin sensitivity. Diabetes 2001;50:150–158.
16. Greenbaum CJ, Cuthbertson D, Krischer JP. Type I diabetes manifested solely by 2-h oral glucose tolerance test criteria. Diabetes 2001;50:470–476.
17. Shaw JE, Zimmet PZ, de Courten M, et al. Impaired fasting glucose or impaired glucose tolerance. What best predicts future diabetes in Mauritius? Diabetes Care 1999;22:399–402.
18. Tominaga M, Eguchi H, Manaka H, Igarashi K, Kato T, Sekikawa A. Impaired glucose tolerance is a risk factor for cardiovascular disease, but not impaired fasting glucose. The Funagata Diabetes Study. Diabetes Care 1999;22:920–924.
19. Tripathy D, Carlsson M, Almgren P, et al. Insulin secretion and insulin sensitivity in relation to glucose tolerance: lessons from the Botnia Study. Diabetes 2000;49:975–980.
20. Reaven GM. Banting Lecture 1988. Role of insulin resistance in human disease. Diabetes 1988;37:1595–1607.
21. DeFronzo RA, Bonadonna RC, Ferrannini E. Pathogenesis of NIDDM. A balanced overview. Diabetes Care 1992;15:318–368.
22. Ipp E. Impaired glucose tolerance: the irrepressible alpha-cell? Diabetes Care 2000;23:569–570.
23. Kahn SE. Clinical review 135: the importance of beta-cell failure in the development and progression of type 2 diabetes. J Clin Endocrinol Metab 2001;86:4047–4058.
24. Weyer C, Bogardus C, Mott DM, Pratley RE. The natural history of insulin secretory dysfunction and insulin resistance in the pathogenesis of type 2 diabetes mellitus. J Clin Invest 1999;104:787–794.
25. Stolk RP, Pols HA, Lamberts SW, de Jong PT, Hofman A, Grobbee DE. Diabetes mellitus, impaired glucose tolerance, and hyperinsulinemia in an elderly population. The Rotterdam Study. Am J Epidemiol 1997;145:24–32.
26. Rewers M, Hamman RF. Risk factors for non-insulin-dependent diabetes. In: Harris ML, Cowie CC, Stern MF, Boyko EJ, Reiber GE, Bennett PH, eds. Diabetes in America, 2nd ed. NIH publication no. 95-1468. NIH, Bethesda, MD, 1995, pp. 179–220.
27. Lee ET, Howard BV, Savage PJ, et al. Diabetes and impaired glucose tolerance in three American Indian populations aged 45–74 years. Diabetes Care 1995;18:599–610.
28. Wing RR, Goldstein MG, Acton KJ, et al. Behavioral science research in diabetes: lifestyle changes related to obesity, eating behavior, and physical activity. Diabetes Care 2001;24:117–123.
29. Kjos SL, Buchanan TA. Gestational diabetes mellitus. N Engl J Med 1999;341:1749–1756.
30. Hu FB, Manson JE, Stampfer MJ, et al. Diet, lifestyle, and the risk of type 2 diabetes mellitus in women. N Engl J Med 2001;345:790–797.
31. Harris MI, Eastman RC, Cowie CC, Flegal KM, Eberhardt MS. Racial and ethnic differences in glycemic control of adults with type 2 diabetes. Diabetes Care 1999;22:403–408.
32. Haffner SM, Hazuda HP, Mitchell BD, et al. Increased incidence of type II diabetes mellitus in Mexican Americans. Diabetes Care 1991;14:102–108.
33. Fujimoto WY. Diabetes in Asian and Pacific Islander Americans. In: Harris MI, ed. Diabetes in America. NIH publication no. 95-1468. National Institutes of Health, Bethesda, MD, 1995, pp. 661–681.

34. National Institute of Diabetes and Digestive and Kidney Diseases. Diabetes Statistics 1995. NIH publication no. 96. National Institutes of Health, Bethesda, MD, 1995, pp. 3926.
35. Bergman RN, Watanabe R, Rebrin K, Ader M, Steil G. Toward an integrated phenotype in pre-NIDDM. Diabet Med 1996;13:S67–S77.
36. Best JD, Kahn SE, Ader M, Watanabe RM, Ni TC, Bergman RN. Role of glucose effectiveness in the determination of glucose tolerance. Diabetes Care 1996;19:1018–1030.
37. Manson JE, Rimm EB, Stampfer MJ, et al. Physical activity and incidence of non-insulin-dependent diabetes mellitus in women. Lancet 1991;338:774–778.
38. Manson JE, Nathan DM, Krolweski AS, et al. A prospective study of exercise and incidence of diabetes among US male physicians. JAMA 1992;268:63–67.
39. Helmrich SP, Ragland DR, Leung RW, et al. Physical activity and reduced occurrence of non-insulin-dependent diabetes mellitus. N Engl J Med 1991;325:147–152.
40. Hamman RF. Genetic and enviromental determinants of non-insulin-dependent diabetes mellitus (NIDDM). Diabetes Metab Rev 1992;8:287–338.
41. DeFronzo RA. Lilly lecture 1987. The triumvirate: β-cell, muscle, liver. A collusion responsible for NIDDM. Diabetes 1988;37:667–687.
42. Knowler WC, Narayan KM, Hanson RL, et al. Preventing non-insulin-dependent diabetes. Diabetes 1995;44:483–488.
43. Campbell PJ, Carlson MG. Impact of obesity on insulin action in NIDDM. Diabetes 1993;42:405–410.
44. Wing RR, Blair EH, Bononi P, et al. Caloric restriction per se is a significant factor in improvements in glycemic control and insulin sensitivity during weight loss in obese NIDDM patients. Diabetes Care 1994;17:30–36.
45. Henry RR, Wallace P, Olefsky JM. Effects of weight loss on mechanisms of hyperglycemia in obese non-insulin-dependent diabetes mellitus. Diabetes 1986;35:990–998.
46. Maron DJ, Fair JM, Haskelll WL. Saturated fat intake and insulin resistance in men with coronary artery disease. Circulation 1991;84:2020–2027.
47. Parillo M, Rivellese AA, Ciardullo AV, et al. A high-monounsaturated-fat/low-carbohydrate diet improves peripheral insulin sensitivity in non-insulin dependent diabetic patients. Metabolism 1992;41:1373–1378.
48. Kriska AM, Bennett PH. An epidemiological perspective of the relationship between physical activity and NIDDM: from activity assessment to intervention. Diabetes Metab Rev 1992;8:355–372.
49. Eriksson KF, Lindgarde F. Prevention of type 2 (non-insulin dependent) diabetes mellitus by diet and physical exercise: the 6-year Malmö feasibility study. Diabetologia 1991;34:891–898.
50. Tritos NA, Mantzoros CS. Clinical review 97: syndromes of severe insulin resistance. J Clin Endocrinol Metab 1998;83:3025–3030.
51. Barrett-Connor E. Epidemiology, obesity, and non-insulin-dependent diabetes mellitus. Epidemiol Rev 1989;11:172–181.
52. Strauss RS, Pollack HA. Epidemic increase in childhood overweight, 1986–1998. JAMA 2001;286:2845–2848.
53. Jones KL, Arslanian S, Peterokova VA, Park J-S, Tomlinson MJ. Effect of metformin in pediatric patients with type 2 diabetes. Diabetes Care 2002;25:89-94.
54. Samos LF, Roos BA. Diabetes mellitus in older persons. Med Clin North Am 1998;82:791–803.
55. Ford ES, Giles, WH, Dietz WH. Prevalence of the metabolic syndrome among US adults: findings from the Third National Health and Nutrition Examination Survey. JAMA 2002;287:356–360.
56. Kahn SE, Porte D Jr. Pathophysiology of type II diabetes mellitus. In: Porte D Jr, Sherwin RS, eds. Diabetes Mellitus. Appleton & Lange, Stamford, CT, 1996, pp. 487–512.

57. Levy J, Atkinson AB, Bell PM, McCance DR, Hadden DR. β-cell deterioration determines the onset and rate of progression of secondary dietary failure in type 2 diabetes mellitus: the 10-year follow-up of the Belfast Diet Study. Diabetes Med 1996;15:290–296.
58. Polonsky KS, Given BD, Hirsch LJ, et al. Abnormal patterns of insulin secretion in non-insulin-dependent diabetes mellitus. N Engl J Med 1988;318:1231–1239.
59. Polonsky KS, Sturis J, Bell GI. Non-insulin-dependent diabetes mellitus—a genetically programmed failure of the beta cell to compensate for insulin resistance. N Engl J Med 1996;334:777–783.
60. Ward WK, Wallum BJ, Beard JC, Taborsky GJ Jr, Porte D Jr. Reduction of glycemic potentiation: a sensitive indicator of β-cell loss in partially pancreatectomized dogs. Diabetes 1988;37:723–729.
61. Goldfine ID. The insulin receptor; molecular biology and transmembrane signaling. Endocr Rev 1987;8:235–255.
62. Kahn, CR. Banting Lecture. Insulin action, diabetogenes, and the cause of type II diabetes. Diabetes 1994;43:1066–1084.
63. Lee, JS, Pilch, PF. The insulin receptor—structure, function, and signaling. Am J Physiol 1994;266:C319–C334.
64. Czech MP, Corvera S. Signaling mechanisms that regulate glucose transport. J Biol Chem 1999;274:1865–1868.
65. White M, Kahn CR. The insulin signaling system. J Biol Chem 1994;269:1–4.
66. White MF. The IRS-signaling system: a network of docking proteins that mediate insulin and cytokine action. Recent Prog Horm Res 1998;53:119–138.
67. Pessin JE, Saltiel AR. Signaling pathways in insulin action: molecular targets of insulin resistance. J Clin Invest 2000;106:165–169.
68. Kido Y, Nakae J, Accili D. Clinical review 125: the insulin receptor and its cellular targets. J Clin Endocrinol Metab 2001;86:972–979.
69. Taylor SI, Kadowaki T, Kadowaki H, Accili C, Cama A, McKeon C. Mutations in insulin receptor gene in insulin resistant patients. Diabetes Care 1990;13:257–279.
70. Taylor SI, Cama A, Accili D, et al. Mutations in the insulin receptor gene. Endocr Rev 1992;13:566–595.
71. O'Rahilly S, Moller DE. Mutant insulin receptors in syndromes of insulin resistance. Clin Endocrinol 1992;36:121–132.
72. Watson RT, Pessin JE. Subcellular compartmentalization and trafficking of the insulin-responsive glucose transporter, GLUT4. Exp Cell Res 2001;271:75–83.
73. Saltiel AR. Diverse signaling pathways in the cellular actions of insulin. Am J Physiol 1996;270:E375–E385.
74. Watson RT Pessin JE. Intracellular organization of insulin signaling and GLUT4 translocation. Recent Prog Horm Res 2001;56:175–193.
75. Kim YB, Nikoulina SE, Ciaraldi TP, Henry RR, Kahn BB. Normal insulin-dependent activation of Akt/protein kinase B, with diminished activation of phosphoinositide 3-kinase, in muscle in type 2 diabetes. J Clin Invest 1999;104:733–741.
76. Araki E, Lipes MA, Patti ME, et al. Alternative pathway of insulin signaling in mice with targeted disruption of the IRS-1 gene. Nature 1994;372,186–190.
77. Tamemoto H, Kadowaki T, Tobe K, et al. 1994. Insulin resistance and growth retardation in mice lacking insulin receptor substrate-1. Nature 372:182–186.
78. Kubota N, Tobe K, Terauchi Y, et al. Disruption of insulin receptor substrate 2 causes type 2 diabetes because of liver insulin resistance and lack of compensatory beta-cell hyperplasia. Diabetes 2000;49:1880-1889.
79. Hotamisligil GS. Mechanisms of TNF-alpha-induced insulin resistance. Exp Clin Endocrinol Diabetes 1999;107:119–125.

80. Yuan M, Konstantopoulos N, Lee J, et al. Reversal of obesity- and diet-induced insulin resistance with salicylates or targeted disruption of Ixkbeta. Science 2001;293:1673–1677.
81. Kim JK, Kim YJ, Fillmore JJ, et al. Prevention of fat-induced insulin resistance by salicylate. J Clin Invest 2001;108:437–446.
82. Kulkarni RN, Bruning JC, Winnay JN, Postic C, Magnuson MA, Kahn CR. Tissue-specific knockout of the insulin receptor in pancreatic beta cells creates an insulin secretory defect similar to that in type 2 diabetes. Cell 1999;96:329–339.
83. Medalie JH, Papeir CM, Goldbourt U, Herman JB. Major factors in the development of diabetes mellitus in 10,000 men. Arch Intern Med 1975;135:811–817.
84. Gulli G, Ferrannini E, Stern M, Haffner SM, DeFronzo RA. The metabolic profile of NIDDM is fully established in glucose-tolerant offspring of two Mexican American parents. Diabetes 1992;41:1575–1586.
85. Haffner SM. Risk factors for non-insulin-dependent diabetes mellitus. J Hypertens 1995;13:S73–S76.
86. Eastman RC, Cowie CC, Harris MI. Undiagnosed diabetes or impaired glucose tolerance and cardiovascular risk. Diabetes Care 1997;20:127–128.
87. Balkau B, Eschwege E, Papoz L, et al. Risk factors for early death in non-insulin-dependent diabetes and men with known glucose tolerance status. BMJ 1993;207:295–299.
88. Sadd MF, Knowler WC, Pettitt DJ, Nelson RG, Bennett PH. The natural history of impaired glucose tolerance in Pima Indians. N Engl J Med 1988;319:1500–1506.
89. Alarcon de la Lastra C, Barranco MD, Motilva V, Herrerias JM. Mediterranean diet and health: biological importance of olive oil. Curr Pharm Des 2001;7:933–950.
90. Chandalia M, Garg A, Lutjohann D, von Bergmann K, Grundy SM, Brinkley LJ. Beneficial effects of high dietary fiber intake in patients with type 2 diabetes mellitus. N Engl J Med 2000;342:1392–1398.
91. Savage PJ, Bennion LJ, Flock EV, et al. Diet-induced improvement of abnormalities in insulin and glucagon secretion and in insulin receptor binding in diabetes mellitus. J Clin Endocrinol Metab 1979;48:999–1007.
92. Eriksson KF, Saltin B, Lindgarde F. Increased skeletal muscle capillary density precedes diabetes development in men with impaired glucose tolerance. A 15-year follow-up. Diabetes 1994;43:805–808.
93. Pan XR, Li GW, Hu YH, et al. Effects of diet and exercise in preventing NIDDM in people with impaired glucose tolerance. The Da Qing IGT and Diabetes Study. Diabetes Care 1997;20:537–544.
94. Wing RR, Venditti E, Jakicic JM, Polley BA, Lang W. Lifestyle intervention in overweight individuals with a family history of diabetes. Diabetes Care 1998;21:350–359.
95. Scheen AJ, Letiexhe MR, Lefebvre PJ. Effects of metformin in obese patients with impaired glucose tolerance. Diabetes Metab Rev 1995;11(Suppl 1):S69–S80.
96. Schoonjans K, Auwerx J. Thiazolidinediones: an update. Lancet 2000;355:1008–1010.
97. Mayer-Davis EJ. Low-fat diets for diabetes prevention. Diabetes Care 2001;24:613–614.
98. O'Dea K. Marked improvement in carbohydrate and lipid metabolism in diabetic Australian aborigines after temporary reversion to traditional lifestyle. Diabetes 1984;33:596–603.
99. Madigan C, Ryan M, Owens D, Collins P, Tomkin GH. Dietary unsaturated fatty acids in type 2 diabetes: higher levels of postprandial lipoprotein on a linoleic acid-rich sunflower oil diet compared with an oleic acid-rich olive oil diet. Diabetes Care 2000;23:1472–1477.
100. Lillioja S. Impaired glucose tolerance in Pima Indians. Diabet Med 1996;13:S127–S132.
101. Sundquist J, Winkleby MA. Cardiovascular risk factors in Mexican American adults: a transcultural analysis of NHANES III, 1988–1994. Am J Public Health 1999;89:723–730.
102. Sundquist J, Winkleby MA, Pudaric S. Cardiovascular disease risk factors among older black, Mexican-American, and white women and men: an analysis of NHANES III, 1988–

1994. Third National Health and Nutrition Examination Survey. J Am Geriatr Soc 2001;49:109–116.

103. Swinburn BA, Metcalf PA, Ley SJ. Long-term (5-year) effects of a reduced-fat diet intervention in individuals with glucose intolerance. Diabetes Care 2001;24:619–624.

104. Long SD, O'Brien K, MacDonald KG, Jr, et al. Weight loss in severely obese subjects prevents the progression of impaired glucose tolerance to type II diabetes. A longitudinal interventional study. Diabetes Care 1994;17:372–375.

105. Bourn DM. The potential for lifestyle change to influence the progression of impaired glucose tolerance to non-insulin-dependent diabetes mellitus. Diabet Med 1996;13:938–945.

106. Lewis V. Polycystic ovary syndrome. A diagnostic challenge. Obstet Gynecol Clin North Am 2001;28:1–20.

107. Zacur HA. Polycystic ovary syndrome, hyperandrogenism, and insulin resistance. Obstet Gynecol Clin North Am 2001;28:21–33.

108. Franks S. Polycystic ovary syndrome. N Engl J Med 1995;333:853–861.

109. Dunaif A. Insulin action in the polycystic ovary syndrome. Endocrinol Metab Clin North Am 1999;28:341–359.

110. Legro RS. Diabetes prevalence and risk factors in polycystic ovary syndrome. Obstet Gynecol Clin North Am 2001;28:99–109.

111. Nelson VL, Qin Kn K, Rosenfield RL, et al. The biochemical basis for increased testosterone production in theca cells propagated from patients with polycystic ovary syndrome. J Clin Endocrinol Metab 2001;86:5925–5933.

112. Larsson H, Ahren B. Androgen activity as a risk factor for impaired glucose tolerance in postmenopausal women. Diabetes Care 1996;19:1399–1403.

113. Talbott EO, Zborowski JV, Sutton-Tyrrell K, McHugh-Pemu KP, Guzick DS. Cardiovascular risk in women with polycystic ovary syndrome. Obstet Gynecol Clin North Am 2001;28:111–133, vii.

114. DeFronzo RA, Goodman AM. Efficacy of metformin in patients with non-insulin-dependent diabetes mellitus. N Engl J Med 1995;333:541–549.

115. Bailey CJ, Turner RC. Metformin. N Engl J Med 1995;334:574–579.

116. Stumvoll M, Nurjhan N, Perrieloo G, et al. Metabolic effects of metformin in non-insulin-dependent diabetes mellitus. N Engl J Med 1995;333:550–554.

117. Bressler R, Johnson D. New pharmacological approaches to therapy of NIDDM. Diabetes Care 1992;15:792–805.

118. Iuorno MJ, Nestler JE. Insulin-lowering drugs in polycystic ovary syndrome. Obstet Gynecol Clin North Am 2001;28:153–164.

119. Ehrmann DA, Barnes RB, Rosenfield RL, Cavaghan MK, Imperial J. Prevalence of impaired glucose tolerance and diabetes in women with polycystic ovary syndrome. Diabetes Care 1999;22:141–146.

120. Velazquez EM, Mendoza S, Hamer T, Sosa F, Glueck CJ. Metformin therapy in polycystic ovary syndrome reduces hyperinsulinemia, insulin resistance, hyperandrogenemia, and systolic blood pressure, while facilitating normal menses and pregnancy. Metabolism 1994;43:647–654.

121. Hoeger K. Obesity and weight loss in polycystic ovary syndrome. Obstet Gynecol Clin North Am 2001;28:85-97, vi-vii.

122. Lindeman RD, Romero LJ, Hundley R, et al. Prevalences of type 2 diabetes, the insulin resistance syndrome, and coronary heart disease in an elderly, biethnic population. Diabetes Care 1998;21:959–966.

123. Weitzman S. Impaired fasting glucose is not a risk factor for cardiovascular mortality. Diabetes Care 1999;22:2104.

124. Raji A, Seely EW, Arky RA, Simonson DC. Body fat distribution and insulin resistance in healthy Asian Indians and Caucasians. J Clin Endocrinol Metab 2001;86:5366–5371.
125. Arner P. Not all fat is alike. Lancet 1998;351:1301–1302.
126. Kulkarni RN, Wang ZL, Wang RM, et al. Leptin reapidly suppresses insulin release from insulinoma cells, rat and human islets, in vivo, in mice. J Clin Invest 100:2729–2736, 1997.
127. Steppan CM, Bailey ST, Bhat S, et al. The hormone resistin links obesity to diabetes. Nature 2001;409:307–312.
128. Steppan CM, Bailey ST, Bhat S, et al. The hormone resistin links obesity to diabetes. Nature 2001;409:307–312.
129. Steppan CM, Lazar MA. Resistin and obesity-associated insulin resistance. Trends Endocrinol Metab 2002;13:18–23.
130. Combs TP, Berg AH, Obici S, Scherer PE, Rossetti L. Endogenous glucose production is inhibited by the adipose-derived protein Acrp30. J Clin Invest 2001;108:1875–1881.
131. Berg AH, Combs TP, Du X, Brownlee M, Scherer PE. The adipocyte-secreted protein Acrp30 enhances hepatic insulin action. Nat Med 2001;7:947–953.
132. Antonucci T, Whitcomb R, McLain R, Lockwood D, Norris RM. Impaired glucose tolerance is normalized by treatment with the thiazolidinedione troglitazone. Diabetes Care 1997;20:188–193.
133. Krentz AJ, Bailey CJ, Melander A. Thiazolidinediones for type 2 diabetes. New agents reduce insulin resistance but need long term clinical trials. BMJ 2000;321:252–253.
134. Olefsky JM. Treatment of insulin resistance with peroxisome proliferator-activated receptor gamma agonists. J Clin Invest 2000;106:467–472.
135. Festa A, D'Agostino R, Jr., Mykkanen L, et al. Relative contribution of insulin and its precursors to fibrinogen and PAI-1 in a large population with different states of glucose tolerance. The Insulin Resistance Atherosclerosis Study (IRAS). Arterioscler Thromb Vasc Biol 1999;19:562–568.
136. Festa A, D'Agostino R Jr, Mykkanen L, Tracy R, Howard BV, Haffner SM. Low-density lipoprotein particle size is inversely related to plasminogen activator inhibitor-1 levels. The Insulin Resistance Atherosclerosis Study. Arterioscler Thromb Vasc Biol 1999;19:605–610.
137. Haffner SM, D'Agostino R, Jr., Mykkanen L, et al. Insulin sensitivity in subjects with type 2 diabetes. Relationship to cardiovascular risk factors: the Insulin Resistance Atherosclerosis Study. Diabetes Care 1999;22:562–568.
138. Lindahl B, Nilsson TK, Jansson JH, Asplund K, Hallmans G. Improved fibrinolysis by intense lifestyle intervention. A randomized trial in subjects with impaired glucose tolerance. J Intern Med 1999;246:105–112.
139. Meigs JB, Mittleman MA, Nathan DM, et al. Hyperinsulinemia, hyperglycemia, and impaired hemostasis: the Framingham Offspring Study. JAMA 2000;283:221–228.
140. Bastard JP, Pieroni L, Hainque B. Relationship between plasma plasminogen activator inhibitor 1 and insulin resistance. Diabetes Metab Res Rev 2000;16:192–201.
141. Eastman RC, Cowie CC, Harris MI. Undiagnosed diabetes or impaired glucose tolerance and cardiovascular risk. Diabetes Care 1997;20:127–128.
142. Seibaek M, Sloth C, Vallebo L, et al. Glucose tolerance status and severity of coronary artery disease in men referred to coronary arteriography. Am Heart J 1997;133:622–629.
143. The Diabetes Prevention Program (DPP) Research Group: Reduction in the incidence of type 2 diabetes with lifestyle intervention or metformin. New Engl J Med 2002;346:393–403.
144. The Diabetes Prevention Program (DPP) Research Group: The diabetes prevention program (DPP): Description of lifestyle intervention. Diabetes Care 2002;25:2165–2171.
145. Moore LLVAJ, Wilson P, D'Agostino RB, Finkle WD, Elliso RC. Can sustained weight loss in overweight individuals reduce the risk of diabetes mellitus? Epidemiology 2000;11:269–273.

6 Diabetes Mellitus
Cardiovascular Complications

Willa Hsueh, MD, and Dorothy Martinez, MD

DIABETES IS AN ATHEROSCLEROSIS RISK EQUIVALENT

In contrast to the microvascular complications of diabetes, such as nephropathy and retinopathy, atherosclerosis occurs early in the process of type 2 diabetes. Based on the observation that patients with diabetes without known atherosclerosis have the same 7-yr incidence rate of fatal or nonfatal myocardial infarction (MI) as nondiabetic patients with documented coronary artery disease, the National Cholesterol Education Program (NCEP) has defined diabetes as an "atherosclerosis risk equivalent" (1). This equivalency suggests that atherosclerosis is present at the time the diagnosis of type 2 diabetes is made. Therefore, early in the disease process, therapeutic strategies to prevent or arrest cardiovascular disease must be employed, and appropriate target goals for atherosclerosis risk factors need to be achieved (Table 1). Moreover, because of the well-documented acceleration of atherosclerosis in the diabetic milieu, therapeutic goals in patients with diabetes are more stringent than in patients without diabetes.

Results of the United Kingdom Prospective Diabetes Study (UKPDS) in type 2 diabetes suggest that glucose control, in part, attenuates cardiovascular events and mortality, although the glucose effect profoundly contributes to the devel-

From: *Contemporary Endocrinology: Early Diagnosis and Treatment of Endocrine Disorders*
Edited by: R. S. Bar © Humana Press Inc., Totowa, NJ

Table 1
Therapeutic Goals for Cardiovascular Disease
in Type 2 Diabetes

Measure	Goal
Glucose	HbA1$_c$ < 6.5%
	Fasting glucose < 110 mg/dL
	Postprandial glucose < 140 mg/dL
Lipids	LDL cholesterol < 100 mg/dL
	HDL cholesterol > 45 mg/dL
	Triglycerides < 150 mg/dL
	Non-HDL cholesterol < 30 mg/dL
Blood pressure	130/80 mmHg if no albuminuria
	125/75 mmHg if albuminuria present

HDL, high-density lipoprotein; LDL, low-density lipoprotein.

opment and progression of microvascular complications *(2)*. The mechanisms by which hyperglycemia contributes to the atherosclerotic process remain unknown. Hyperglycemia causes endothelial cell dysfunction, possibly owing to alterations in cell signaling pathways such as protein kinase C β (PKCβ) *(3)*. The formation of advanced glycosylation end products (AGEs) has also been implicated in damage of the vascular wall, although this mechanism has not been confirmed *(4)*. Glycosylation of tissue proteins also appears to enhance oxidation *(4)*. Current recommendations for glycemic control suggested by the American Association of Clinical Endocrinologists (AACE) includes a hemoglobin A1$_c$ (HbA1$_c$) of 6.5%, a fasting glucose of less than 110 mg/dL, and a postprandial glucose of less than 140 mg/dL *(5)*. A current multicenter study Angioplastie Coronaire, Corvasal Diltiazem (ACCORD), is addressing the issue of whether lowering HbA1$_c$ to less than 7% will impact on cardiovascular events and mortality *(6)*.

It is not clear that hypertension accelerates both the micro- and macrovascular complications of diabetes *(2)*. The American Diabetes Association (ADA) and the National Kidney Foundation (NKF) recommend a blood pressure of 130/80 mmHg, as more recent studies have demonstrated that this level of blood pressure is cardiovascular protective *(7)*. If albuminuria or proteinuria are detected, not only is diabetic nephropathy present, but widespread vascular disease is also likely to be present *(7)*. This finding should underscore the importance of aggressive treatment of cardiovascular risk factors. Blood pressure goals in the presence of proteinuria are 125/75 mmHg *(7)*.

Part of the antihypertensive regimen should be aimed at inhibiting the renin-angiotensin system (RAS). Angiotensin II (Ang II) promotes tissue damage by stimulation of inflammation, oxidation, thrombosis, and tissue remodeling and is particularly implicated in diabetic nephropathy, cardiac hypertrophy and failure, and atherosclerosis *(8)*. Although angiotensin-converting enzyme inhibition (ACEI) inhibits the development and progression of diabetic nephropathy in type 1 diabetes *(9)*, it has less of a consistent effect compared with other antihypertensive regimens in type 2 diabetes *(10)*. Two trials with Ang II AT1 receptor blockers (ARBs) have recently shown that these agents inhibit the development and progression of renal disease in patients with type 2 diabetes and that they consistently decrease proteinuria and albuminuria *(11)*. Treatment with one of these ARBs, losartan, was also associated with less heart failure compared with those patients with diabetes treated with traditional antihypertensive agents without RAS inhibition *(11)*. In addition, the recently reported Losartan Intervention for Endpoint Reduction in Hypertension (LIFE) Trial demonstrated that losartan was associated with fewer cardiovascular endpoints in patients with diabetes and hypertension than atenolol, particularly less stroke *(12)*. Thus, inhibition of RAS should be employed early in the diagnosis of diabetes, even before the onset of hypertension or albuminuria, since ACEI (ramipril) is indicated to prevent cardiovascular disease in high-risk patients *(13)*. High risk includes patients with diabetes, which is an atherosclerosis risk equivalent.

The level of low-density lipoprotein (LDL) cholesterol is directly correlated with cardiovascular events and mortality in both primary and secondary prevention studies *(14)*. The ADA and American Heart Association recommendation for LDL cholesterol in patients with diabetes is less than 100 mg/dL. However, the recently reported Heart Protection Study suggests that even lower levels may be even more cardiovascular protective in patients with diabetes and that there are tissue effects of statins beyond cholesterol lowering *(15)*. Lower LDL cholesterol goals may be particularly important in insulin resistance because of the enhanced tendency for LDL cholesterol to be oxidized *(16)*. Low levels of high-density lipoprotein (HDL) cholesterol, which are commonly seen in insulin resistance, constitute another important risk factor for atherosclerosis *(17)*. Currently recommended levels for HDL cholesterol are more than 45 mg/dL *(18)*. The recommended triglyceride level is less than 150 mg/dL *(18)*. The NCEP has also focused on goals for non-HDL cholesterol levels, which represent the cholesterol carried in LDL and very low-density lipoprotein (VLDL) particles (total cholesterol–HDL cholesterol). This measurement is important for people with high triglyceride levels (>150 mg/dL), considered an independent risk factor for coronary artery disease. The non-HDL cholesterol level should be 30 mg/dL or less *(1)*.

IMPAIRED GLUCOSE TOLERANCE IS A DISEASE

The prediabetes state of IGT is associated not only with progression to diabetes but also with increased coronary artery disease mortality; therefore, it should be recognized, diagnosed, and treated early (*see* ref. *1* and Chapter 5 of this book). Moreover, the demonstration that lifestyle intervention can substantially

Table 2
Components of the Metabolic Syndrome

Risk factor	Defining level
Abdominal obesity[a] (waist circumference)[b]	
Men	>102 cm (>40 in.)
Women	>88 cm (>35 in.)
Triglycerides	≥150 mg/dL
High-density lipoprotein cholesterol	
Men	<40 mg/dL
Women	<50 mg/dL
Blood pressure	≥130/≥85 mmHg
Fasting glucose	≥110 mg/dL

[a]Overweight and obesity are associated with insulin resistance and the metabolic syndrome. However, the presence of abdominal obesity is more highly correlated with the metabolic risk factors than is an elevated body mass index (BMI). Therefore, the simple measure of waist circumference is recommended to identify the body weight component of the metabolic syndrome.
[b]Some male patients can develop multiple metabolic risk factors when the waist circumference is only marginally increased, e.g., 94–102 cm (37–40 in.). Such patients may have a strong genetic contribution to insulin resistance, and they should benefit from changes in life habits, like men with categorical increases in waist circumference.
Data from ref. 1.

prevent or delay the progression of IGT to type 2 diabetes underscores the need for early diagnosis (1). The accelerated heart disease in IGT probably stems from the presence of insulin resistance and its associated metabolic syndrome, which are defined in Table 2 according to the NCEP ATP III report (1). Three of five elevated factors, which are easy to measure, constitute the metabolic syndrome. Certain components of the syndrome, such as low HDL, elevated triglycerides, and hypertension, are well-known risk factors for cardiovascular disease. Other components that are less commonly measured in the clinical setting, such as elevated small, dense LDL cholesterol (the moiety that is more susceptible to oxidation) and elevated levels of the prothrombotic factor plasminogen activator inhibitor-1 (PAI-1), correlate with cardiovascular events and mortality (19).

Whether coronary artery disease risk factor goals should be as stringent in IGT as in type 2 diabetes is unknown. However, lowering cholesterol and control of blood pressure has been shown to be effective in slowing the progression of cardiovascular disease in IGT (20). Postprandial glucose levels have also been demonstrated to correlate with cardiovascular events across a European population in the Diabetes Epidemiology: Collaborative Analysis of Diagnostic Criteria in Europe (DECODE) Study *(21)*. This study is clearly different from the DECODE study designed to genotype the population of Iceland. Whether lowering postprandial glucose levels impacts on cardiovascular disease in IGT also remains to be determined.

INSULIN RESISTANCE IS A STATE OF INFLAMMATION

In addition to the fact that components of the metabolic syndrome contribute to cardiovascular disease, increasing data suggests insulin resistance is a proinflammatory state in itself. Adipose tissue secretes substances (adipokines) that decrease insulin-mediated glucose uptake and/or promote vascular inflammation (Table 3). Adipocytokines circulate at higher levels in obese animals or in humans with increased viceral adiposity. Tumor necrosis factor-α (TNF-α) directly suppresses activation of tyrosine kinase on the insulin receptor, resulting in insulin resistance *(22)*. TNF-α levels are not only high in atherosclerotic vessels, promoting inflammation, but are elevated in damaged myocardium and have been implicated in heart failure *(23)*. Adiponectin (Acrp 30) also arises from fat but, in contrast to TNF-α, is low in the circulation of obese humans and animals, enhances insulin-mediated glucose uptake, and inhibits inflammatory responses *(24)*. Leptin is another substance from fat; circulating levels are high in obese subjects *(25)*. Leptin has been shown to regulate appetite and other metabolic functions and has variable effects on insulin mediated glucose uptake *(25)*. Recently leptin has been shown to enhance inflammation and to mediate immune responses *(25)*. Interleukin 6 (IL-6) comes from fat and is a well-known proinflammatory factor *(26)*. The prothrombotic, profibrotic factor PAI-1 is also secreted by adipose tissue; insulin can enhance its secretion from adipose tissue; secretion is regulated by Ang II, insulin, and other factors. PAI-1 is elevated in the circulation of obese subjects, and elevated plasma levels correlate with cardiovascular events *(27)*. Free fatty acids (FFAs) are high in obesity, because of increased lipolysis *(28)*. FFAs affect multiple target organs contributing to diabetes: they decrease insulin-mediated glucose uptake into skeletal muscle, enhance apoptosis of pancreas islet cells, enhance liver glucose production, and contribute to endothelial dysfunction *(28)*. Thus, FFAs may be a major contributor to the diabetic state with vascular damage.

Taken together, increasing evidence suggests that obesity is not only an insulin-resistant state but a proinflammatory state as well. This conclusion is supported by observations demonstrating that highly sensitive C-reactive protein (hs CRP) levels are elevated in insulin resistance. Abundant evidence indicates that hs CRP is a marker of, and possibly a contributory factor to, vascular inflammation. High levels portend a cardiovascular event *(29)*. In addition, high levels of hs CRP occur in IGT and are predictive of the development of diabetes *(29)*.

Table 3
Adipokines (Inflammatory and Metabolic Regulators from Fat)

Adipokines that ↓ insulin-mediated glucose uptake and ↑ inflammation
Tumor necrosis factor-α
Leptin
Angiotensinogen
Resistin
Adipokines that ↑ inflammation, thrombosis
Interleukin-6
Plasminogen activator inhibitor-1
Adipokines that ↑ insulin-mediated glucose uptake and ↓ inflammation
Adiponectin (Acrp-30)

Thus, a vascular inflammatory marker predicts both cardiovascular disease and diabetes.

One of the earliest detectable manifestations for this inflammatory milieu in insulin resistance is endothelial dysfunction Balletshorfer et al. *(30)* demonstrated brachial artery endothelial dysfunction in insulin-resistant, but not insulin-sensitive, relatives of patients with diabetes, even though the relatives had no traditional risk factors for atherosclerosis. We found that Mexican Americans with no traditional risk factors for atherosclerosis who did not even qualify for the ATP III diagnosis of the metabolic syndrome had significant coronary vasomotor dysfunction, primarily endothelium-dependent, as assessed noninvasively by positron emission tomography scanning *(31)*. These observations suggest that endothelial dysfunction occurs early in insulin resistance and can appear independent of the dyslipidemia, hypertension, and hyperglycemia that occurs later in the process of insulin resistance. Therefore, an important issue is the point at which disease begins in insulin resistance, since evidence of target organ change is present before IGT or even the metabolic syndrome appear. Equally important is how we detect endothelial dysfunction and the roles of measurements of hs CRP and circulating adipokines.

THE ROLE OF INSULIN SENSITIZERS

Activation of peroxisome proliferator-activated receptor-γ (PPAR-γ), in adipose tissue restores the adipokine balance to increase insulin sensitivity and to decrease vascular inflammation *(32)*. The decrease in FFAs, TNF-α, leptin, and other adipokines and the reciprocal increase in adiponectin that occurs with PPAR-γ ligand [thiazolidinedione (TZD)] administration probably contributes to the action of these ligands to enhance insulin-mediated glucose uptake. Because of these changes and the decrease in PAI-1 and IL-6, PPAR-γ ligands also appear to attenuate the proinflammatory state. In addition, the ligands directly

Table 4
PPAR-γ Ligands Attenuate Atherosclerosis in Genetically
Modified Mice Models

LDLR$^{-/-}$ on high-fat diet (insulin-resistant diabetes model)
↓ TRO *(34)*
↓ RSG *(35)*
↓ GW7845 *(35)*
LDLR$^{-/-}$ on high-fructose diet (non-insulin-resistant model)
↓ TRO *(34)*
LDLR$^{-/-}$ high fat, Ang II accelerated
↓ RSG *(36)*
↓ Merck L805,645 *(36)*
↓ PIO *(37)*
ApoE$^{-/-}$
↓ TRO *(38)*
↓ RXRα ligand *(39)*

AngII, angiotension II; PIO, pioglitazone; RSG, rosiglitazone; RXR-α, retinoid X receptor-α; TRO, troglitazone.

inhibit inflammatory processes in monocytes/macrophages including cell migration and attachment, intercellular nitric oxide synthase (iNOS), interleukin, matrix metalloproteinase (MMP), and superoxide dismutase (SOD) expression *(33)*. Whether PPAR-γ itself mediates these effects has been questioned, since relatively large doses of ligand have been used to achieve these effects in vitro, and monocytes null for PPAR-γ respond similarly to monocytes that express the receptor *(33)*. Nevertheless, clinical trials are currently in progress to determine whether these effects translate to cardiovascular protection by TZDs in people with diabetes.

In genetically modified mice prone to atherosclerosis, PPAR-γ ligands consistently retard lesion development in both early and aggressive models of vascular injury (Table 4). Much of this effect probably results from the antiinflammatory action of the ligands, since they do not substantially improve the lipid milieu in these rodent models and they attenuate atherosclerosis in models that are not associated with insulin resistance *(34–39)*. In addition to effects in monocyte/macrophages, PPAR-γ ligands decrease MMP, the early growth response-1 gene (Egr-1), and macrophage chemoattractant protein-1 (MCP-1) expression in vascular smooth muscle cells (VSMCs). Egr-1 orchestrates a cascade of inflammatory changes in VSMCs *(40)*, and MCP-1 is a potent stimulator of monocyte migration into the vessel wall *(40)*. Thus, these antiinflammatory effects translate to vascular protection in animal models. In humans, treatment with PPAR-γ ligands both improves endothelial function and retards the progression of carotid intimal medial wall thickness, both markers of vascular damage and atherosclerosis *(41)*. PPAR-γ ligand administration to patients with IGT or type 2 diabetes is also associated with decreases in blood pressure and albuminuria as well as a 30% decrease in hs CRP levels *(42–44)*.

Metformin decreases liver glucose production and has a modest effect on enhancement of insulin-mediated glucose uptake *(45)*. Treatment with metformin is reported to decrease circulating insulin and PAI-1, to lower hs CRP by about 10%, and to have variable effects in reducing blood pressure *(45)*. Other oral antihyperglycemic agents such as sulfonyureas, metiglitanides, and acarbose do not appear to have direct vascular protective effects.

IMPLICATIONS

The fact that obesity is not only intimately associated with insulin resistance and that obese subjects have variable components of the metabolic syndrome, but that obesity is a state of vascular inflammation, now shifts the paradigm to suggest that obesity is a major disease, not just a predisposing factor to diabetes, hypertension, and cardiovascular and other chronic diseases. One approach therefore, is to pursue weight loss aggressively in all obese subjects, but successful weight loss been shown to be extremely difficult *(46)*. It may be useful to target early subjects at high risk for diabetes and cardiovascular disease by defining their inflammatory state. Table 5 lists the chronologic order of changes that occur in obesity ultimately resulting in coronary artery disease as assessed by specific testing. Visceral obesity is more commonly associated with cardiovascular endpoints, so identifying fat distribution may be a first step in identification of high-risk patients. In some patients, such as Asians, substantial abdominal adiposity may be present even with a normal body mass index, so that a scan may be necessary to quantitate visceral adiposity *(47)*. Strong evidence of inflammation or thrombosis such as elevated hs CRP, TNF-α, or PAI-1 in the circulation with concomitant decreased adiponectin levels would strongly support interventions to reduce the proinflammatory state, particularly help in losing weight (Table 6). The presence of dyslipidemia, albuminuria, hyperglycemia, or hypertension should be noted early, and aggressive pharmacologic intervention to reach normalization of these parameters should be pursued. Targeting of vascular inflammation includes early lifestyle changes and earlier use of statins, inhibitors of the RAS, aspirin, and possibly PPAR-γ ligands. Indeed, adolescent obesity is rising in epidemic proportions in the United States, so weight loss programs and weight gain prevention need to be instituted in the teenage years. If evidence of cardiovascular inflammation is present, pharmacologic intervention should be started, perhaps in the 30s and even 20s, depending on the constellation of traditional and nontraditional risk factors present. Clearly, more aggressive treatment of obesity and cardiovascular risk early in the process has important implications for prevention of both diabetes and cardiovascular morbidity and mortality.

Table 5
Possible Chronologic Order of Pathophysiologic Changes in Obesity Leading
to Coronary Artery Disease and Potential Test to Assess Changes

1. Presence of abdominal obesity: waist-to-hip ratio, abdominal CT or MRI (especially Asian populations)
2. Inflammatory state: hs CRP, TNF-α, adiponectin, PAI-1
3. Lipid panel: TG, HDL and LDL cholesterol, possibly s.d. LDL cholesterol
4. Albumin excretion rate
5. Fasting glucose
6. Blood pressure

CT, computed tomography; HDL, high-density lipoprotein; hs CRP, highly sensitive C-reactive protein; LDL, low-density lipoprotein; MRI, magnetic resonance imaging; PAI-1; plasminogen activator inhibitor-1; s.d., small density; TG, triglycerides; TNF-α, tumor necrosi factor-α.

Table 6
Early Intervention in Obesity

Lifestyle changes:	Exercise, diet, and weight loss
	↓
↓ Inflammation:	Statin
	inhibit the rennin-angiotensin system
	PPAR-γ ligands
	ASA

PPAR-γ, peroxisome proliferator-activated receptor-γ.

REFERENCES

1. Expert Panel on Detection, Evaluation, and Treatment of High Blood Cholesterol in Adults, Executive Summary of the Third Report of the National Cholesterol Education Program (NCEP). JAMA 2001;285:2486–2479.
2. UK Prospective Diabetes Study (UKPDS) Group. Intensive blood-glucose control with sulfonylurea or insulin compared with conventional treatment and risk of complications in patients with type 2 diabetes (UKPDS 33). Lancet 1998;352:837–853.
3. King, GL, Shiba T, Oliver L, et al. Cellular and molecular abnormalities in the vascular endothelium of diabetes mellitus. Annu Rev Med 1994;45:179–188.
4. Brownlee M. Advanced glycosylation in diabetes and aging. Annu Rev Med 1995;46: 223–234.
5. The American Association of Clinical Endocrinologists Medical Guidelines for the Management of Diabetes Mellitus. The AACE System of intensive diabetes self-management—2000 update. Endocr Prac 2000;6:43–84.
6. Multi-center study. The ACCORD Study. Angioplastie Coronaire, Corvasal Diltiazem.
7. Bakris GL, Williams M, Dworkin L, et al. Preserving renal function in adults with hypertension and diabetes: a consensus approach. National Kidney Foundation Hypertension and Diabetes Executive Committees Working Group. Am J Kidney Dis 2000;36:646–661.
8. Siragy HM, Bedigian M. Mechanism of action of angiotensin-receptor blocking agents. Curr Hypertens Rep 1999;1:289–295.

9. Lewis EJ, Hunsickur LG, Bain RP, Rolede RD. The effect of angiotensin-converting enzyme inhibition on diabetic nephropathy. The Collaborative Study Group. N Engl J Med 1993;329:1456–1462.

10. Hsueh WA. Treatment of type 2 diabetes nephropathy by blockade of the renin-angiotensin system: a comparison of angiotensin-converting-enzyme inhibitors and angiotensin receptor antagonists. Curr Opinion Pharmacol 2002;2:182–188.

11. Brenner BM. Effects of losartan on renal and cardiovascular outcomes in patients with type 2 diabetes and nephropathy. N Engl J Med 2001;345:861–869.

12. Lindholm LH, Ibsen H, Dahlof B, et al. Cardiovascular morbidity and mortality in patients with diabetes in the Losartan Intervention for Endpoint Reduction in Hypertension study (LIFE): a randomised trial against atenolol. Lancet 2002;359:1004–1010.

13. Dagenois GR, Yusuf S, Bourassa MG, et al. Effects of ramipril on coronary events in high-risk persons: results of the Heart Outcomes Prevention Evaluation Study. Circulation 2001;104:522–526.

14. Waters DD. Are we aggressive enough in lowering cholesterol? Am J Cardiol 2001;88(Suppl 4):10F–15F.

15. MRC/BHF Heart Protection Study of Cholesterol lowering with simvastatin in 20,536 high-risk individuals: a randomised placebo-controlled trial. Lancet 2002;360:7–22.

16. Krauss RM. Dense low density lipoproteins and coronary artery disease. Am J Cardiol 1995;75:53B–57B.

17. Garber AJ. Treatment of dyslipidemia in diabetes. Endocrinol Metab Clin North Am 2001;30:999–1010.

18. American Diabetes Association.Clinical Practice Recommendations. Position Statement: management of dyslipidemia in adults with diabetes. Diabetes Care 2000;23(suppl 1):S57–S60.

19. Reaven GM. Multiple CHD risk factors in type 2 diabetes beyond hyperglycemia. Diabetes Obes Metab 2002;1(suppl 4):S13–18.

20. Pyorala K, Pedersen TR, Kjekshus J, et al. Cholesterol lowering with Simvastatin improves prognosis of diabetic patients with coronary heart disease: a subgroup analysis of the Scandinavian Simvastatin Survival Study (4S). Diabetes Care 1997;20:614–620.

21. Glucose tolerance and mortality: comparison of WHO and American Diabetes Association diagnostic criteria. The DECODE study group. European Diabetes Epidemiology Group. Diabetes Epidemiology: Collaborative Analysis of Diagnostic criteria in Europe. Lancet 1999;354:617–621.

22. Hotamisligil GS, Spiegelman BM. Tumor necrosis factor alpha: key component of the obesity-diabetes link. Diabetes 1994;43:1271–1278.

23. Torre-Amione G, Kapadia S, Lee J, et al. Tumor necrosis factor alpha and tumor necrosis factor receptor in the failing human heart. Circulation 1996;93:704–711.

24. Ouchi N, Kihara S, Arita Y, et al. Novel modulator for endothelial adhesion molecules: adipocyte-derived plasma protein adiponectin. Circulation 1999;100:2473–2476.

25. Mantzoros CS. The role of leptin in human obesity and disease: a review of current evidence. Ann Intern Med 1999;130:671–680.

26. Papanicolau DA, Wilder RL, Manolagos SC, Chrousos GP. 1998 The pathophysiologic roles of interleukin-6 in human disease. Ann Intern Med 128:127–137.

27. Juhan-Vague I, Alessi MC. 1997 PAI-1, obesity, insulin resistance and risk of cardiovascular events. Thromb Haemost 78:656–660.

28. Steinberg HO, Tarshoby M, Monestel R, et al. Elevated circulating free fatty acid levels impair endothelium-dependent vasodilation. J Clin Invest 1997;100:1230–1239.

29. Fichtlscherer S, Zeiher AM. Endothelial dysfunction in acute coronary syndromes: association with elevated C-reacrive protein levels. Ann Intern Med 2000;32:515–518.

30. Balletshofer BM, Rittig K, Enderle MD, et al. Endothelial dysfunction is detectable in young normotensive first-degree relatives of subjects with type 2 diabetes in association with insulin resistance. Circulation 2000;101:1780–1784.
31. Quiñones MJ, Pamploni MH, et al. Insulin resistance in healthy Mexican-Americans in associated with coronary artery endothelial dysfunction. Diabetes 2000;49(suppl 1):A–146.
32. Loviscach M, Rehman N, Carter, L, et al. Distribution of peroxisome proliferator-activated receptors (PPARS) in human skeletal muscle and adipose tissue: relation to insulin action. Diabetologia 2000;43:304–311.
33. Wakino S, Law RE, Hsueh WA. Vascular protective effects by activation of nuclear receptor PPAR gamma. J Diabet Complic 2002;16:46–49.
34. Collins AR, Meehan WP, Kintscher U, et al. Troglitazone inhibits formation of early atherosclerotic lesions in diabetic and nondiabetic low density lipoprotein receptor-deficient mice. Arteriocler Thromb Vasc Biol 2001;21:365–371.
35. Li AC, Brown KK, Silvestre MJ, Willson TM, Palinski W, Glass CK. Peroxisome proliferator-activated receptor gamma ligands inhibit development of atherosclerosis in LDL receptor deficient mice. J Clin Invest 2000;106:523–531.
36. Collins AR, et al. Peroxisome proliferator-activated receptor gamma ligands attenuated angiotensin II accelerated attenuation in male LDL receptor deficient (LDLR$^{-/-}$) mice. Diabetes 2001;50(suppl 2):A72.
37. Collins AR, et al. Pioglitazone attenuated angiotensin II NL-NAME accelerated attenuated LDLR–/–. Diabetes 2002;51(suppl 2):A155.
38. Chen Z, Ishibashi S, Perrey S, et al. Troglitazone inhibits atherosclerosis in apolipoprotein E knockout mice: pleiotropic effects on CD36 expression and HDL. Arterioscler Thromb Vasc Biol 2001;21:372–377.
39. Claudel T, Leibowitz MD, Fievet C, et al. Reduction of atherosclerosis in apolipoprotein E knockout mice by activation of a retinoid X receptor. Proc Natl Acad Sci USA 2001;98:2610–2615.
40. Hsueh WA, Law RE. PPARgamma and atherosclerosis: effects on cell growth and movement. Arterioscler Thromb Vasc Biol 2001;21:1891–1895.
41. Koshiyama H, Shimono D, Kuwamura N, Minamikawa J, Nakamura Y. Rapid communication:inhibitory effect of pioglitazone on carotid arterial wall thickness in type 2 diabetes. J Clin Endocrinol Metab 2001;86:3452–3456.
42. Imano E, kanda T, Nakatani Y, et al. Effect of troglitazone on microalbuminuria in patients with incipient diabetic nephropathy. Diabetes Care 1998;21:2135–2139.
43. Ogihara T, Rakugi II, Ikegami H, Mikami H, Mauso K. Enhancement of insulin sensitivity by troglitazone lowers blood pressure in diabetic hypertensives. Am J Hypertens 1995;8:316–320.
44. Aljada A, Gary R, Ghanim H, et al. Nuclear factor-kappa B suppressive and inhibitor-kappa B stimulating effects of troglitazone in obese patients with type 2 diabetes: evidence of an antiinflammatory action? J Clin Endocrin Metab 2001;86:3250–3256.
45. Chu NV. Differential effects of metformin and troglitazone on cardiovascular risk factors in patients with type 2 diabetes. Diabetes Care 2002;25:542–549.
46. Scheen AJ. Results of obesity treatment. Ann Endocrinol 2002;63:163–170.
47. Raji A. Body fat distribution and insulin resistance in healthy Asian Indians and Caucasians. J Clin Endocrinol Metab 2001;86:5366–5371.

7 Obesity
A Challenging Global Epidemic

Ngozi E. Erondu, MD, PhD

CONTENTS

INTRODUCTION

Obesity can be defined as a condition of abnormal or excessive adiposity (>25% of total body weight for men and >30% for women); it results from a chronic imbalance between energy intake and energy expenditure. Although there is some disagreement about its classification as a disease *(1–3)*, there is a consensus regarding the worldwide increase in the prevalence of obesity and obesity-related diseases. A recently convened consultation by the World Health Organization (WHO) concluded that obesity is a rapidly growing global epidemic that is replacing the more traditional public health concerns such as undernutrition and infectious diseases as the most significant contributor to ill health *(4)*.

Since a comprehensive, in-depth review of obesity cannot be provided in a single book chapter, it is hoped that the reader will be inspired to consult the many excellent textbooks, monographs, and reviews on this subject *(4–12)*. This chapter begins with a brief overview of the classification of obesity, followed by a discussion of the prevalence and trends of both adult and pediatric obesity in different regions of the world. The health and economic impact of obesity is considered next, followed by an overview of strategies for prevention. Lastly,

From: *Contemporary Endocrinology: Early Diagnosis and Treatment of Endocrine Disorders*
Edited by: R. S. Bar © Humana Press Inc., Totowa, NJ

current and future treatment modalities are discussed, followed by a few concluding remarks.

CLASSIFICATION

As stated above, obesity is defined as excessive accumulation of body fat. Since body fat is difficult to measure directly, several attempts have been made to devise or identify clinically useful surrogate measures. Currently, body mass index (BMI; body mass in kilograms divided by the square of the height in meters) is an acceptable index of obesity, and has been shown in epidemiologic studies to predict risk of obesity-related morbidity and mortality reasonably. In the guidelines adopted by the National Heart, Lung, and Blood Institute (NHLBI) of the National Institutes of Health (NIH) and WHO, obesity is defined as a BMI of 30 kg/m^2 or more; overweight is defined as a BMI of 25 kg/m^2 or more. As shown in Table 1, the risk of comorbidities rises progressively with increasing obesity. It should be noted that the relationship between BMI and body fat content can vary by age, gender, ethnicity, body build, and body proportion *(4,5,13,14)*. Thus, a given BMI may not correspond to the same degree of adiposity across all patient groups. In addition, the increased health risks associated with obesity occur in people with lower BMIs in the Asia-Pacific region *(5)*. This fact is reflected in the proposed alternative classification system for the region (Table 2), where obesity is defined as a BMI of 25 kg/m^2 or more.

Several published studies have also demonstrated the association of fat distribution (in particular central or visceral obesity), with increased risk for the metabolic complications of obesity, such as insulin resistance, type 2 diabetes mellitus, hypertension, and dyslipidemia *(15–26)*. Although the link(s) between visceral obesity and obesity-related comorbidities have not been thoroughly clarified, a number of pathophysiologic mechanisms have been postulated. For example, dysregulation of the hypothalamic-pituitary-adrenal axis could lead to Cushing's disease of the omentum, which would result in visceral obesity as well as an increase in circulating free fatty acid levels *(27,28)*. The increased free fatty acids not only promote hypertriglyceridemia and lipoprotein abnormalities but may also contribute to insulin resistance/hyperinsulinemia and glucose intolerance, which in a permissive genetic setting results in type 2 diabetes mellitus *(29)*. Hyperinsulinemia, by altering the function of atrial natriuretic factor and activating the renin-angiotensin-aldosterone and sympathetic nervous systems, combined with the vascular effects of cortisol, has been postulated to contribute to hypertension *(30–32)*. Other endocrinopathies that have been seen in obese individuals, such as abnormalities of growth hormone and the sex steroid axis, are also likely to amplify the effects of cortisol. Despite the lack of a clear understanding of the pathogenetic/pathophysiologic links between obesity and its comorbidities, it is generally accepted that visceral obesity is associated with increased risk for metabolic disorders.

Table 1
1998 NHLBI Clinical Guidelines on the Identification, Evaluation,
and Treatment of Overweight and Obesity in Adults

Classification	BMI (kg/m²)	Obesity class	Disease risk relative to normal weight and waist circumference[a]	
			Men: ≤102 cm (≤40 in.) Women: ≤88 cm (≤35 in.)	Men: >102 cm (>40 in.) Women: >88 cm (>35 in.)
Underweight[b]	< 18.5	—		
Normal[c]	18.5–24.9	—	Average	Increased
Overweight	25.0–29.9	—	Increased	High
Obesity	30.0–34.9	I	High	Very high
	35–39.9	II	Very high	Very high
Extreme obesity	≥40	III	Extremely high	Extremely high

BMI, body mass indes; NHLBI, National Heart, Lung, and Blood Institute.
[a]Disease risk for type 2 diabetes, hypertension, and cardiovascular disease.
[b]Low risk for obesity-related comorbidities but risk of other clinical problems is increased.
[c]Increased waist circumference is a marker for increased risk even in persons of normal weight.
From ref. 6.

Table 2
Comorbidities Risk Associated with Different Levels of BMI
and Suggested Waist Circumference in Adult Asians

Classification	BMI (kg/m²)	Risk of comorbidities	
		Waist circumference (cm)	
		<90 (men) <80 (women)	≥90 (men) ≥80 (women)
Underweight	<18.5	Low (but increased risk of other clinical problems)	Average
Normal range	18.5–22.9	Average	Increased
Overweight	23–24.9	Increased	Moderate
Obese I	25–29.9	Moderate	Severe
Obese II	≥30	Severe	Very severe

BMI, body mass index.
From World Health Organization/International Association for the Study of Obesity/International Obesity Taskforce. The Asia-Pacific Perspective: redefining obesity and its treatment. Available at: http://www.idi.org.au/obesity_report.htm.

Over the years, a number of anthropometric measurements have been developed to identify individuals with increased health risks owing to visceral obesity. Waist circumference (WC) is generally regarded as the most useful (albeit crude) measure of increased abdominal fat content and has been shown in numerous studies to correlate with increased obesity-related morbidity *(4–6)*. This is reflected in the adoption of WC by the WHO and NHLBI for risk categorization in obese subjects (Table 1). There was, however, an acknowledgment that populations differ in the level of risk associated with a particular WC, and so the values in this table, which were based on a study in the Netherlands, are most applicable to Caucasians. As shown in Table 2, lower WC cutoff values have been suggested for Asians, because they not only tend to have increased abdominal obesity for any given BMI, they also have an absolute increase in risk at any particular WC *(5)*.

PREVALENCE

Comparison of obesity rates on a global scale is complicated by a number of factors, including differences in study populations and obesity classification systems and the use of unreliable, self-reported weight and height measurements to calculate BMI. One illustration of this difficulty is the reported increase in the 1989 prevalence of obesity in northern China from 6 to 15% when the BMI cutoff point was reduced from 27 to 25 kg/m^2 *(4,5)*. Similarly in the United States over the 1988–1994 period, the prevalence of obesity in men fell from 31.7 to 19.9% when the BMI cutoff point was changed from 27.8 to 30 kg/m^2 *(4)*. Regional variation in the prevalence of obesity within individual countries also adds another level of complexity. However, projects such as the WHO MONICA (MONItoring of trends and determinants in CArdiovascular diseases) study, in which the data were collected in the same time periods, age-standardized, and based on weights and heights measured with identical protocols, are particularly valuable for comparison purposes. Thus, despite the limited availability of suitable country-level data, it is clear that the prevalence of obesity is rising to epidemic proportions at an alarming rate in both developed and developing countries. The estimated number of obese adults worldwide (BMI $\geq$ 30 kg/m^2) rose from 200 million in 1995 to over 300 million in 2000 *(33)*.

Africa and the Middle East

AFRICA

In contrast to most industrialized nations, the emphasis in this region has been on undernutrition and food security, resulting in the paucity of data on the current prevalence of obesity. However, some regional studies indicate a growing prevalence of obesity in certain socioeconomic groups. This is illustrated by the high prevalence of obesity (44 and 33%) found in black women in the Cape Peninsula of the Republic of South Africa and among urban women 35 years or older in

Table 3
Obesity Prevalence (BMI≥ 30 kg/m^2) in Selected Countries
in Africa and the Middle East

Country	Year	Age (yr)	Prevalence of obesity (%)	
			Men	Women
Africa				
Gambia (Urban)[a]	1996/97	35+		33
Ghana	1987/88	20+	0.9	
Mali	1991	20+	0.8	
Mauritius	1987	25–74	3.4	10.2
	1992		5.3	15
Rodrigues				
Creoles	1992	25–69	10	31
South Africa (Cape Peninsula) Blacks	1990	15–64	8	44
Tanzania	1986/89	35–64	0.6	3.6
Middle East				
Bahrain	1991–92	20–65		
Urban			9.5	30.3
Rural			6.5	11.2
Kuwait	1994	18+	32	44
Saudi Arabia	1990	15+		
Urban			18	28
Rural			12	18
United Arab Emirates	1992	17+	16	38

BMI, body mass index.
[a]Data from ref. 34.
Adapted from ref. 4.

Gambia, respectively (34). Furthermore, as shown in Table 3, there was a dramatic increase in obesity prevalence in Mauritius over a 5-yr period in both men and women aged 25–74.

THE MIDDLE EAST

With the exception of Saudi Arabia, nationally representative data have not been well documented in this region. However, the limited data available indicate a higher prevalence of obesity in women in this region than that reported in the West. The United Arab Emirates, Bahrain (urban), Saudi Arabia (urban), and Kuwait all have female obesity rates above 25% (Table 3).

The Americas and Europe

THE AMERICAS

Not surprisingly, the most comprehensive data in this region come from the United States, and these are based on data from the National Health Examination Survey (NHES 1960–62), the National Health and Nutrition Examination Survey I (NHANES I, 1971–74), NHANES II (1976–1980), and NHANES III (1988–94). More than half of U.S. adults are overweight (55% with BMI ≥ 25 kg/m^2) and nearly one-fourth are obese (22% with BMI ≥ 30 kg/m^2). It should be noted that detailed analysis of the data reveals that black women and other racial/ethnic minorities have particularly high rates of obesity compared with Caucasians. For example in the 20+ age group, the prevalence of overweight (BMI ≥ 25 kg/m^2) is 65.8, 65.9, and 49.2% for black, Mexican, and white women, respectively.

As depicted in Table 4, Canada also has a worsening obesity problem, although it is not as bad as the situation in the United States. In the 1980s, there was a dramatic increase in the prevalence of obesity in the United States, which is reflected by the much larger increase between the third and fourth surveys. Unfortunately, this trend has continued in the 1990s, as has been noted in more recent surveys like the Behavioral Risk Factor Surveillance System (BRFSS) *(36)*. In these cross-sectional telephone surveys of noninstitutionalized adults aged 18 yr or older conducted by the Centers for Disease Control and Prevention and state health departments, a number of troubling facts have emerged. For example, the prevalence of obesity (based on self-reported weight and height) in U.S. adults increased from 12.0 to 19.8% in 2000, reflecting an increase of 61%. Furthermore, in 1991, none of the 45 participating states had rates of 20% or higher, and only 4 of the states had rates of 15% or higher; however, by 2000, 22 states had rates of 20% or higher, and 49 states had rates 15% or higher. Unfortunately, the real picture is likely to be worse, since people tend to underestimate their weights in self-reported surveys. In addition, those individuals who do not own a telephone (and consequently would not have participated) are likely to have low socioeconomic status (SES), which confers a greater probable prevalence of obesity.

In Brazil (Table 4), one of the few Latin American countries to have conducted nationally representative surveys, obesity is on the rise, especially among low-income and urban populations. A similar picture is emerging in the Caribbean, Central America, and the rest of South America *(4,37,38)*.

EUROPE

Current obesity prevalence data from individual national studies suggest a range of 10–20% for men, and 10–25% for women. However, the most comprehensive set of obesity prevalence data in Europe is from the WHO MONICA

Table 4

Trends in Obesity (BMI $\geq$ 30 kg/m^2) in Selected Countries
in the Americas and Europe

| Country | Year | Age (yr) | Prevalence of obesity (%) | |
			Men	Women
Americas				
Brazil	1975	25–64	3.1	8.2
	1989		5.9	13.3
Chile[a]	1988	>15	6	14
	1992		11	24
Canada[b]	1981	20–64	9	8
	1996		14	12
USA	1960	20–74	10	15
	1973		11.6	16.1
	1978		12.0	14.8
	1991		19.7	24.7
Europe				
England	1980	16–64	6	8
	1986/87		7	12
	1997		17	20
Finland	1978/9	20–75	10	10
	1985/7		12	10
	1991/3		14	11
Former East	1985	25–65	13.7	22.2
Germany	1992		20.5	26.8
Netherlands	1987	20–59	6	8.5
	1991		7.5	8.8
	1995		8.4	8.3
Sweden	1980/81	16–84	4.9	8.7
	1988/89		5.3	9.1

[a]Study conducted in the city of Santiago ref. *38*.
[b]Data from ref. *35*.
Adapted from ref. *4*.

project *(4)*. Although the surveys were conducted in selected cities rather than nationally, the data were collected in an identical fashion, which provides a high degree of confidence in making comparisons between countries over time. All the same, it is worth noting that there is a wide variation in the prevalence of obesity between and within these countries. In general, there has been an increase of 10–40% in prevalence in most of European countries from the 1980s to the 1990s. As shown in Table 4, the most dramatic increase occurred in England, where a doubling of the obesity prevalence occurred in both men and women. On the other hand, there was little or no change in countries such as Sweden, Finland, and the Netherlands.

Asia-Pacific

The prevalence of obesity in this region is highest in the Pacific Islands (up to 75% of adult women and 60% of adult men in urban Samoa). It is in the range of 10–15% in the general population of Australia and New Zealand but is much lower (<5%) in Japan and China. As previously stated, Asian investigators have suggested that the BMI cutoff point for obesity be lowered from 30 or more to 25 kg/m^2 or more. This recommendation was based on the fact that obesity-related comorbidities occur at much lower BMI values than those seen in Caucasians. Adoption of this new classification system will have a great impact on the prevalence estimates in this region of the world. In fact, considering that the populations of some of the Asian countries (China and India) are in the billions, even small changes in the BMI cutoff points will increase the world estimate of obesity prevalence by several hundred million.

The prevalence and trend data on obesity from selected countries in this region are summarized in Table 5, revealing the impact of changes in BMI cutoff points (China and Japan). It is also obvious that there has been a dramatic rise in the already high prevalence in the Polynesian and Micronesian societies of this region. Equally significant is the approx 2.4-fold increase in male obesity in Japan from 1976 to 1993.

Childhood Obesity

No review of the global obesity epidemic would be complete without mention of the emerging critical problem of childhood obesity. However, such a discussion is hampered by the lack of consistency and agreement among different studies over the definition of obesity *(39–45)*. Different percentile cutoff points, based on age-specific local or national percentile distributions for weight, height, or BMI, are often used. Although the International Obesity Task Force (IOTF) has recently published "standards" for childhood overweight and obesity *(46)*, their universal applicability remains controversial *(47)*. Nevertheless, irrespective of the method used, all studies have generally reported a high prevalence of obesity in children and adolescents. The data from a number of such studies are summarized in Table 6.

Ethnic differences in prevalence rates have also been observed, and they tend to parallel what has been reported for adults. For example, in the United States, the prevalence is highest in Mexican-American children, intermediate among non-Hispanic black children, and lowest in non-Hispanic white children *(42)*. In New Zealand, the highest prevalence was found in Pacific Island and Maori children; it was intermediate among Europeans and lowest in children of Asian

Table 5
Trends in Obesity (BMI ≥ 30 kg/m^2) in Selected Asia-Pacific Countries

Country	BMI cutoff	Year	Age (yr)	Prevalence of obesity (%)	
				Men	Women
Australia		1980	25–64	9.3	8.0
		1983		9.1	10.5
		1989		11.5	13.2
China	27	1989	20–45	1.7	4.3
		1991		2.9	4.3
China	30	1989	20–45	0.3	0.9
		1991		0.4	0.9
India (Urban Delhi middle class)	30	1997	40–60	3.2	14.3
Japan	26.4	1976	20+	7.1	12.3
		1993		11.8	12.0
Japan	30	1976	20+	0.7	2.8
		1993		1.8	2.6
New Zealand	30	1989	18–64	10	13
Papua New Guinea					
Urban	30	1991	25–69	36.6	54.3
Rural				23.9	18.6
Samoa					
Urban	30	1978	25–69	38.8	59.1
		1991		58.4	76.8
Rural	30	1978	25–69	17.7	37.0
		1991		41.5	59.2

BMI, body mass index.
Adapted from ref. 4.

descent (44). In addition, lower SES is positively correlated with high obesity prevalence in the United States and other industrialized countries.

As already stated, childhood obesity is not limited to the industrialized nations. In China, the overall prevalence of obesity among preschool children (aged 2–6 yr) increased from 4.2% in 1989 to 6.4% in 1997 (48). This trend reflects the dramatic increase in urban areas, where the prevalence in the same age group increased from 1.5% in 1989 to 12.6% in 1997 (Table 6). It is also remarkable that in several developing countries there is a juxtaposition of obesity and undernourishment (49). For example, the percentage of overweight children in North Africa (8%) and Eastern Asia (4.3%) slightly exceeds the percentage of undernourished children in both regions (7 and 3.4%, respectively). It is quite alarming to note that improvements in the standard of living in the developing world are accompanied by increased prevalence of childhood obesity (45,48). In other

Table 6
Prevalence of Childhood Obesity in Selected Countries

Country	Year	Age (yr)	Prevalence of obesity (%) Males	Females
Canada[a]	1981	7–13	2	2
	1996		10	9
China				
Rural[b]	1989	2–6	5.2	
	1997		4.8	
Urban[b]	1989	2–6	1.5	
	1997		12.6	
England[d]	1984	4–11	0.6	1.3
	1994		1.7	2.6
Russia[c]	1992	6–9	13.9	13.5
Scotland[d]	1984	4–11	0.9	1.8
	1994		2.1	3.2
Taiwan[e]	1980–82	12–15	12.4	10.1
	1994–96		16.4	11.1
Thailand[f]	1997	2nd and 3rd graders		
Rural			7.4	
Urban			23	
UK[g]	1989	3–4	5.4	
	1998		9.2	
US[c]	1993	6–9	11.4	12.7

[a]Obesity was defined by IOTF standards *(35)*.

[b]Obesity was defined by IOTF standards *(48)*.

[c]Obesity was defined as BMI ≥ 95th percentile *(45)*.

[d]Obesity was defined by IOTF standards *(40)*.

[e]Obesity was defined by body weight >120% of ideal body weight within age- and gender-specific strata *(41)*.

[f]Obesity was defined as > 97th percentile of weight-for-height using Thai national standards *(43)*.

[g]Obesity was defined by age- and gender-specific BMI > 95th percentile using British growth reference charts *(39)*.

words, there is a negative correlation between SES and obesity prevalence, which is not the case in the developed countries. The global nature of the progressive rise in childhood obesity rates and the potential impact on the health of children and adults are obvious. Thus, plans for reversing the global public health crisis associated with obesity must surely include the control of childhood obesity.

CONSEQUENCES

The rising epidemic of obesity has been appropriately declared a global public health threat by WHO. As is discussed below, several cross-sectional and prospective studies across various populations have provided evidence linking obesity to substantial health and economic costs.

Mortality

The controversy surrounding the relationship between obesity and mortality stems mainly from the fact that not all studies have confirmed the association between the two. However, it is widely believed that certain factors contribute to the negative studies: failure to control for smoking or occult/overt illness; inappropriately controlling for medical conditions such as hypertension and hyperglycemia (which are in fact related to obesity); and the use of BMI as a surrogate for obesity *(12)*. For example, in a recent population-based cohort study of 6296 elderly men and women in the Netherlands, WC showed a better correlation with mortality than did BMI *(50)*. In any case, it is clear that obesity (defined as a BMI $\geq$ 30 kg/m^2) is associated with a high risk of premature death. Two prospective studies (1960–1972 and 1982–1996) of participants in the American Cancer Society's Cancer Preventive Study concluded that men and women with a BMI of 30 or more had approximately 50–100% higher mortality than those with a BMI of less than 25 *(51,52)*. In an analysis of data from six prospective cohort studies (the Alameda Community Health Study, the Framingham Heart Study, the Tecumseh Community Health Study, the American Cancer Society Cancer Prevention Study I, the Nurses' Health Study, and the NHANES I Epidemiologic Follow-up Study), Allison et al. *(53)* estimated that approximately 280,000 deaths per year can be attributed to obesity among U.S. adults. They also reported that more than 80% of the obesity-attributable deaths occurred in individuals with a BMI of 30 kg/m^2 or more.

Comorbidities

The spectrum of obesity-related diseases ranges from type 2 diabetes mellitus (DM) and cardiovascular disease to osteoarthritis and gallbladder disease. The relative risk of a number of these health problems associated with obesity is shown in Table 7 and Fig. 1.

TYPE 2 DIABETES MELLITUS

Must et al. *(54)* used data from NHANES III to show that the prevalence of DM increased with increasing weight category (Fig. 1A), a relationship that was evident across racial, ethnic, and gender lines. Analysis of another U.S. study

Table 7
Relative Risk of Health Problems Associated with Obesity

Greatly increased (relative risk much greater than 3)	Moderately increased (relative risk 2–3)	Slightly increased (relative risk 1–2)
Type 2 diabetes	CHD	Certain cancers
Gallbladder disease	Hypertension	Reproductive hormone abnormalities
Dyslipidemia	Osteoarthritis	
Insulin resistance	Hyperuricemia and gout	Polycystic ovarian syndrome
Dyspnea/Hypoventilation		Impaired fertility
Sleep apnea		Low back pain
		Increased anesthetic risk
		Fetal defects

CHD, coronary heart disease.
Adapted from ref. 4.

(BRFSS) revealed that every 1-kg increase in self-reported weight was associated with a 9% increase in the prevalence of DM for the 1991–1998 period (36). Remarkably, from 1999 to 2000, the average weight of U.S. adults increased by 0.5%, whereas the prevalence of DM increased by about 6% (36). Similar increases in diabetes risk in the obese population have been reported in studies conducted in Asia, Europe, and the Middle East. As previously noted, fat distribution (i.e., visceral obesity) is an important contributor and in many instances a strong predictor of the risk for developing DM.

HYPERTENSION

Several studies, including the Atherosclerosis Risk in Communities (ARIC) Study, the Framingham Heart Study, the Nurses' Health Study, and NHANES, have shown that weight gain is clearly associated with increases in blood pressure, an association that has been observed in both developed and developing countries (55,56). In fact, in the analysis by Must et al. (54), hypertension was the most common obesity-related comorbidity and its prevalence showed a strong increase with increasing BMI class (Fig. 1B).

Fig. 1. (opposite page) The prevalence of type 2 diabetes mellitus (**A**) and Hypertension (**B**) by BMI class. BMI is expressed in kg/m². [Adapted from an analysis of the NHANES III data by Must et al. (54).]

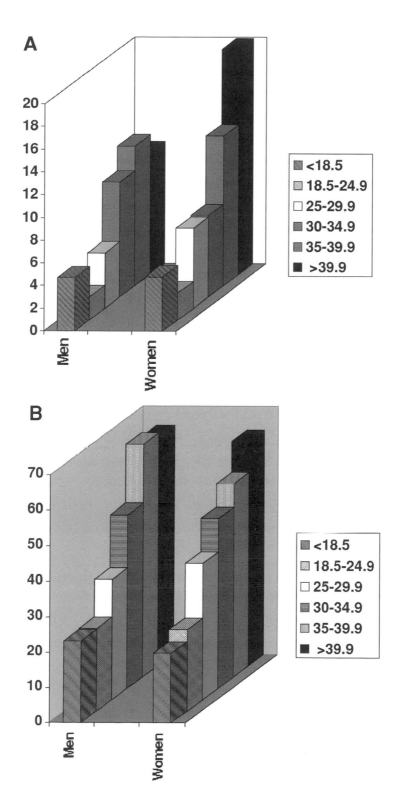

DYSLIPIDEMIA

The lipid abnormality most commonly associated with obesity is low high-density lipoprotein (HDL) cholesterol with hypertriglyceridemia, a finding that is more profound in visceral obesity *(57,58)*. The small dense (atherogenic) low-density lipoprotein (LDL) particles associated with this abnormality contribute to the increased cardiovascular risk that is associated with obesity. Not surprisingly, more stringent criteria for the recognition of low HDL (<40 mg/dL for men and <50 mg/dL for women) and high triglycerides (>150 mg/dL) were proposed in the recent guidelines issued by the National Cholesterol Education Program *(59)*.

CARDIOVASCULAR DISEASE

Cardiovascular disease, which includes coronary heart disease (CHD), cerebrovascular disease (stroke), and peripheral vascular disease, is the most significant problem associated with obesity. This is reflected in the recent "call to action" issued by the American Heart Association in response to the obesity epidemic *(60)*. Although the increased cardiovascular disease risk results partly from the impact of obesity on dyslipidemia, hypertension, insulin resistance, and impaired glucose tolerance or frank DM *(61,62)*, longer term studies have shown that obesity is also important as an independent risk factor for CHD *(63,64)*.

GALLBLADDER DISEASE

Data from the Nurses' Health Study suggest that the risk for gallstones increases with higher body weight *(65)*, which is also reflected in the analysis done by Must et al. *(54)*. The same picture has been seen elsewhere *(66)*, although it should be noted that transnational comparisons are complicated because the demographics of the study populations tend to be different as well as nonrepresentative. It is worth mentioning that rapid weight loss is also associated with an increased risk for the development of gallstones *(4)*.

OSTEOARTHRITIS

The association of osteoarthritis with increasing BMI was also evident in the study by Must et al. *(54)*. From a purely mechanical viewpoint, it is logical that obesity would be associated with an increased risk of joint dysfunction. However, there is also an inflammatory component involved in this process, presumably owing to the release of cytokines; this would explain the observed increase in osteoarthritis of the hands with obesity, even though the joints are not weight-bearing *(67)*.

CANCER

Several studies have found an association between obesity and an increased risk for various cancers, particularly those that are gastrointestinal or hormone-dependent. Examples include cancer of the colon, stomach, gallbladder, prostate, breast, endometrium, ovary, cervix, and kidney *(68–70)*. In a recent meta-analysis,

Bengstrom et al. *(71)* estimated that excess body mass accounts for 5% of all cancers in the European Union, or 72,000 cases of cancer annually. Along the same lines, a panel of experts who recently reviewed over 4000 studies on this subject concluded that 30–40% of all cases of cancer (3–4 million cases of cancer per year worldwide) could be prevented by better diets together with maintenance of physical activity and appropriate body weight *(72)*.

PULMONARY DYSFUNCTION

Obesity, especially of the upper body, is a risk factor for pulmonary diseases such as obstructive sleep apnea and Pickwickian syndrome (obesity-hypoventilation). If left unchecked, the pulmonary dysfunction can over time cause right-sided heart failure or lead to sudden death secondary to an arrhythmia during sleep *(73)*.

ENDOCRINE DYSFUNCTION

Hormonal abnormalities associated with obesity include hyperinsulinemia and insulin resistance, hypogonadism (in males), hyperandrogenism and ovulatory dysfunction (in females), decreased growth hormone levels, and dysregulation of cortisol metabolism *(74)*. These findings are particularly present in visceral obesity and, as discussed above, are believed to underlie many of the metabolic abnormalities associated with obesity.

PSYCHOSOCIAL PROBLEMS

Psychological problems associated with obesity include depression, low self-esteem, and distorted body image; societal issues include unemployment, discrimination, isolation, and marital stress *(75)*. Women, especially those with physical ailments, are usually the most affected. In addition, there are interesting cultural differences; for example, although African-American women are two to three times more likely to be obese than white women in the United States, they (African-American women) face less social pressure regarding their body weight.

Economic Cost

Based on an estimated proportion of disease prevalence attributable to obesity, Wolf and Colditz *(76)* calculated that the total cost attributable to obesity in 1995 in the United States was $99.2 billion. Approximately $52 billion was direct medical cost, accounting for nearly 6% of the national health expenditure in the United States. It is noteworthy that this figure was recently revised to 9.4%. Available estimates of the direct costs attributable to obesity (as percent of national health care costs) around the globe include approx 2% for France and Australia, 2.4% for Canada, and 4% for the Netherlands *(77)*. Although no estimates are currently available from the developing world, the data from the Western world illustrate that the impact of this disease on health care resources in the developing countries will be quite severe.

Childhood Obesity

As discussed in the Childhood Obesity section above, childhood obesity has reached epidemic proportions and continues to rise worldwide. Unfortunately, obesity-associated disease risk factors present in adults also manifest in obese children. For example, approximately 60% of overweight children in the Bogalusa Heart Study had one cardiovascular risk factor such as hypertension, hyperlipidemia, or hyperinsulinemia, and more than 20% of overweight children had two or more risk factors (78). Equally alarming is a study conducted in the Cincinnati area, which revealed a tenfold increase between 1982 and 1994 in the incidence of type 2 DM among adolescents (79). In fact, type 2 DM was reported to account for nearly 40% of all cases of new-onset DM in this age group. Furthermore, children are especially vulnerable to the psychological and behavioral consequences of obesity. Other comorbidities afflicting this age group include orthopedic and neurologic problems, sleep apnea, and hepatic and gastrointestinal dysfunction. One of the most alarming aspects of this disease in children is the known potential for the persistence of obesity and its associated health risks into adulthood (80,81).

PREVENTION

The staggering health and socioeconomic burden imposed globally by obesity makes the case for urgent action, and, like all public health problems, prevention should be the cornerstone of such efforts. However, an understanding of the causes of obesity (especially the factors driving the current global epidemic) will considerably enhance the probability of success of any intervention.

Etiologic Classification

As previously stated, the underlying cause of obesity in most cases is the chronic energy imbalance resulting from excessive energy intake relative to energy expenditure. However, this positive energy balance is a consequence of a complex interaction between environmental/societal influences (that affect dietary and physical activity) and the biologic/genetic milieu. Although the genetic contribution has been estimated from population studies to be as high as 40–70%, genetic factors cannot fully explain the current obesity epidemic. It is obvious that the rapid increases in obesity rates have occurred in too short a time for there to have been significant genetic changes within populations.

It is equally pertinent to note that specific and identifiable etiologies can only be ascribed to a minority of cases of obesity and, as such, do not significantly contribute to the current global obesity problem. However, it is important to be aware of these specific causes during the clinical evaluation of obesity since a number of these cases will be amenable to appropriate therapies. Examples include endocrinopathies such as insulinoma, Cushing's syndrome, hypothyroidism, hypogonadism, polycystic ovarian syndrome; hypothalamic lesions secondary to trauma, surgery, or primary or metastatic tumor; genetic syndromes like leptin deficiency, leptin receptor/melanocortin receptor defects, Prader-Willi, Bardet-Biedl, and Down's; and drugs such as insulin, sulfonylureas, glucocorticoids, antiepileptics, antipsychotics, and depoprovera.

Factors Underlying the Current Epidemic

As is discussed below, the key features of the global obesity epidemic mainly reflect the influence of environmental and societal factors on dietary and physical activity patterns. There has been a convergence toward increased consumption of an energy-dense (usually high-fat) diet and a transition to a more sedentary lifestyle.

GLOBAL ECONOMY

The industrialization and consequent globalization of the food economy have led to the increased availability of unhealthy and relatively cheap food products. To make matters worse, the food industry has engaged in aggressive marketing and advertising campaigns that have resulted in the consumption of ever increasing portions of energy-dense, relatively nutrient-poor foods (82). An analysis of data from NHANES III revealed that 33% of U.S. adults consume 45% of their daily energy from "junk food" (83). Worse, 77–85% of 2–19-yr-old Americans exceed the recommended intake of total fat, and 91–93% exceed the recommended intake of saturated fat (84).

SOCIOECONOMIC STATUS

Several studies have shown that obesity is more prevalent among those of low SES in developed countries, whereas the reverse is the case in the developing world. Interestingly, as the less developed countries undergo economic growth and attain higher levels of affluence, the positive relationship between SES and obesity is replaced by the negative relationship seen in modern societies.

It is not surprising that minority ethnic groups in developed countries are more susceptible to obesity since poverty is common in these populations. Families from the lower SES groups have more unemployment and live in unsafe neighborhoods, which could result in less physical activity and more television watching. Unfortunately, they also tend to consume a cheap, energy-dense diet with a high fat content, thereby facilitating the development of obesity. Limited education is another contributory factor, which makes it less likely for these individuals to follow dietary recommendations and adhere to dietary guidelines.

In developing countries, the consequences of poverty are different: people in the low SES are more likely to be engaged in heavy manual labor and tend to have limited funds for food. Undernutrition rather than obesity is the problem in this group. On the other hand, the emerging middle class in these countries tends to live in an urban environment with fewer ties to traditional values including the usual diet. Members of this relatively well-to-do class also have more money to indulge in junk food, have access to public/private transportation, and have jobs that are less demanding in terms of physical activity, all of which would contribute to the development of obesity.

CULTURAL NORMS

Cultural values are important determinants of people's behavior as it relates to food intake and physical activity. For example, the macronutrient composition of the diet varies from place to place, as does the attitude toward physical activity. Equally relevant is the body shape ideal in a given society, as exemplified in many developing countries where "fatness" is viewed as a sign of health and prosperity, vs the developed countries where the "anorexic" body image is portrayed as the ideal in the mass media.

Childhood Obesity

As is the case in adults, increase in energy intake and decrease in physical activity are the primary environmental influences on childhood obesity. A number of studies have documented that the increase in obesity prevalence has paralleled the increased consumption of junk foods/snacks and decreased physical activity in this age group (85–87). Incidentally, children are especially vulnerable since most decisions regarding diet and physical activity are beyond their control. For example, parental concerns over safety have tended to limit time for recreational activity and to limit activities such as walking or bicycling to school. One obvious consequence is longer periods of television viewing, which leads to prolonged/unsupervised exposure to direct advertisement of foods and drinks, most of which are high in fat and/or simple sugars.

Critical Periods of Increased Susceptibility

To assist with intervention strategies, certain periods of life at which an individual is especially vulnerable to weight gain have been identified.

- Prenatal—based on the postulate that early undernutrition may alter regulation of food intake, thereby predisposing to later obesity.
- Adiposity rebound—early timing of the second increase in BMI (normally between the ages of 5 and 7 yr).
- Adolescence—obesity at this stage significantly increases the risk for adult obesity as well as adult morbidity (even if subsequent weight is normalized).
- Early adulthood—partly owing to reduced physical activity.
- Pregnancy—wide range of weight gain after pregnancy.
- Menopause—combination of reduction in physical activity and hormonal changes.

Strategies for Prevention

It is worth repeating the WHO position that obesity is a serious global public health problem, requiring urgent action. As a result of the very limited success of current therapies, prevention is likely to be more cost-effective and to have a greater impact in the long run. The overall goal, in simple terms, would be to help the public adopt a healthy diet and engage in an adequate amount of physical activity. A key element for a successful program will be *early detection* to facilitate effective intervention at a number of age/BMI levels. First, primordial prevention would prevent individuals with desirable BMIs from developing obesity. Second, primary prevention would aim to prevent individuals at risk (overweight/preobese category) from becoming obese. Finally, secondary prevention would attempt to prevent worsening of obesity and comorbidities in already obese individuals. A number of organizations, including WHO and the IOTF, have been examining this issue in recent years. Some of the measures that would address a fair number of the societal/environmental factors that are driving the current global epidemic of childhood and adult obesity are given below.

Public/Family/Individual

- Provision of good prenatal nutrition and health care as well as avoidance of excessive maternal weight gain.
- Provision of a balanced diet and avoidance of excess high-calorie snacks in infancy.
- Provision of adequate nutrition and physical education to preschool and school-aged children.
- Maintenance of a healthy lifestyle through adolescence and adulthood.
- Promotion of walking and cycling as means of transportation.

Food Industry/Government

- Production and promotion of food products low in dietary fat and energy.
- Improvements in the quality of food labeling as well as the institution of pricing practices that encourage the purchase of healthy foods.
- Development and adoption of appropriate standards and guidelines for healthy nutrition.
- Regulation of food marketing and advertising practices, especially those aimed at children.
- Promotion of water rather than sugar-loaded beverages as the main daily drink.

Healthcare/Media/Employers

- Provision of adequate training in obesity care to physicians and other health care professionals.
- Provision of medical insurance coverage for the prevention and treatment of obesity.

- Institution of well-designed public health campaign(s) to educate the public.
- Promotion of healthy foods/lifestyles/body image in the mass media.
- Provision of local recreational/exercise facilities.
- Provision of flexible working arrangements to allow time for adequate physical activity.

It must be emphasized that the success of such programs will depend heavily on cooperative and complementary efforts by governments, international agencies, the food industry, media, employers, health care professionals, the insurance industry, and the public at large.

CURRENT AND FUTURE THERAPIES

As discussed previously, the health and economic consequences of obesity are considerable to the individual patient and to society at large. It is therefore not surprising that clinical guidelines for the management of obesity have been published by several organizations including NHLBI, the North American Association for the Study of Obesity, the American Association of Clinical Endocrinologists, the Scottish Intercollegiate Guidelines Network, and the Royal College of Physicians of London. In general, treatment is recommended for individuals with a BMI of 30 kg/m^2 or more as well as for individuals with a BMI between 25 and 29.9 kg/m^2 or a high-risk WC if associated with two or more risk factors/comorbidities. The recommended goal of therapy is the loss and long-term maintenance of at least a 5–10% reduction in body weight, as studies have shown that a modest reduction in weight is associated with a marked improvement in risk factors and comorbidities *(4–6)*. Because of the complex nature of this disease, the obvious and logical therapeutic approach (diet, exercise, and behavior modification) is successful in only a minority of patients. Surgery is reserved for those individuals with extreme or clinically severe obesity (BMI ≥ 40 kg/m^2), an intervention that is not without significant risk.

The limited success achieved with diet/exercise coupled with the realization that obesity is a chronic disease requiring lifelong treatment has fueled the intense drive to develop an effective drug therapy. Unfortunately, this attempt has received a lot of negative press for a variety of reasons, ranging from the inappropriate use of thyroid hormone, diuretics, and addictive sympathomimetics to the withdrawal of fenfluramine/dexfenfluramine owing to associated valvular heart disease and pulmonary hypertension *(88,89)*. Although a few have questioned the wisdom of using pharmacologic agents to treat obesity *(90)*, most health care professionals and experts in this field lament the lack of safe and effective drug(s) to complement lifestyle modifications (diet/exercise). Despite the many challenges inherent in this enterprise, recent advances in the understanding of the mechanisms/pathways that regulate/modulate appetite and energy expenditure (albeit studied mostly in rodents) have provided a number of potential targets. Antiobesity drugs can be classified into those that (1) suppress appetite (anorectics), (2) alter metabolism or nutrient partitioning, and (3) increase energy expenditure.

Anorectics

The use of these drugs results in a reduction in caloric intake, leading to a loss in body weight. A number of centrally acting anorectic agents may also increase energy expenditure.

CATECHOLAMINERGIC AGENTS

These agents act by increasing the release of noradrenaline and/or block its reuptake into neurons of the hypothalamus, an area of the brain that plays a central role in energy homeostasis. Their side-effect profile, which includes central nervous system stimulation and abuse/addiction potential, has limited their use. Amphetamine and phenylpropanolamine are no longer in use; phentermine is restricted to short-term use (maximum of 3 mo), and mazindol is approved for use in extreme obesity and only in Japan.

SEROTONINERGIC AGENTS

Members of this class, such as fenfluramine and dexfenfluramine, which act by enhancing the release and blocking the reuptake of serotonin, were withdrawn from the market in the late 1990s because of valvular heart disease and pulmonary hypertension. Some antidepressants such as fluoxetine and sertraline inhibit serotonin reuptake but do not enhance serotonin release from nerve terminals, which may explain the absence of any valvular heart disease or pulmonary hypertension associated with their use. Although they are not approved for the treatment of obesity, off-label use has demonstrated the induction of weight loss in some obese patients. However, this effect may be transient, as significant weight regain has been reported after several months of treatment with fluoxetine *(91)*.

SEROTONIN-NORADRENALINE REUPTAKE INHIBITORS

Sibutramine, a serotonin-noradrenaline reuptake inhibitor that also has dopamine reuptake inhibitory properties, is one of two drugs currently approved for the long-term treatment of obesity. The drug undergoes extensive first-pass metabolism, with formation of two metabolites, M1 (a secondary amine) and M2 (a primary amine), which mediate the pharmacologic activity of the parent molecule *(92)*. The inhibition of serotonin reuptake by these metabolites enhances satiety, thereby decreasing caloric intake, while the effect on noradrenaline reuptake enhances sympathetic outflow and is believed to cause an increase in energy expenditure *(93)*. There is no evidence of increased serotonin release, which may explain why no valvular heart disease has been associated with its use. However, the increased sympathetic activity was associated with tachycardia and elevation of systolic/diastolic blood pressure in clinical trials.

Table 8
Selected Long-Term Clinical Studies with Sibutramine

Study	Duration (wk)	Dose (mg/d)	Initial weight (kg)	Weight loss (%)	Comments
Bray et al.,	24	0	95	−1.2	Dose range finding
1999 (98)		1	94	−2.7	
		5	94	−3.9	
		10	91	−6.1	
		15	93	−7.4	
		20	93	−8.8	
		30	95	−9.4	
Apfelbaum	52	0	97.7	+0.2	Weight maintenance after
et al.,		10	95.7	−6.1	4 wk of VLCD
1999 (95)					
James et al.,	104	0	102.6	−4.6	Weight maintenance after
2000 (94)		10	102.6	−9.6	24 wk of treatment with
					sibutramine 10 mg/d
Dujovne et	24	0	102	−0.6	Improvements in HDL
al., 2001		20	99.7	−4.9	cholesterol and
(97)					triglycerides
Smith et al.,	52	0	87	−1.8	Primary care setting
2001 (99)		10	87	−5.0	
		15	87	−7.3	
Wirth and	48	0	98.2	+0.2	Patients who lost at least
Krause		15 (intermittent)	98.2	−3.5	2 kg or 2% after 4 wk
2001 (96)		15 (continuous)	98.6	−4.0	of treatment with 15 mg
					sibutramine.

HDL, high-density lipoprotein; VLCD, very low-calorie diet.

This led to sibutramine being contraindicated in patients with congestive heart failure, coronary artery disease, arrhythmias, stroke, and uncontrolled or poorly controlled hypertension.

The effectiveness of sibutramine in inducing weight loss and achieving weight maintenance has been demonstrated in several clinical trials. A number of long-term clinical studies in humans are summarized in Table 8. Maximal weight loss, usually less than 10% of baseline body weight, is achieved within 6 mo and is maintained over 12 mo. In one European multicenter study (94), obese patients who had lost more than 5% of their body weight (an average of 11.3 kg) after 6 mo of treatment with 10 mg/d of sibutramine, were randomized to receive placebo or 10 mg/d sibutramine. The dose of the drug was increased to 20 mg/d if weight regain occurred. At the end of the 18-mo follow-up period, the placebo group had regained weight to –4.7 kg, whereas the sibutramine group showed only a slight weight regain to –10.2 kg, compared with the –11.3-kg weight change from baseline after 6 mo of sibutramine treatment for both groups. Similar results were observed in another study (95), in which the initial weight loss was induced with 4 wk of a very low calorie diet. In a recently published multicenter study conducted in Germany (96), 1001 patients who had weight loss of at least 2% or 2 kg after 4 wk of treatment with sibutramine (15 mg/d) were randomized to receive continuous placebo (wk 5–48) or sibutramine 15 mg/d (wk 1–48), or intermittent sibutramine 15 mg/d (wk 1–12, 19–30, and 37–48, with placebo during all other weeks). At the end of the study, both the continuous and intermittent sibutramine therapies were shown to be statistically equivalent, although there was greater weight loss with the continuous treatment group.

Other beneficial endpoints reported for sibutramine include reductions in WC and visceral adipose tissue as well as improvements in triglycerides and HDL cholesterol. It should be noted that these changes were similar in magnitude to those observed in patients who succeeded in losing weight while on placebo (97).

BUPROPRION

This is an antidepressant drug that is also used as a smoking cessation aid. It presumably acts by inhibiting the reuptake of dopamine and possibly noradrenaline but has little or no effect on serotonin reuptake. The results of a 26-wk multicenter, randomized, placebo-controlled study in obese subjects with mild to moderate depression were presented at the 2001 meeting of the North American Association for the Study of Obesity (NAASO) in Quebec, Canada. Subjects who received buproprion in a sustained release form had a 4.6% weight loss from baseline, compared with the placebo group, which had a 1.8% weight loss. Further studies will be needed to show that this agent is sufficiently safe and effective to be developed as an antiobesity agent.

TOPIRAMATE

During clinical trials evaluating the use of topiramate as a treatment for patients with epilepsy, it was noted that the drug reduced body weight in humans. Topiramate is a sodium channel blocker that also stimulates γ-aminobutyric acid receptors and antagonizes glutamate receptors. Although the precise mechanism of weight loss induction in humans has not been established, its efficacy was sufficiently robust for the manufacturers (Johnson & Johnson, New Brunswick, NJ) to initiate phase III obesity trials with the compound. However, the studies were discontinued in early 2002 in order to develop a controlled release formulation, apparently to enhance its tolerability. The major question remains whether the side-effect profile will be sufficiently improved to allow continued development of the drug.

Cannabinoids

There are at least two cannabinoid receptors, one of which (CB_2R) is largely expressed in the periphery and does not appear to be involved in the regulation of energy homeostasis. On the other hand, CB_1R is predominantly localized in the brain and is expressed in the hypothalamus, amygdala, hippocampus, basal ganglia, cerebral cortex, and cerebellum *(100)*. Activation of CB_1R by agonists such as tetrahydrocannabinol (THC) stimulates appetite, which is reflected in the approval of THC for treating AIDS-associated anorexia. Thus, antagonism of this pathway would be expected to reduce food intake and ultimately result in weight loss. In fact, a CB_1R antagonist (SR 141716) synthesized by Sanofi Synthelabo (Paris, France), has been shown to reduce hunger, caloric intake, and body weight in overweight or obese men *(101)*. Phase III human trials have been initiated with this compound. Although only minor gastrointestinal adverse events were observed in the phase II studies, some concern remains about potential central nervous system side effects associated with this pathway.

Histaminergic Agents

Intracerebroventricular (ICV) administration of histamine decreases food consumption, whereas histamine antagonists increase food intake in animals *(102)*. Four histamine receptor subtypes have been characterized; the available experimental data indicate that the modulation of feeding behavior by histamine is predominantly mediated via the H_1 and H_3 receptors *(103)*. H_3 receptors are located presynaptically, where they function as autoreceptors, regulating histamine release. Currently, H_3 receptor antagonism is considered a better therapeutic target than H_1 receptor agonism, but there is some concern regarding the potential impact of H_3 receptor antagonism on water intake *(104)*.

Leptin

Leptin is a 146-amino acid protein mainly produced by adipocytes; its circulating levels reflect, to a great extent, the degree of adiposity or the amount of energy stored in adipose tissue *(105)*. Although leptin has pleiotropic actions including neuroendocrine, metabolic, reproductive, hematopoietic, and metabolic regulation, its role in energy balance has received the most attention. It is the product of the OB gene, which is mutated in the genetically obese (*ob/ob*) mouse; its receptor is mutated in the diabetic (*db/db*) mouse and the fatty (*fa/fa*) rat, which are also obese. Mutations in either leptin or its receptor, although quite rare, have been reported in humans; these result in hyperphagia and early-onset obesity *(106,107)*. Binding of the peptide to its receptor on hypothalamic neurons leads to increased expression of anorexigenic (appetite-suppressing) peptides, such as melanocyte-stimulating hormone (α-MSH), cocaine- and amphetamine-regulated transcript (CART), and corticotropin-releasing hormone (CRH) and to decreased expression of orexigenic (appetite-stimulating) peptides such as neuropeptide Y (NPY), melanin-concentrating hormone (MCH), and agouti-related peptide (AgRP). Evidence from several studies indicates that leptin-induced reduction in body weight results from a decrease in appetite and an increase in energy expenditure *(105)*.

The dramatic response of the *ob/ob* mouse and a leptin-deficient child to exogenous leptin led to the mistaken belief that a cure for human obesity had been found *(108,109)*. It soon became apparent that the vast majority of obese humans are not leptin-deficient but do in fact have very high circulating levels of the protein. This has led to introduction of the concept that human obesity is a state of leptin resistance, sometimes compared with the insulin resistance seen in the early phases of type 2 DM, when hyperglycemia persists despite hyperinsulinemia. The mechanistic basis of the resistance remains poorly understood but may include impairment of leptin transport across the blood-brain barrier as well as abnormalities of leptin receptor signaling *(110)*. Thus far, clinical trials in humans using both short- and long-acting formulations of leptin have produced disappointing results *(111,112)*. These setbacks notwithstanding, there is no doubt that the discovery of leptin was not only a major scientific accomplishment but has led to a tremendous growth in our understanding of the neuroendocrine pathways involved in energy homeostasis.

CILIARY NEUROTROPHIC FACTOR

Ciliary neurotrophic factor (CNTF) is a growth factor that was observed to induce weight loss during clinical trials on patients with amyotrophic lateral sclerosis (Lou Gehrig's disease). It has been suggested that CNTF acts via a leptin-like pathway to suppress appetite, leading to weight loss. The initial clinical studies revealed significant adverse experiences such as nausea, antibody production, and reactivation of herpetic lesions *(113)*. A recombinant version, named Axokine™ (Regeneron, Tarrytown, NY), is said to be less immunogenic and less likely to cause nausea at the low doses being tested.

In phase II studies, 12 wk of treatment with Axokine™ was reported to induce an average of 10 lb more weight loss than placebo. Interestingly, the weight loss was sustained for about 9 mo after discontinuation of drug therapy, a finding that could reflect the induction of irreversible changes in the neuronal pathways that regulate energy homeostasis. The publication of data from phase II as well as the ongoing phase III studies is eagerly awaited, and will hopefully shed more light on the mechanism of action, efficacy, and side-effect profile of this molecule.

NEUROPEPTIDES

Since the discovery of leptin in the 1990s, there has been a dramatic increase in the number of peptides implicated in the regulation/modulation of energy balance. Although this has increased the number of potential targets, it has also highlighted one of the biggest problems in developing an antiobesity drug—the presence of multiple redundant mechanisms for maintaining body weight. Many of these peptides affect food intake when injected into various parts of the brain such as the hypothalamus or the ventricles; others affect both food intake and energy expenditure. The receptors for many of the neuropeptides have been identified and shown to belong to the G-protein-coupled class of receptors. Both the peptides and their cognate receptors are widely distributed in the brain, especially in those regions known to be involved in body weight regulation, like the hypothalamus. The overall strategy for drug development is to develop antagonists to pathways involving orexigenic peptides and agonists to the pathways that involve anorexigenic peptides.

Neuropeptide Y. NPY is a 36-amino acid peptide that is highly conserved across species and is one of the most potent stimulators of appetite known. Five NPY receptors (Y-1, -2, -4, -5, and -6) have been cloned, but only the Y-1 and Y-5 receptors are thought to mediate the NPY-induced modulation of energy homeostasis *(114)*. Chronic central administration of NPY leads to weight gain in rodents, whereas antisense oligonucleotides or NPY antibodies significantly decrease feeding *(115)*. NPY also decreases thermogenesis and uncoupling protein 1 in brown adipose tissue and increases white fat storage *(114)*. Thus, NPY regulates energy balance via effects on both appetite and energy expenditure. Additional support for the role of NPY includes the observed increase in NPY levels with starvation and in genetically obese rodent models such as *fa/fa* rats, *db/db* mice, and *ob/ob* mice.

Surprisingly, NPY$^{-/-}$, Y1R$^{-/-}$ and Y5R$^{-/-}$ mice are not lean and remain susceptible to diet-induced obesity, presumably as a consequence of compensatory mechanisms or redundant inputs from non-NPY pathways *(115–118)*. However, in NPY$^{-/-}$ mice, the degree of obesity is reduced when the *ob* gene is coexpressed, indicating that NPY antagonists could be most effective when leptin levels are low. Despite several years of research, there are still no published studies in humans supporting the effectiveness of NPY antagonism in the treatment of obesity. Potential liabilities include the increased seizure activity/alcohol preference exhibited by NPY$^{-/-}$ mice, as well as possible interference with NPY-mediated effects on anxiogenesis and circadian rhythm.

Melanin-Concentrating Hormone. MCH is a 19-amino acid cyclic peptide whose mRNA is predominantly expressed in the lateral hypothalamus and the zona incerta *(119)*. Several studies in rodents have demonstrated the orexigenic nature of this pathway. Unlike NPY-deficient mice, pro-MCH and MCH1 receptor-deficient mice are lean and hypophagic and have increased metabolic rate *(120)*. Hypothalamic MCH mRNA levels are elevated in *ob/ob* and fasted mice, presumably as a result of the removal of the inhibiting effects of leptin on MCH mRNA expression. In addition, chronic ICV infusion of MCH causes hyperphagia and obesity, as does overexpression of the prohormone of the MCH precursor in transgenic mice *(121)*. Based on the rodent data, it appears that MCH1 receptor antagonists would be effective antiobesity agents. However, this remains to be demonstrated in humans, who have the additional complexity of possessing a second receptor, MCH2R, with an undetermined role in energy homeostasis.

Other Orexigenic Neuropeptides. *Galanin* is a 29-amino acid peptide that is widely distributed in the central and peripheral nervous systems as well as in endocrine organs. The highest mRNA expression is in the hypothalamus and median eminence, and central administration has been shown to stimulate food intake in rodents *(122)*. However, galanin knockout mice are not lean, and there have been some studies in rodents showing that chronic administration failed to induce sustained increase in food intake and body weight *(123)*. Thus more work remains to be done to validate this pathway.

Orexin-A and *-B*, which are also called *hypocretins*, are derived from the same precursor molecule, prepro-orexin peptide. These peptides and their receptors OX1 and OX2 are widely distributed in regions of the brain involved in modulating energy homeostasis. ICV injection of these peptides elicits an increase in food intake but to a much lesser degree than is observed with NPY *(124)*. However, it is becoming apparent that this pathway is involved in much more than the regulation of energy balance. For example, most cases of human narcolepsy are associated with a deficiency of these peptides in the cerebrospinal fluid or in the brain *(125)*. In addition, a mutation that caused an impairment of peptide processing and trafficking was found in a young child with severe narcolepsy *(126)*. Thus, it is possible that antagonism of this pathway could have undesirable effects on the sleep-wake cycle.

Melanocortins. α-*MSH* is one of several peptides derived from pro-opiomelanocortin (POMC); it reduces body weight by decreasing appetite and increasing metabolic rate. There are five melanocortin receptors (MCRs), but only MC-3R and MC-4R, which are highly expressed in the hypothalamus, are believed to be involved in energy homeostasis *(127)*. As previously stated, this pathway is downstream of leptin. Mutations involving POMC processing or the MC-4R signaling pathway are associated with obesity in humans as well as rodents, thus providing the rationale for the development of MC-4R agonists as antiobesity agents *(127,128)*. Recently, it was reported that 6 wk of intranasal treatment with a peptide melanocortin receptor agonist induced a reduction in body adiposity in lean subjects *(129)*. However, it is critical to develop a highly selective agonist for this purpose, as highlighted by the fact that a nonselective melanocortin agonist (MT II) caused penile erection in the absence of sexual stimulation *(130)*. Several groups in academia and industry are actively engaged in attempts to develop such a compound *(131)*.

Other Anorexigenic Peptides. *Bombesin* is a 14-amino acid peptide that was originally isolated from the skin of the European frog, *Bombina bombina*. In mammals, two bombesin-like peptides, neuromedin B (NM-B) and gastrin-releasing peptide (GRP), have been identified and are believed to play a role in the regulation of energy homeostasis *(132)*. The NM-B-preferring receptor (BB1) and the GRP-preferring receptor (BB2) are widely distributed in the central nervous system and gastrointestinal tract, and the third receptor (BRS-3) is restricted to the central nervous system, notably the hypothalamus. Although the natural ligand for BRS-3 has not been identified, there is more interest in it since BRS-3$^{-/-}$ mice (unlike BB1$^{-/-}$ and BB2–/– mice) are obese and have other features consistent with the metabolic syndrome *(133)*.

CRH is a 41-amino acid peptide that is involved in many physiologic processes including adrenocorticotropic hormone production, depression, anxiety, memory, learning, and energy homeostasis *(134)*. Chronic infusion of CRH into the brains of animals inhibits food intake and activates the sympathetic nervous system, thereby reducing body weight *(135)*. In a recent study, peripheral administration of CRH to healthy men and women resulted in an increase in resting energy expenditure *(136)*. However, it appears that the CRH type 2 receptor, which has a higher affinity for urocortin (another member of the CRH family), is a better target, as activation of this receptor decreases food intake without the undesirable effects such as anxiogenesis seen with CRH *(137)*.

Neurons containing *cocaine-amphetamine-regulated transcript* (CART) are present in several hypothalamic nuclei and in the arcuate nucleus coexpress POMC mRNA *(138)*. As previously stated, this gene is upregulated by leptin. It is therefore not surprising that its mRNA is reduced in states of leptin deficiency such as fasted rats and *ob/ob* mice. It is hoped that the identification and characterization of the cognate receptor for CART will advance a development program in this area.

GASTROINTESTINAL PEPTIDES

Ghrelin is an acylated 28-amino acid peptide that is predominantly produced by the stomach, and stimulates the release of growth hormone (GH) from the pituitary gland. Results of studies in rodents and humans indicate that this peptide also has potent orexigenic activity, presumably via activation of the NPY pathway. For example, peripheral administration of ghrelin stimulates appetite in humans *(139)*, whereas its orexigenic effect in rats was abolished by an NPY-1R antagonist *(140)*. One would therefore predict that ghrelin receptor antagonists would be efficacious in appetite reduction and consequently in body weight reduction. However, infusion of ghrelin produced beneficial hemodynamic effects in patients with congestive heart failure *(141)*. Thus, potential liabilities of a ghrelin antagonist include potentially deleterious effects on the cardiovascular system and on GH release.

Glucagon-like peptide-1 (GLP-1) was originally identified as one of the products of the processing of preproglucagon in the intestine, where it functions as an incretin—inducing glucose-dependent insulin release from pancreatic β-cells. In addition, it was shown to inhibit gastric motility, delay nutrient absorption, and induce satiety. Subsequently, GLP-1 expression was detected in the central nervous system, especially in the hypothalamus, and it has been demonstrated in rodents that both central and peripheral administration of this peptide increases energy expenditure and decreases food intake, resulting in a reduction in body weight *(142)*.

In a meta-analysis of several studies involving the intravenous administration of the peptide in humans, Verdich et al. *(143)* concluded that the infusion reduces energy intake in a dose-dependent manner in both obese and lean subjects. There is considerable interest in this pathway for the development of antiobesity and antidiabetic drugs. A number of approaches have been adopted to overcome a major limitation owing to the extremely short half-life of the peptide; these include the identification of long-acting GLP-1 analogs/mimetics, selective inhibition of the degrading enzyme dipeptidyl peptidase IV (DPP-IV) and the synthesis of DPP-IV-resistant analogs.

Cholecystokinin (CCK) is released in response to meals, especially those rich in lipids and protein. It binds to two receptors, CCK_A and CCK_B, which are primarily located in the gastrointestinal tract and brain, respectively. The anorectic effects of the peptide are mediated via vagal signals from the brain that are triggered after activation of the CCK_A receptors. Validation of this pathway as a target for anti-obesity therapy comes from both rodent and human studies, including the obese phenotype of the $CCK_A^{-/-}$ mouse *(144)* and the induction of satiety and the reduction in food intake following infusion of CCK in obese humans *(145)*. It remains to be seen whether chronic use of CCK_A receptor agonists will be associated with adverse effects such as gallstones, pancreatitis, and nausea.

Drugs That Alter Metabolism or Nutrient Partitioning

Included in this class are drugs that interfere with nutrient (especially fat) absorption such as orlistat and compounds that target metabolic pathways, particularly lipid metabolism.

INHIBITION OF FAT ABSORPTION

Orlistat, an inhibitor of gastric and pancreatic lipases, is the second drug currently approved for the long-term treatment of obesity. It is a synthetic derivative of lipstatin, which is produced by *Streptomyces toxitricini (146)*. Inhibition of lipase activity decreases fat absorption by about 30%, leading to maintenance of a caloric deficit over the long term, which would then result in a reduction in body weight. There is negligible systemic absorption of orally administered drug, and there have been no reported clinically significant interactions with several drugs including warfarin, digoxin, pravastatin, nifedipine, phenytoin, glyburide, and oral contraceptive pills *(146)*.

The efficacy of orlistat has been demonstrated in several clinical studies, some of which are summarized in Table 9. On average, 1–2 yr of treatment with the

Table 9
Selected Long-Term Clinical Studies with Orlistat

Study	Duration (wk)	Dose (mg tid)	Initial weight (kg)	Weight loss at 52 wk (%)	Comments
Hollander et al., 1998 (147)	52	0 120	99.7 99.6	−4.3 −6.2	Obese patients with type 2 diabetes
Sjostrom et al., 1998 (148)	104	0 120	99.8 99.1	−6.1 −10.2	European multicenter study
Davidson et al., 1999 (149)	104	0 120	100.6 100.7	−5.8 −8.8	U.S. multicenter study
Finer et al., 2000 (150)	52	0 120	98.4 95.7	−5.4 −8.5	Multicenter study in the UK
Hauptman et al., 2000 (151)	104	0 60 120	101.8 100.4 100.5	−4.1 −7.1 −7.9	Primary care setting
Muls et al., 2001 (152)	24	0 120	91.2 90.2	−3.9 −6.9	Obese patients with hyper-cholesterolemia

drug produced an 8–10% body weight loss, compared with a loss of 4–6% in the placebo-treated groups. In all these studies, the combination of orlistat and diet was more effective than placebo plus diet in inducing and maintaining weight loss. More importantly, the use of this drug led to significant improvements in obesity-related risk factors such as blood pressure, glycemic control, and lipid profile. However, there have been concerns related to the gastrointestinal adverse effects, which include abdominal pain, fecal incontinence with oily stools, flatulence, nausea, vomiting, and malabsorption of fat-soluble vitamins. Thus, the drug is contraindicated in chronic malabsorption and cholestasis.

FATTY ACID SYNTHASE INHIBITION

Fatty acid synthase (FAS) catalyzes the synthesis of palmitic acid from malonyl coenzyme A (CoA), which means that enzyme inhibition will result in accumulation of malonyl CoA. In rodents, central and peripheral administration of C-75, a FAS inhibitor, has profound effects on food intake and body weight, presumably by interacting with hypothalamic pathways such as NPY/AgRP

(153). It has been proposed that the accumulation of malonyl CoA and possibly long-chain fatty acyl CoA in hypothalamic neurons constitutes the molecular basis for the appetite-suppressing effect of C-75. The next phase is the synthesis of safe and potent FAS inhibitors for testing in rodents and hopefully in humans.

ACETYL-COA CARBOXYLASE INHIBITION

Acetyl-CoA carboxylase (ACC), which is comprised of two isoenzymes encoded by separate genes, catalyzes the carboxylation of acetyl CoA to form malonyl CoA. ACC1 is mainly expressed in the liver and adipose tissue, whereas ACC2 is enriched in the heart and skeletal muscle, where it is believed to function in the outer membrane of the mitochondria. Unlike FAS inhibition, ACC inhibition will be expected to lower malonyl CoA levels, which probably accounts for the hyperphagia exhibited by ACC2$^{-/-}$ mice *(154)*. However, these mice are also lean and have reduced adiposity and body weight, providing a rationale for the potential use of ACC2 inhibitors as antiobesity drugs. Potential liabilities include cardiac toxicity, hyperphagia (secondary to low malonyl CoA) interfering with the antiobesity effects, and the difficulty in synthesizing selective inhibitors.

ADIPONECTIN

This is an adipocyte-derived protein (additional names include AdipoQ, Acrp30, apM1, and GBP28) that is reduced in obese mice and humans *(155)*. A number of rodent experiments have provided evidence regarding the modulation of fat metabolism, insulin sensitivity, and energy homeostasis by this protein. For example, injection of adiponectin into obese or lipoatrophic mice decreased blood glucose levels and reduced insulin resistance *(156,157)*. In addition, treatment of mice with a recombinant globular head fragment of adiponectin produced an increase in fatty acid oxidation as well as body weight reduction without affecting food intake *(158)*. Results of ongoing studies will provide much-needed clarity on the suitability of this target for obesity and DM therapy.

GROWTH HORMONE

Obese individuals secrete less GH than normal weight individuals, and administration of this hormone to GH-deficient individuals leads to enhanced lipolysis, increase in metabolic rate, and improvements in fat distribution *(159)*. However, chronic GH treatment in humans is associated with impaired glucose homeostasis and other undesirable effects that have reduced enthusiasm for the use of the hormone in long-term treatment of obesity *(160)*. Interestingly, AOD9604 (Metabolic Pharmaceuticals, Melbourne, Australia), a C-terminal fragment of GH (acting via a GH-receptor-independent mechanism), stimulated lipolysis, increased fat oxidation and induced weight loss in obese mice after 14 d of treatment *(161)*. Furthermore, a recent press release claimed that weekly intravenous administration of this peptide to obese humans produced what was described as positive results in terms of safety, tolerability, and weight reduction. In addition, the fat breakdown and weight reduction reportedly occurred after single intravenous doses. More information will be needed to evaluate these results and validate this approach for the long-term treatment of human obesity.

Drugs that Increase Energy Expenditure

β-Adrenergic agonism has been recognized as an appropriate target since the resultant catecholamine release would be expected to increase metabolic rate and consequently energy expenditure. However, the adverse cardiac effects seen with thyroid hormone and other sympathomimetics such as ephedrine and caffeine have highlighted the potential dangers associated with this approach (8,11). Recently, a number of major pharmaceutical companies have filed patents on selective thyroid hormone receptor modulators, indicating renewed interest in this mechanism. It may well be that the selectivity of these new compounds will lead to an acceptable safety profile to complement their presumed efficacy. It is worth mentioning that β3-adrenergic receptor agonist research has yet to bear fruit, despite years of positive results in mice, confirming the adage that mice are neither men nor women.

Another target of interest is the *uncoupling of electron transport from ATP synthesis*, which is mediated by three mitochondrial uncoupling proteins (UCP1-3), and would be expected to result in thermogenesis (162). However, attempts to validate this target have produced conflicting results.

CONCLUSIONS

The declaration by WHO, the U.S. Surgeon General, and several national medical and scientific organizations that obesity is a global epidemic requiring urgent action is a major first step in this "battle of the bulge." We can now begin to understand and confront the medical, economic, and social consequences of the disease. It is hoped that this chapter has painted an appropriately balanced picture, reflecting not only on the enormity of this challenge but also the numerous advances that have been made in recent years.

This is certainly an exciting period in the field of obesity research and management, especially with the influx of many young, more molecularly oriented scientists engaged in dissecting the pathways involved in energy homeostasis. Based on past experience, a note of caution is, however, necessary. The development of a single magic bullet that is sufficiently safe and efficacious for most obese patients is unlikely. In the final analysis, prevention, especially *early prevention*, is our best chance. This will require a concerted effort by all of us: individual citizens, governments, international agencies, the food industry, media, employers, health care professionals and the insurance industry.

ACKNOWLEDGMENTS

I would like to thank my daughters, Mgbechi and Chioma, for their invaluable assistance with word processing, and Dr. Keith Kaufman for reading the manuscript.

REFERENCES

1. Downey M. Obesity as a disease entity. Am Heart J 2001;142:1091–1094.
2. Heshka S, Allison DB. Is obesity a disease? Int J Obes 2001;25:1401–1404.
3. Kopelman PG, Finer N. Reply: Is obesity a disease? Int J. Obes 2001;25:1405–1406.
4. World Health Organization. Obesity: Preventing and Managing the Global Epidemic. Report of a WHO Consultation on Obesity, Geneva, 3–5 June, 1997. World Health Organization, Geneva, 1998, WHO/NUT/NCD/98.1.
5. World Health Organization/International Association for the Study of Obesity/International Obesity Taskforce. The Asia-Pacific perspective: redefining obesity and its treatment. Available at: http://www.idi.org.au/obesityreport.htm.
6. National Institutes of Health. Clinical guidelines on the identification, evaluation, and treatment of overweight and obesity in adults: the evidence report. NIH, NHLBI, June, 1998.
7. Bray GA, Bouchard C, James WPT, eds. Handbook on Obesity. Marcel Dekker, New York, 1998.
8. Bray GA, Greenway FL. Current and potential drugs for treatment of obesity. Endocr Rev 1999;20:805–875.
9. Bjorntop P, Lockwood DH, Heffner TG eds. Obesity: pathology and therapy. Springer Verlag, New York, 2000.
10. Bjorntorp P, ed. International Textbook of Obesity. John Wiley & Sons, New York, 2001.
11. Clapham JC, Arch JRS, Tadayyon M. Anti-obesity drugs: a critical review of current therapies and future opportunities. Pharmacol Therap 2001;89:81–121.
12. Visscher TLS, Seidell JC. The public health impact of obesity. Annu Rev Public Health 2001;22:355–375.
13. Gallagher D, Visser M, Sepulveda D, Pierson RN, Harris T, Heymsfield SB. How useful is body mass index for comparison of body fatness across age, sex, and ethnic groups? Am J Epidemiol 1996;143:228–229.
14. Deurenberg P, Yap M, van Staveren WA. Body mass index and percent body fat: a meta analysis among different ethnic groups. Int J Obes 1998;22:1164–1171.
15. Lundgren H, Bengtsson C, Blohme G, Lapidus L, Sjostrom L. Adiposity and adipose tissue distribution in relation to incidence of diabetes in women: results from a prospective population study in Gothenburg, Sweden. Int J Obes 1989;13:413–423.
16. Cassano P, Rosner B, Vokonas P, Weiss S. Obesity and body fat distribution in relation to the incidence of non-insulin-dependent diabetes mellitus. Am J Epidemiol 1992;136:1474–1486.
17. Filipovsky J, Ducimetiere P, Darne B, Richard J. Abdominal body mass distribution and elevated blood pressure are associated with increased risk of death from cardiovascular diseases and cancer in middle-aged men. The results of a 15- to 20-year follow-up in the Paris prospective study. Int J Obes 1993;17:197–203.
18. Chan JM, Rimm EB, Colditz GA, Stampfer MJ, Willet WC. Obesity, fat distribution and weight gain as risk factors for clinical diabetes in men. Diabetes Care 1994;17:961–969.
19. Bjorntorp P. Body fat distribution, insulin resistance and metabolic diseases. Nutrition 1997;13:795–803.
20. Carey VJ, Walters EE, Colditz GA, et al. Body fat distribution and risk of non-insulin-dependent diabetes mellitus in women. The Nurses' Health Study. Am J Epidemiol 1997;145:614–619.

21. Kissebah A. Central obesity: measurement and metabolic effects. Diabetes Rev 1997;5:8–20.
22. Reeder BA, Senthilselvan A, Despres J-P, et al. The association of cardiovascular risk factors with abdominal obesity in Canada. Can Med Assoc J 1997;157:S39–S45.
23. Rexrode KM, Carey VJ, Hennekens CH, et al. Abdominal adiposity and coronary heart disease in women. JAMA 1998;280:1843–1848.
24. Ho SC, Chen YM, Woo JLF, Leung SSF, Lam TH, Janus ED. Association between simple anthropometric indices and cardiovascular risk factors. Int J Obes 2001;25:1689–1697.
25. Takami R, Takeda N, Hayashi M, et al. Body fatness and fat distribution as predictors of metabolic abnormalities and early carotid atherosclerosis. Diabetes Care 2001;24:1248–1252.
26. Henandez-Ono A, Monter-Carreola G, Zamora-Gonzalez J, et al. Association of visceral fat with coronary risk factors in a population-based sample of postmenopausal women. Int J Obes 2002;26:33–39.
27. Bujalska IJ, Kumar S, Stewart PM. Does central obesity reflect 'Cushing's disease of the omentum'? Lancet 1997;349:1210–1213.
28. Bjorntorp P. Neuroendocrine perturbations as a cause of insulin resistance. Diabetes Metab Res Rev 1999;15:427–441.
29. Busetto L. Visceral obesity and the metabolic syndrome: effects of weight loss. Nutr Metab Cardiovasc Dis 2001;11:195-204.
30. Dessi-Fulgheri P, Sarzani R, Rappelli A. The natriuretic peptide system in obesity-related hypertension: new pathophysiological aspects. J Nephrol 1998;11:296–299.
31. Redon J. Hypertension in obesity. Nutr Metab Cardiovasc Dis 2001;11:344–353.
32. Rocchini AP. Obesity hypertension. Am J Hypertens 2002;15:50S–52S.
33. WHO: Controlling the global obesity epidemic. Available at http://www.who.int/nut/obs.htm.
34. van der Sande MAB, Ceesay SM, Milligan PJM, et al. Obesity and undernutrition and cardiovascular risk in rural and urban Gambian communities. Am J Public Health 2001;91:1641–1644.
35. Tremblay MS, Katzmarzyk PT, Willms JD. Temporal trends in overweight and obesity in Canada, 1981–1996. Int J Obes 2002;26:538–543.
36. Mokdad AH, Bowman BA, Ford ES, Vinicor F, Marks JS, Koplan JP. The continuing epidemics of obesity and diabetes in the United States. JAMA 2001;286:1195–1200.
37. Popkin BM. The nutrition transition and obesity in the developing world. J Nutr 2001;131:871S–873S.
38. Uauy R, Albala C, Kain J. Obesity trends in Latin America: transiting from under-to over-weight. J Nutr 2001;131:893S–899S.
39. Bundred P, Kitchiner D, Buchan I. Prevalence of overweight and obese children between 1989 and 1998: population based series of cross sectional studies. BMJ 2001; 322:1–4.
40. Chinn S, Rona RJ. Prevalence and trends in overweight and obesity in three cross sectional studies of British children. BMJ 2001;322:24–26.
41. Chu N-F. Prevalence and trends of obesity among school children in Taiwan—the Taipei Children Heart Study. Int J Obes 2001;25:170–176.
42. Park MK, Menard SW and Schoolfield J. Prevalence of overweight in a triethnic pediatric population of San Antonio, Texas. Int J Obes 2001;25:409–416.
43. Sakamoto N, Wansorn, S, Tontisirin K, Marui E. A social epidemiologic study of obesity among preschool children in Thailand. Int J Obes 2001;25:389–394.
44. Tyrell VJ, Richards GE, Hofman P, Gillies GF, Robinson E, Cutfield WS. Obesity in Auckland school children: a comparison of the body mass index and percentage body fat as the diagnostic criterion. Int J Obes 2001;25:164–169.
45. Wang Y. Cross-national comparison of childhood obesity: the epidemic and the relationship between obesity and socioeconomic status. Int J Epidemiol 2001;30:1129–1136.
46. Cole TJ, Bellizzi MC, Flegal KM, Dietz WH. Establishing a standard definition for child overweight and obesity worldwide: international survey. BMJ 2000;320:1240–1243.

47. Deurenberg P. Universal cut-off BMI points for obesity are not appropriate. Br J Nutr 2001;85:135–136.
48. Luo J, Hu FB. Time trends of obesity in pre-school children in China from 1989 to 1997. Int J Obes 2002;26:553–558.
49. De Onis M, Blossner M. Prevalence and trends of overweight among pre-school children in developing countries. Am J Clin Nutr 2000;72:1032–1039.
50. Visscher TLS, Seidell JC, Molarius A, van der Kuip, Hofman A, Witteman JCM. A comparison of body mass index, waist-hip ratio and waist circumference as predictors of all-cause mortality among the elderly: the Rotterdam study. Int J Obes 2001;25:1730–1735.
51. Stevens J, Cai J, Pamuk ER, Williamson DF, Thin MJ, Wood JL. The effect of age on the association between body-mass index and mortality. N Engl J Med 1998;338:1–7.
52. Calle EE, Thun MJ, Petreli JM, Rodrigues C, Heath CW. Body-mass index and mortality in a prospective cohort of US adults. N Engl J Med 1999;341:1097–1105.
53. Allison DB, Fontaine KR, Manson JE, Stevens J, Van Itallie TB. Annual death attributable to obesity in the United States. JAMA 1999;282:1530–1538.
54. Must A, Spadano J, Coakley EH, Field AE, Colditz G, Dietz WH. The disease burden associated with overweight and obesity. JAMA 1999;282:1523–1529.
55. Doll S, Paccaud F, Bovet P, Burnier M and Wietlisbach V.Body mass index, abdominal adiposity and blood pressure: consistency of their association across developing and developed countries. Int J Obes 2002;26:48–57.
56. Juhaeri, Stevens J, Chambless LE, et al. Associations between weight gain and incident hypertension in a bi-ethnic cohort: the Atherosclerosis Risk in Communities Study. Int J Obes 2002;26:58–64.
57. Despres JP. Lipoprotein metabolism in visceral obesity. Int J Obes 1991;15(suppl 2):45–52.
58. Khaidhiar L, Blackburn GL. Obesity assessment. Am Heart J 2001;142:1095–1101.
59. Adult Treatment Panel III. Executive summary of the third report of the National Cholesterol Education Program (NCEP) Expert Panel on Detection, Evaluation, and Treatment of High Blood Cholesterol in Adults. JAMA 2001;285:2486–2497.
60. Eckel RH, Krauss RM. American Heart Association call to action: obesity as a major risk factor for coronary heart disease. Circulation 1998;97:2099–2100.
61. Deurenberg-Yap M, Chew Sk, Lin VFP, Tan BY, van Staveren WA, Duerenberg P. Relationships between indices of obesity and its comorbidities in multi-ethnic Singapore. Int J Obes 2001;25:1554–1562.
62. Anderson JW, Konz EC. Obesity and disease management. Obes Res 2001;9 (Suppl 4):326S–334S.
63. Shaper AG, Wannamethee SG, Walker M. Body weight: implications for the prevention of coronary heart disease, stroke, and diabetes melllitus in a cohort of middle aged men. BMJ 1997;314:1311–1317.
64. Jousilahti P, Tuomilehto J, Vartiainen E, Pekkanen J, Puska P. Body weight, Cardiovascular risk factors and coronary mortality: 15 year follow-up of middle-aged men and women in eastern Finland. Circulation1996;93:1372–1379.
65. Stampfer MJ, Maclure MK, Colditz GA, Manson JE, Willet WC. Risk of symptomatic gallstones in women with severe obesity. Am J Clin Nutr 1992;55:652–658.
66. Acalovschi MV, Blendea D, Pascu M, Georoceaunu A, Badea RI, Prelipceanu M. Risk of asymptomatic and symptomatic gallstones in moderately obese women: a longitudinal follow-up study. Am J Gastroenterol 1997;92:127–131.
67. Cicuttini FM, Baker JR, Spector TD. The association of obesity with osteoarthritis of the hand knee in women: a twin study. J Rheumatol 1996;23:1221–1226.
68. Garfinkel L. Overweight and cancer. Ann Intern Med 1985;103:1034–1036.
69. Moller H, Mellemgard A, Ludvig K, Olsen JH. Obesity and cancer risk; a Danish record linkage study. Eur J Cancer 1994;30A:344–350.

70. Chow W-H, Gridley G, Fraumeni JF, Jarvholm B. Obesity, hypertension and the risk of kidney cancer in men. N Engl J Med 2000;343:1305–1311.
71. Bergstrom A, Pisani P, Tenet V, et al. Overweight as an avoidable cause of cancer in Europe. Int J Cancer 2001;91:421–430.
72. World Cancer Research Fund. Food, Nutrition and the Prevention of Cancer: A Global Perspective. American Institute Cancer Research, Washington, DC, 1997.
73. Rossner S, Longerstrand L, Persson HE, Sachs C. The sleep apnea syndrome of obesity: risk of sudden death. J Intern Med 1991;230:135–142.
74. Pasquali R, Vicennati V. Obesity and hormonal abnormalities. In: Bjorntorp P, ed. International Textbook of Obesity. John Wiley & Sons, New York, 2001, pp. 225–239.
75. Sullivan M, Karlsson J, Sjostrom L, et al. Swedish obese subjects (SOS)—an intervention study of obesity. Baseline evaluation of health and psychosocial functioning in the first 1743 subjects examined. Int J Obes Relat Metab Disord 1993;17:503–512.
76. Wolf AM, Colditz GA. Current estimates of the economic cost of obesity in the United States. Obes Res 1998;6:97–106.
77. IOTF. Economic cost of obesity. Available at: http://www.obesite.chaire.ulaval.ca/IOTF.htm.
78. Freedman DS, Dietz WH, Srinivasan SR, Berenson GS. The relation of overweight to cardiovascular risk factors among children and adolescents: the Bogalusa Heart Study. Pediatrics 1999;103:1175–1182.
79. Pinhas-Hamiel O, Dolan LM, Daniels SR, et al. Increased incidence of non-insulin dependent diabetes mellitus among adolescents. J Pediatr 1996;126:608–615.
80. Goran MI. Metabolic precursors and effects of obesity in children: a decade of progress, 1990–1999. Am J Clin Nutr 2001;73:158–171.
81. Steinberger J, Moran A, Hong C-P, Jacobs D, Sinaiko AR. Adiposity in childhood predicts obesity and insulin resistance in young adulthood. J Pediatr 2001;138:469–473.
82. Young LR, Nestle M. The contribution of expanding portion sizes to the US obesity epidemic. Am J Public Health 2002;92:246–249.
83. Kant AK, Schatzkin A, Graubard BI, Schairer C. Consumption of energy-dense, nutrient-poor foods by adult Americans: nutritional and health implications: the third National Health and Nutrition Examination Survey, 1988–1994. Am J Clin Nutr 2000;72:929–936.
84. Kennedy E, Goldberg J. What are American children eating? Implications for public policy. Nutr Rev 1995;53:111–126.
85. Crespo CJ, Smit E, Troiano RP, et al. Television watching, energy intake and obesity in US children: results from the Third National Health and Nutrition Examination Survey, 1988–1994. Arch Pediatr Adolesc Med 2001;155:360–365.
86. Dietz WH. The obesity epidemic in young children: reduce television viewing and promote playing. BMJ 2001;322:313–314.
87. Williams CL. Can childhood obesity be prevented? In: Bendich A, Deckelbaum RJ, eds. Primary and Secondary Preventive Nutrition. Humana, Totowa, NJ, 2001, pp. 185–203.
88. Abenhaim L, Moride Y, Brenot F, et al. Appetite suppressant drugs and the risk of primary pulmonary hypertension. N Engl J Med 1996;335: 609–616.
89. Cannistra LB, Davis SM, Bauman AG. Valvular heart disease associated with dexfenfluramine. N Engl J Med 1997;337:636–639.
90. Kassirer JP, Angell M. Losing weight—an ill-fated New Year's resolution. N Engl J Med 1998;338:52–54.
91. Daubress J, Kolanowski J, Krzentowski M, et al. Usefulness of fluoxetine in obese non-insulin dependent diabetics: a multicenter study. Obes Res 1996;4:391–396.
92. Hind ID, Mangham JE, Ghani SP, Haddock RE, Earratt CJ, Jones RW. Sibutramine pharmacokinetics in young and elderly healthy subjects. Eur J Clin Phrmacol 1999;54:847–849.

93. Hansen DL, Toubro S, Stock MJ, Macdonald IA, Astrup A. Thermogenic effects of subutramine in humans. Am J Clin Nutr 1998;68:1180–1186.
94. James WPT, Astrup A, Finer N, et al. Effect of sibutramine on weight maintenance after weight loss: a randomized trial. Lancet 2000; 356:2119–2125.
95. Apfelbaum M, Vague P, Ziegler O, Hanotin C, Thomas F, Leutenegger E. Long-term maintenance of weight loss after a very-low-calorie diet: a randomized blinded trial of the efficacy and tolerability of sibutramine. Am J Med 1999;106:179–184.
96. Wirth A, Krause J. Long-term weight loss with sibutramine: a randomized trial. JAMA 2001;286:1331–1339.
97. Dujovne CA, Zavoral JA, Rowe A, Mendel CM. Effects of sibutramine on body weight and serum lipids: a double-blind, randomized, placebo-controlled study in 322 overweight and obese patients with dyslipidemia. Am Heart J 2001;142:489–497.
98. Bray GA, Blackburn GL, Ferguson JM, et al. Sibutramine produces dose-related weight loss. Obes Res. 1999;7:189–198.
99. Smith IG, Goulder MA. Randomized placebo-controlled trial of long-term treatment with sibutramine in mild to moderate obesity. J Fam Pract 2001;50:505–512
100. Guzman M, Sanchez C. Effects of cannabinoids on energy metabolism. Life Sci 1997;65:657–664.
101. Heshmati HM, Caplain H, Bellisle F, et al. SR14176, a selective cannabinoid CB1 receptor antagonist, reduces hunger, caloric intake, and body weight in overweight or obese men. Obes Res 2001;9(suppl 3):70S.
102. Masaki T, Yoshimatsu H, Chiba S, Watanabe T, Sakata T. Central infusion of histamine reduces fat accumulation and upregulates UCP family in leptin-resistant obese mice. Diabetes 2001;50:376–384.
103. Sakata T, Yoshimatsu H, Kurokawa M. Hypothalamic neuronal histamine—implications of its homeostatic control of energy metabolism. Nutrition 1997;13:403–411.
104. Lecklin A, Etuseppala P, Stark H, Tuomisto L. Effects of intracerebroventricularly infused histamine and selective H-1, H-2 and H-3 agonists on food and water intake and urine flow in Wistar rats. Brain Res 1998;793:279–288.
105. Ahima RS, Flier JS. Leptin. Annu Rev Physiol 2000;62:413–437.
106. Montague CT, Farooqi IS, Whitehead JP, et al. Congenital leptin deficiency is associated with severe early-onset obesity in humans. Nature 1997;387:903–908.
107. Clement K, Vaisse C, Lahlou N, et al. A mutation in the human leptin receptor gene causes obesity and pituitary dysfunction. Nature 1998;392:398–401.
108. Pelleymounter MA, Cullen MJ, Baker MB, Hecht R, et al. Effects of the obese gene product on body weight regulation in ob/ob mice. Science 1995;265:540–543.
109. Farooqi IS, Jebb SA, Langmack G, et al. Effects of recombinant therapy in a child with congenital leptin deficiency. N Engl J Med 1999;341:879–884.
110. Caro JF, Kolaczynski JW, Nyce MR, et al. Decreased cerebrospinal-fluid/serum leptin ratio in obesity: A possible mechanism for leptin resistance. Lancet 1996;348:159–161.
111. Heymsfield SB, Greenberg AS, Fujioka K, et al. Recombinant leptin for weight loss in obese and lean adults: a randomized, controlled, dose-escalation trial. JAMA 1999;282:1568–1575.
112. Hukshorn CJ, Saris WHM, Westerterp-Plantenga MS, Farid AR, Smith FJ, Campfield LA. Weekly subcutaneous pegylated recombinant native human leptin (PEG-OB) administration in obese men. J Clin Endocrinol Metab 2000;85:4003–4009.
113. ALS CNTF Treatment Study Group. A double-blind placebo controlled clinical trial of subcutaneous recombinant human ciliary neurotrophic factor (rHCNTF) in amyotrophic lateral sclerosis. Neurology 1996;46:1244–1249.
114. Hwa JJ, Witten MB, Williams P, et al. Activation of the NPY Y5 receptor regulates both feeding and energy expenditure. Am J Physiol 1999;46:R1428–R1434.

115. Hulsey MG, Pless CM, Martin RJ. ICV administration of anti-corticotropin-releasing factor antisense oligonucleotide: effects on feeding behavior and body weight. Regul Pept 1995;59:241–246.

116. Palmiter RD, Erickson JC, Hollopeter G, Baraban SC, Schwartz MW. Life without neuropeptide Y. Rec Prog Horm Res 1998;53:163–198.

117. Marsh DJ, Hollopeter G, Kafer KE, Palmiter RD. Role of the Y5 neuropeptide Y receptor in feeding and obesity. Nat Med 1998;4:718–721.

118. Pedrazzini T, Seydoux J, Kunstner P, et al. Cardiovascular response, feeding behavior and locomotor activity in mice lacking the NPY Y1 receptor. Nat Med 1998;4:722–726.

119. Bittencourt JC, Elias CF. Melanin-concentrating hormone and neuropeptide EI projections from the lateral hypothalamic area and zona incerta to the medial septal nucleus and spinal cord, a study using multiple neuronal tracers. Brain Res 1998;806:1–19.

120. Shimada M, Tritos NA, Lowell BB, Flier JS, Maratos-Flier E. Mice lacking melanin-concentrating hormone are hypophagic and lean. Nature 1998;396:670–674.

121. Ludwig DS, Tritos NA, Mastaitis JW, et al. Melanin-concentrating hormone overexpression in transgenic mice leads to obesity and insulin resistance. J Clin Invest 2001;107:379–386.

122. Crawley JN. Biological actions of galanin. Regul Pept 1995;59:1–16.

123. Wynick D, Small CJ, Bloom SR, Pachnis V. Targeted disruption of murine galanin gene. Ann NY Acad Sci 1998;863:22–47.

124. Arch JRS, Haynes AC, Cai X, et al. Orexins, new neuropeptide receptor targets for anti-obesity drugs? Int J Obes 1999;23:S16–S17.

125. Nishino S, Ripley B, Overeem S, Lammers GJ, Mignot E. Hypocretin (orexin) deficiency in human narcolepsy. Lancet 2000;355:39–40.

126. Peyron C, Faraco J, Rogers W, et al. A mutation in a case of early onset narcolepsy and a generalized absence of hypocretin peptides in human narcoleptic brains. Nat Med 2000;6:991–997.

127. Wardlaw SL. Obesity as a neuroendocrine disease: lessons to be learned from pro-opiomelanocortin and melanocortin receptor mutations in mice and men. J Clin Endocrinol Metab 2001;86:1442–1446.

128. Wisse BE, Schwartz MW. Role of melanocortins in control of obesity. Lancet 2001;857–859.

129. Fehm HL, Rudiger S, Werner K, McGregor GP, Bickel U, Born J. The melanocortin melanocyte-stimulating hormone/adrenocorticotropin$_{4-10}$ decreases body fat in humans. J Clin Endocrinol Metab 2001;86:1144–1148.

130. Wessells H, Levine N, Hadley ME, Dorr R, Hruby V. Melanocortin receptor agonists, penile erection, and sexual motivation: human studies with Melanotan II. Int J Impot Res 2000;12(suppl 4):S74–S79.

131. Wilkberg JES. Melanocortin receptors: new opportunities in drug discovery. Exp Opin Ther Patents 2001;11:61–76.

132. Merali Z, Kateb CC. Rapid alterations of hypothalamic and hippocampal bombesin-like peptide levels with feeding status. Am J Physiol 1993;265:R420–R425.

133. Yamada K, Wada E, Wada K. Bombesin-like peptides: studies on food intake and social behaviour with receptor knock-out mice. Ann Med 2000;32:519–529.

134. Behan DP, Grigoriadis DE, Lovenberg T, et al. Neurobiology of corticotropin releasing factor (CRF) receptors and CRF-binding protein: implications for the treatment of CNS disorders. Mol Psychiatry 1996;1:265–277.

135. Arase K, York DA, Shimizu H, Shargill N, Bray GA. Effects of corticotropin-releasing factor on food intake and brown adipose tissue thermogenesis in rats. Am J Physiol 1988;255:E255–E259.

136. Smith SR, de Jonge L, Pellymounter M, et al. Peripheral administration of human corticotropin-releasing hormone: a novel method to increase energy expenditure and fat oxidation in man. J Clin Endocrinol Metab 2001;86:1991–1998.

137. Spina M, Merlo-Pich E, Chan RK, et al. Appetite-suppressing effects of urocortin, a CRF-related neuropeptide. Science 1996;273:1561–1564.
138. Kristensen P, Judge ME, Thim L, et al. Hypothalamic CART is a new anorectic peptide regulated by leptin. Nature 1998;393:72–76.
139. Broglio F, Arvat E, Benso A, et al . Ghrelin, a natural GH secretagogue produced by the stomach, induces hyperglycemia and reduces insulin secretion in humans. J Clin Endocrinol Metab 2001;86:5083–5086.
140. Shintani M, Ogawa Y, Ebihara K, et al. Ghrelin, an endogenous growth hormone secreta-gogue, is a novel orexigenic peptide that antagonizes leptin action through the activation of hypothalamic neuropeptide Y/Y1 receptor pathway. Diabetes 2001;50:227–232.
141. Nagaya N, Miyatake K, Uematsu M, et al. Hemodynamic, renal, and hormonal effects of ghrelin infusion in patients with chronic heart failure. J Clin Endocrinol Metab 2001;86:5854–5859.
142. Tang-Christensen M, Larsen PJ, Goke R, et al. Central administration of GLP-1-(7-36) amide inhibits food and water intake in rats. Am J Physiol 1996;271:R848–R856.
143. Verdich C, Flint A, Gutzwiller J-P, et al. A meta-analysis of the effect of glucagon-like peptide-1 (7-36) amide on ad libitum energy intake in humans. J Clin Endocrinol Metab 2001;86:4382–4389.
144. Moran TH, Katz LF, Plata-Salaman CR, Schwartz GJ. Disordered food intake and obesity in rats lacking cholecystokinin A receptor. Am J Physiol 1998;274:R618–R625.
145. Bray GA. Afferent signals regulating food intake. Proc Nutr Soc 2000;59:373–384.
146. Lucas KH, Kaplan-Machlis B. Orlistat—a novel weight loss therapy. Ann Pharmacother 2001;35:314–328.
147. Hollander PA, Elbein SC, Hirsch IB, et al. Role of orlistat in the treatment of obese patients with type 2 diabetes: a 1 year randomized double-blind study. Diabetes Care 1998;21:1288–1294.
148. Sjostrom L, Rissanen A, Andersen T, et al. Randomised placebo-controlled trial of orlistat for weight loss and prevention of weight regain in obese patients. Lancet 1998;352:167–173.
149. Davidson MH, Hauptman J, DiGirolamo M, et al. Weight control and risk factor reduction in obese subjects treated for 2 years with Orlistat: a randomized controlled trial. JAMA 1999;281:235–242.
150. Finer N, James WPT, Kopelman PG, Lean MEJ, Williams G. One-year treatment of obesity: a randomized, double-blind, placebo-controlled, multicentre study of orlistat, a gastrointes-tinal lipase inhibitor. Int J Obes 2000;24:306–313.
151. Hauptman J, Lucas C, Boldrin MN, et al. Orlistat in the long-term treatment of obesity in primary care settings. Arch Fam Med 2000;9:160–167.
152. Muls E, Kolanowski J, Scheen A, et al. The effects of Orlistat on weight and on serum lipids in obese patients with hypercholesterolemia: a randomized, double-blind, placebo-con-trolled, multicentre study. Int J Obes 2001;25:1713–1721.
153. Loftus TM, Jaworsky DE, Frehywot GL, et al. Reduced food intake and body weight in mice treated with fatty acid synthase inhibitors. Science 2000;288:2379–2381.
154. Abu-Elheiga L, Matzuk MM, Abo-Hashema KAH, Wakil SJ. Continuous fatty acid oxidation and reduced fat storage in mice lacking acetyl-CoA carboxylase 2. Science 2001;291:2613–2616.
155. Kahn BB, Flier JS. Obesity and insulin resistance. J Clin Invest 2000;106:473–481.
156. Yamauchi T, Kamon J, Waki H, et al. The fat-derived hormone adiponectin reverses insulin resistance associated with both lipoatrophy and obesity. Nat Med 2001;7:941–946.
157. Berg AH, Combs TP, Du X, Brownlee M, Scherer PE. The adipocyte-secreted protein Acrp30 enhances hepatic insulin action. Nat Med 2001;7:947–953.
158. Fruebis J, Tsao TS, Javorschi S, et al. Proteolytic cleavage product of 30-kDa adipocyte complement-related protein increases fatty acid oxidation in muscle and causes weight loss in mice. Proc Natl Acad Sci USA 2001;98:2005–2010.

159. Gertner JM. Growth hormone actions on fat distribution and metabolism. Horm Res 38:41–43.
160. Spryer G, Ellard S, Hattersley A. Growth-hormone treatment and risk of diabetes. Lancet 2000;355:1913–1914.
161. Heffernan MA, Thorburn AW, Fam B, et al. Increase of fat oxidation and weight loss in obese mice caused by chronic treatment with human growth hormone or a modified C-terminal fragment. Int J Obes 2001;25:1442–1449.
162. Collins S, Cao W, Daniel KW, et al. Adrenoceptors, uncoupling proteins, and energy expenditure. Exp Biol Med 2001;226:982–990.

8   Dyslipidemia

Darcy Putz, MD, and
Udaya M. Kabadi, MD, FRCP(C), FACP, FACE

INTRODUCTION

Cardiovascular disease has reached epidemic proportions in the United States and throughout the world and is the leading cause of death in both men and women in the United States. For this reason, intense and extensive research efforts have been carried out to identify risk factors for coronary artery disease in order to develop preventive and treatment strategies. These investigations have demonstrated that alterations in lipid metabolism adversely affect coronary health. Fortunately, these risk factors involving lipids are amenable to modification through dietary interventions and pharmacologic therapies.

LIPID STRUCTURE AND FUNCTION

Understanding lipid structure and metabolism is integral to a knowledge of the lipid contribution to atherogenesis. Lipids are hydrophobic and insoluble in plasma and therefore cannot be transported individually in circulation. Thus, they are bound to a protein forming a lipoprotein molecule, in which they remain at the hydrophobic center surrounded by a hydrophilic shell containing phospholipids, free cholesterol, and proteins. The proteins of the hydrophilic outer shell

From: *Contemporary Endocrinology: Early Diagnosis and Treatment of Endocrine Disorders*
Edited by: R. S. Bar © Humana Press Inc., Totowa, NJ

Table 1
Characteristics of Apoproteins

Apoprotein	Lipoprotein	Function
Apo A-1	HDL, chylomicrons	LCAT activator
Apo A-II	HDL, chylomicrons	Unknown
Apo A-IV	HDL, chylomicrons	Unknown
Apo B-48	Chylomicrons	Assembly of chylomicrons in the small intestine
Apo B-100	VLDL, IDL, LDL	Ligand for LDL receptor
Apo C-I	Chylomicrons, VLDL, IDL, HDL	Inhibition of hepatic uptake of VLDL and chylomicron remnants
Apo C-II	Chylomicrons, VLDL, IDL, HDL	Activates lipoprotein lipase
Apo C-III	Chylomicrons, VLDL, IDL, HDL	Inhibits lipoprotein lipase
Apo E	Chylomicrons, VLDL, IDL, HDL	Ligand for LDL receptor
Apo(a)	Lp(a)	Covalently links with apo B to create Lp(a)

HDL, high-density lipoprotein; IDL, intermediate-density lipoprotien; LCAT, lecithin/cholesterol acyl transferase; Lp(a), lipoprotein (a); VLDL, very low-density lipoprotein.
Data from ref. *1*.

are called apoproteins and serve as either cofactors for enzymes required for lipoprotein metabolism or as ligands for receptors. The functions of the apoproteins and their associations with specific lipoproteins are summarized in Table 1 *(1)*.

There are five recognized lipoproteins categorized according to molecular weight, size, individual lipid content, and biochemical function (Table 2). All lipoproteins carry cholesterol, triglycerides, phospholipids, and apoproteins in different proportions. The largest and the least dense of the lipoproteins is the chylomicron, with triglycerides as the major constituent of its hydrophobic core. The very low-density lipoprotein (VLDL) is slightly smaller and denser, with a smaller amount of triglycerides and a greater amount of cholesterol compared with chylomicrons. The intermediate-density lipoprotein (IDL) contains both triglycerides and cholesterol esters, with a slightly higher concentration of the former. The low-density lipoprotein (LDL) and the high-density lipoprotein (HDL) carry primarily cholesterol in the hydrophobic core *(2)*. However, the major content of HDL is apoproteins.

In addition to the classically defined lipoproteins described above, yet another lipoprotein form has been identified as a risk factor in the initiation and the promotion of early aggressive atherosclerosis. Lipoprotein (a) (Lp[a]) is an LDL molecule with an apoprotein B (apo B) on its surface linked covalently to an

Table 2
Characterisitics of Lipoproteins

Lipoprotein	Density (g/dL)	TG (%)	Cholesterol (%)	Phospholipids (%)
Chylomicrons	0.95	80–95	2–7	3–9
VLDL	0.95-1.006	55–80	5–15	10–20
IDL	1.006–1.019	20–50	20–40	15–25
LDL	1.019–1.063	5–15	40–50	20–25
HDL	1.063–1.21	5–10	15–25	20–30

TG, triglycerides. For other abbreviations, see Table 1 footnote.
Data from ref. *1*.

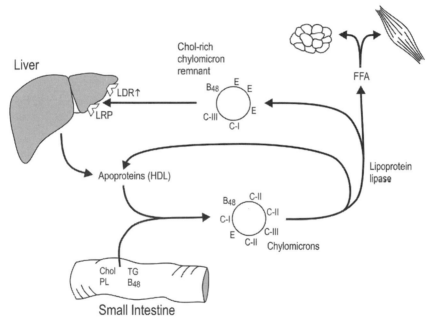

Fig 1. Transport of chylomicron and chylomicron remnants following dietary ingestion of nutrients. Chol, cholesterol; FFA, free fatty acids; HDL, high-density lipoprotien; LDR, LDL receptor; LRP, lipoprotein receptor-related protein; PL, phospholipid; TG, triglycerides.

apoprotein a. Increased levels of Lp(a) appear to accelerate the atherosclerotic process independently of other risk factors *(3)*.

There are two pathways by which the body acquires and then metabolizes lipids. In the exogenous pathway (Fig. 1), dietary cholesterol and free fatty acids derived from dietary fats are absorbed by the intestinal cells. Within the intestinal cell, cholesterol is esterified and the free fatty acids combine to synthesize triglycerides. Chylomicrons are assembled from the triglycerides and apop B-48, C-

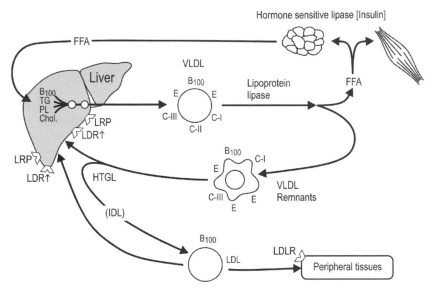

Fig. 2. Endogenous metabolic cascade for very low-density lipoprotien (VLDL), intermidiate-density lipoprotein (IDL), and low-density lipoprotein (LDL). LDLR, LDL receptor. For other abbreviations, see Fig. 1 legend.

II, and E. The chylomicrons are released into the circulation. The enzyme lipo-protein lipase (LPL) secreted by portal venous endothelium plays a key role in the subsequent metabolism of chylomicrons. This LPL uses apoprotein C-II as a cofactor, hydrolyzes the triglyceride core of the chylomicron, and converts it into the chylomicron remnant and free fatty acids, which are subsequently used by adipose and muscle tissue. The chylomicron remnant is cleared from the circulation by hepatocytes via the LDL receptor and apo E ligand action *(1)*.

The endogenous pathway of lipids involves the synthesis and metabolism of VLDL, LDL, and HDL (Fig. 2). The VLDL molecule is generated in the liver and contains primarily triglycerides at its core, whereas apo B-100, C-II, and E are found on its surface. Like chylomicrons, the triglyceride core is hydrolyzed to free fatty acids by hormone-sensitive LPL, with the key hormone being insulin. The VLDL remnant is then cleared from the circulation by hepatocytes or con-verted to LDL by the removal of additional triglyceride content by hepatic lipase. The LDL particle retains apo B-100 but loses the rest of the apoproteins *(1)*. Subsequently, the LDL molecule is removed from circulation by hepatocytes and any other nucleated cell. Within the cell, the LDL is hydrolyzed to free cholesterol, which is used to make cell membranes and hormones, or is esterified and stored. The production of cellular cholesterol *de novo* by hydroxy-methylglutaryl-coenzyme A (HMG-CoA) reductase and the regulation of LDL receptors are mediated by a feedback loop. An increase in cellular cholesterol downregulates HMG-CoA reductase and LDL receptors on the cell surface and *vice versa (2)*.

HDL cholesterol formation occurs in the intestine and the liver. The initial HDL molecule consists of phospholipids and apoproteins and acquires the requisite outer shell components, including more apoproteins, free cholesterol, and phospholipids, from the hydrolysis of VLDL and chylomicrons. The acquired free cholesterol is then esterified by an enzyme, lecithin/cholesterol acyl transferase (LCAT), and converted to LDL and triglyceride-rich lipoproteins, which are subsequently transferred back to hepatocytes. HDL also transports cholesterol to the adrenal glands and to the gonads for the synthesis of steroid hormones. The surplus free cholesterol in peripheral tissues is also collected by the HDL molecule and then converted to LDL and to triglyceride-rich lipoproteins and transported back to the liver. Finally, HDL acts as a carrier of apoproteins, which contribute to the synthesis of VLDL and chylomicrons *(2)*.

PRIMARY DISORDERS OF LIPID METABOLISM

Lipid derangements have traditionally been classified according to their Frederickson phenotype. In this classification system, phenotype I is characterized by elevated chylomicrons and a triglyceride level in the 99th percentile. Phenotype IIa includes subjects with total cholesterol levels in the 90th percentile with elevated LDL and triglyceride levels; phenotype IIb manifests as total cholesterol in the 90th percentile, with elevated LDL, VLDL, and apo B levels. Both total cholesterol and triglyceride levels are above the 90th percentile in subjects with phenotype III, whereas the VLDL and chylomicron levels are elevated. Phenotype IV is characterized by elevated concentrations of VLDL, with the total cholesterol and/or the triglyceride levels higher than the 90th percentile. The triglyceride levels in phenotype V are in the 99th percentile, with both elevated chylomicrons and VLDL levels *(4)*. However, recently, this traditional classification system has been overshadowed by a newer one based on better defined specific characteristics and patterns.

Primary Hypertriglyceridemia

FAMILIAL COMBINED HYPERLIPIDEMIA

Familial combined hyperlipidemia (FCH) is a common disorder probably inherited in an autosomal dominant fashion. Epidemiologic studies have shown that 1–2% of the general population suffer from this genetic defect and that it accounts for one-half of all cases of familial coronary artery disease *(5)*. Unfortunately, these subjects present with no overt physical manifestations of hyperlipidemia such as xanthomata. The mechanism of this disorder involves the overproduction of apo B-100 with consequential increase in VLDL and LDL, leading to significant phenotypic variations. In some patients, both hypertriglyceridemia and hypercholesterolemia ensue, whereas in others an isolated elevation of either VLDL or LDL occurs. This variability is thought to be related to the degree of the decreased function of lipoprotein lipase, the enzyme responsible for the hydrolysis of the triglyceride core of both VLDL and chylomicron *(1)*.

DISORDERS OF LIPOPROTEIN LIPASE DEFICIENCY OR APO C-II DEFICIENCY

These disorders appear to be transmitted via an autosomal recessive gene. The clinical manifestations include eruptive xanthomas, hepatomegaly, and splenomegaly. These patients complain of abdominal pain and may develop pancreatitis. Lipemia retinalis has been noted in children and adolescents with this disorder. The degree of hypertriglyceridemia is severe, with levels frequently exceeding 2000 mg/dL. The lipemia in this disorder is exacerbated by estrogens and pregnancy *(2)*. The laboratory diagnosis in these disorders is based on demonstration of chylomicronemia. However, older adult subjects may also manifest elevated levels of VLDL with decreased concentrations of both LDL and HDL *(2)*.

MIXED HYPERTRIGLYCERIDEMIA

In these disorders, the pathophysiologic mechanisms are not well defined. The clinical presentations depend on the degree of lipemia. Most patients manifest abdominal pain and pancreatitis, as well as eruptive xanthomas and lipemia retinalis. In some patients, associations with insulin resistance, hypertension, hyperuricemia, and obesity have been described *(2)*. The laboratory diagnosis is characterized by elevated levels of VLDL, representing endogenously generated lipids, and by chylomicrons, representing exogenously acquired lipids. The degree of lipemia is variable but is clearly exacerbated by alcohol intake, administration of estrogens, uncontrolled diabetes, and obesity *(2)*.

FAMILIAL DYSBETALIPOPROTEINEMIA

Familial dysbetalipoproteinemia (FD) is an autosomal recessive disorder that manifests with specific clinical findings such as tuberous xanthomas on the extensor surfaces of the elbow and knee and xanthomas of the palmar creases exhibiting an orange hue. The mechanism of disease involves apo E, a ligand for the removal of triglyceride-rich lipoproteins from the circulation. In FD, patients are homozygous for the expression of apo E2, which has a lower affinity for the LDL receptor than other apo E proteins. Consequently, VLDL and chylomicron remnants are not readily cleared and therefore accumulate in the circulation *(2)*.

Primary Disorders of LDL Metabolism

FAMILIAL HYPERCHOLESTEROLEMIA

Familial hypercholesterolemia (FH) is a common disorder occurring in 1 in every 500 people in the United States *(2)*. The clinical manifestations include tendinous xanthomatosis most commonly involving the Achilles, the patellar, and the extensor tendons of the hands. Subjects may also have xanthelasma, arcus corneae, and premature coronary artery disease. The defect in FH involves the LDL receptor. A variety of mutations can occur that lead to the absence of or a functional defect in the LDL receptor. In some subjects, the synthesis of the LDL receptor is defective. In others, the transport of the receptor to the cell surface is inhibited, whereas in still others, the LDL receptor is on the cell surface but does not bind or internalize LDL lipoproteins. Typically, the serum cholesterol level ranges from 260 to 400mg/dL (2).

FAMILIAL DEFECTIVE APO B-100

This disorder is autosomal dominant. Its clinical manifestations are similar to those of FH and include tendon xanthomas and premature coronary artery disease. In this disease, the LDL receptor is normal. However, apo B-100, the ligand for the LDL receptor, is dysfunctional. Consequently, LDL is not cleared readily from the circulation, resulting in elevated LDL cholesterol levels (2).

Lp(a) HYPERLIPOPROTEINEMIA

As previously described, Lp(a) is an LDL molecule in which the apo B protein is bound to apolipoprotein (a). Increased amounts of Lp(a) have been associated with coronary artery disease and unstable angina. Plasma levels of Lp(a) greater than 30 mg/dL are predictive of an increased risk for premature coronary artery disease (6).

SMALL, DENSE LDL PHENOTYPE

LDL cholesterol can be classified into phenotype A and phenotype B based on its size, density, and composition. LDL phenotype A molecules are larger, fluffy, and therefore less dense than phenotype B molecules. The phenotype B is associated with a greater risk of coronary artery disease. The amount of LDL phenotype B in the circulation seems to be determined by both genetic and environmental factors (7) such as diets rich in saturated fats and cholesterol.

PHYTOSTEROLEMIA (β-SITOSTEROLEMIA)

In this disorder, patients readily absorb phytosterols and cholesterol in abnormally large concentrations from the intestine, causing cholesterol levels as high as 700 mg/dL, with a predominance of LDL. Tendinous and tuberous xanthomas, premature coronary artery disease, polyarthritis, and a leukocytoclastic vasculitis are the most common manifestations of this disorder (2).

CEREBROTENDINOUS XANTHOMATOSIS

The synthesis of bile acids is defective in this disorder, which results in increased cholesterol levels and consequent accumulation of cholesterol in peripheral tissues. Progressive neurologic dysfunction resulting in dementia, spasticity, and ataxia typically ensue by the fifth decade, as well as premature coronary artery disease, cataracts, and tendinous xanthomas (2).

ABETALIPOPROTEINEMIA

Homozygotes for this disorder have essentially no apo B present in the serum secondary to a mutation in the synthesis or secretion of the apoprotein. Consequently, HDL is the only measurable cholesterol in circulation, and total cholesterol levels are typically less than 90 mg/dL. This severe deficiency in VLDL, LDL, and chylomicrons results in acanthocytic red blood cells, retinal degeneration, malabsorption of fat-soluble vitamins, and progressive neurologic degeneration, which is usually present by late childhood *(2)*.

Primary Disorders of HDL Metabolism

TANGIER DISEASE

This disorder of HDL metabolism is autosomal recessive and very rare. Patients have a very low HDL level, elevated triglycerides, and low LDL levels. Clinically, the disorder is detected in childhood or early adulthood during a routine physical exam or during assessment of a sore throat because of the typical large orange tonsils. These patients also manifest a peripheral neuropathy, hepatosplenomegaly and premature coronary artery disease *(8)*.

FAMILIAL HDL DEFICIENCY

This disorder is autosomal dominant and manifests as a serum HDL below the 50th percentile for age and gender. There are none of the systemic manifestations associated with Tangier disease *(8)*, except premature coronary artery disease.

SECONDARY CAUSES OF DYSLIPIDEMIA

The presence of dyslipidemia must be documented on more than one occasion and after a 10–12 h overnight fast in order to pursue further evaluation. Before considering a definitive therapy with antihyperlipidemic agents, secondary causes must be excluded (Table 3). Treatment with antihyperlipidemic drugs without correction of secondary causes is likely to be less than successful. The vast majority of secondary causes can be excluded with a detailed medical history, a thorough physical exam, and routine laboratory tests. A history of high saturated fat intake, alcohol binging, persistent abdominal pain, polyuria, nocturia, use of certain drugs, i.e., β-blockers or diuretics, the presence of various xanthomata, edema, jaundice, and obesity on examination; simple laboratory tests such as fasting glucose, creatinine, liver profile, thyroid-stimulating hormone, urine dipstick for protein, and bilirubin help to identify the most common secondary causes of abnormal lipid metabolism.

Diabetes Mellitus

The increased frequency of premature coronary events in subjects with diabetes is widely recognized. Although this accelerated rate of atherosclerosis is not

Table 3
Secondary Causes of Dyslipidemia

Diabetes mellitus
Hypothyroidism
Nephrotic syndrome
Chronic renal failure
Obstructive Liver Disease
Chronic use of certain medications (see in text for details)
Obesity
Diet rich in saturated fats
Syndrome X
Alcohol
Acute pancreatitis
Renal dialysis and transplantation
Dysgammaglobulinemia
Glycogen storage disorders
Porphyria

well understood, derangements in serum lipoproteins certainly play a role. Typically, subjects with both type 1 and type 2 diabetes manifest hypertriglyceridemia and low HDL levels. This metabolic abnormality occurs with hyperglycemia and seems to improve and sometimes normalize when euglycemia is attained and maintained. Moreover, abnormalities of LDL metabolism are also frequently noted in subjects with type 2 diabetes (9).

The mechanism of hypertriglyceridemia in diabetes appears to involve enhanced synthesis of triglycerides from abundantly present circulating free fatty acids because of unrestricted lipolysis owing to lack of insulin in type 1 diabetes and to insulin resistance in type 2 diabetes. Furthermore, decreased activity of insulin-dependent hormone-sensitive LPL leads to decreased metabolism and clearance of VLDL, a triglyceride-rich lipoprotein. The LDL cholesterol in type 2 diabetes is more commonly phenotype B, and is therefore, associated with a greater risk of atherosclerosis. Finally, the low HDL concentration occurs because of several metabolic derangements. Inhibition in the conversion of VLDL in the metabolic cascade may be one mechanism. Alternatively, HDL in diabetes contains more triglyceride at its core, with formation of a larger molecule causing interference in the accurate measurement of HDL. Additionally, triglyceride-enriched HDL is prone to hepatic lipase activity, with production of smaller HDL particles that are more readily cleared from the circulation (9), causing the decline in its concentration.

Hypothyroidism

In patients with hypothyroidism, the lipoprotein abnormality most commonly seen is an elevated LDL level, although elevated levels of triglycerides and Lp(a) have also been reported *(10)*. The mechanism of the lipid derangement is attributed to the decrease in the excretion of cholesterol through the biliary tree and the inhibition in the activity of hepatic lipase. With thyroid replacement therapy, the elevation in various lipids usually resolves unless other contributing factors such as diabetes or primary lipid disorders coexist *(2)*.

Nephrotic Syndrome

Lipoprotein abnormalities in nephrotic syndrome consist of an elevation in both LDL and Lp(a) levels. The HDL cholesterol in nephrotic syndrome has a greater subfraction of HDL3, which is less antiatherogenic than HDL2. The mechanism of these abnormalities is not well defined. Increased hepatic synthesis of apo B-containing lipoproteins, a decrease in LPL activity, and decreased LDL receptor-mediated clearance of LDL *(11)* have been implicated.

Chronic Renal Failure

Chronic renal failure (CRF) lipoprotein abnormalities are characterized by hypertriglyceridemia and a reduced HDL. The LDL particles in CRF tend to be of the phenotype B variety and therefore are more atherogenic. Atherogenicity is further enhanced by elevated Lp(a) levels. Decreased activity of both LPL and hepatic lipase are presumed to induce decreased clearance of triglyceride-rich lipoproteins. Unfortunately, these abnormalities do not resolve with the institution of dialysis or transplantation *(11)*.

Obstructive Liver Disease

Primary biliary cirrhosis and other cholestatic liver disorders are associated with abnormalities in lipid metabolism. Classically, elevated LDL and decreased HDL levels are noted in the advanced stages of the disease *(12)*, with cholesterol deposition manifesting as planar xanthomas and possibly also as peripheral neuropathies *(2)*.

Drugs

Many patients with hyperlipidemia frequently suffer from other comorbid disorders and therefore receive complicated regimens of medications. Several of these medications contribute to lipid abnormalities. The most frequently implicated drugs are diuretics, β-blockers, sex steroids, glucocorticoids, cyclosporine, retinoids, and antiretrovirals.

Hydrochlorothiazide and chorthalidone have both been shown to induce adverse effects on lipid profiles, causing increases in both the LDL and triglyceride levels. βblockers raise the triglycerides and also appear to lower the HDL level. The steroid hormones have variable effects on lipid metabolism. Anabolic androgens decrease the HDL and increase the LDL levels, but physiologic replacement of testosterone, administered topically as a patch or gel, does not appear to have a significant effect on lipids. Unopposed estrogen therapy, especially in the supraphysiologic doses associated with oral contraceptives, may cause a significant elevation in triglycerides in women susceptible to or demonstrating underlying lipid abnormalities, whereas the selective estrogen receptor modulator raloxifene decreases LDL and increases triglyceride levels. Cyclosporine administration used in subjects with transplants is also associated with variable forms of dyslipidemia, with raised LDL and triglycerides being the most frequent. Oral retinoids are documented to raise triglyceride and LDL levels and lower HDL levels *(13)*. Most recently, the antiretrovirals have been recognized to cause both hypertriglyceridemia and hypercholesterolemia *(14)*. Finally, although these drug-induced dyslipidemias are well documented, the exact mechanisms remain to be elucidated.

DIAGNOSIS

Clinical Features

Most patients with lipid abnormalities do not present with clinical manifestations. However, the presence of certain clinical manifestations prompt evaluation of serum lipids in an individual patient. Xanthelasma, tendinous xanthomas, palmar xanthomas, orange tonsils, lipemia retinalis, and arcus corneae may indicate a specific lipid disorder. Recurrent abdominal pain may also indicate the presence of markedly elevated triglyceride levels.

SCREENING

The National Cholesterol Education Panel (NCEP) recently published its updated guidelines on the detection, evaluation, and treatment of hyperlipidemia *(15)*. These guidelines recommend the determination of a complete lipid profile, including total cholesterol, HDL, LDL, and triglyceride levels after an overnight 10–12 h fast, in all adults 20 yr of age or older at intervals of 5 yr. As an alternative, a serum total cholesterol and HDL level may be determined in nonfasting patients. However, if a total cholesterol level of more than 200 mg/dL or an HDL level of less than 40 mg/dL is noted in a nonfasting state, a full lipid profile must be obtained in order to design management strategies. The NCEP recommends that the risk factors for coronary artery disease be evaluated and used with the LDL level to determine the intensity of treatment. The highest risk category encompasses subjects with known coronary artery disease or those with coronary artery disease risk equivalents such as diabetes, current cigarette smoking,

Table 4
Risk Factors for Coronary Artery Disease (Leading to Screening for Dyslipidemia)[a]

Everyone at age 20 yr or older should be screened every 5 yr
Physical exam findings suggestive of abnormal lipids such as xanthelasma, xanthomas,
    or arcus corneae
Diabetes or impaired glucose tolerance
Visceral obesity
Chronic use of medications that alter lipid metabolism (diuretics, β-blockers, sex steroids,
    glucocorticoids, cyclosporine, retinoids, antiretrovirals)
Cigarette smoking
Hypertension (blood pressure > 140/90 mmHg or on antihypertensive agents)
Previous history of low HDL (< 40 mg/dL)
Family history of premature coronary artery disease (male first-degree relative younger
    than 55 yr and female first-degree relative younger than 65 yr)
Age: (men 45yr old or more and women 55 yr old or more)

HDL, high-density lipoprotein.
[a]The screening test of choice would be a fasting lipid profile obtained after a 10–12 h fast.

hypertension, low HDL, a family history of premature coronary artery disease, age, and gender (Table 4). Moreover, the 10-yr risk of coronary artery disease may be examined by the Framingham risk assessment criteria described in the new NCEP guidelines (15). A subject with two major risk factors and a 10-yr risk of 20% or higher belongs to the highest risk category and should receive the most intensive therapeutic regimen, with a target LDL of less than 100 mg/dL (15). The intermediate-risk category includes subjects with at least two major risk factors for coronary artery disease but with a 10-yr risk of less than 20% based on risk stratification (15). The recommended therapeutic goals for this population are somewhat less stringent with an LDL target of less than 130 mg/dL. Finally, the lowest risk category has less than two major risk factors for coronary artery disease and the desirable LDL concentration of less than 160 mg/dL.

MANAGEMENT OF DYSLIPIDEMIA

Rationale

Without a doubt, coronary artery disease is associated with significant morbidity and mortality. Therefore, researchers have spent tremendous amounts of time and resources in arriving at interventions to prevent or delay the onset and retard the progression of this disease. Most of these research efforts have been directed toward lowering LDL levels, since elevated LDL concentrations have been clearly linked to coronary artery disease.

Prior to the introduction of statins or HMG CoA-reductase inhibitors, three major clinical trials attempting primary prevention of coronary artery disease through the use of other LDL-lowering medications were conducted. The World Health Organization (WHO) Cooperative Trial, using clofibrate to reduce serum cholesterol levels (16), documented a 20% reduction in first major coronary events and a 25% reduction in nonfatal myocardial infarctions. However, the all-cause mortality rate was significantly higher in the clofibrate-treated group, raising concerns regarding safety. Another trial, the Lipid Research Clinics Coronary Primary Prevention Trial, demonstrated the efficacy of cholestyramine in reducing the number of coronary artery disease deaths (–24%) and the number of nonfatal myocardial infarctions (–19%), with no significant rise in the all-cause mortality (17). In the later Helsinki Heart Study in 1987 (18), gemfibrozil was shown to be efficacious in the primary prevention of coronary artery disease, with a decline in events of 34%. However, once again, the overall mortality in the treatment group remained the same as that in the control group.

With the advent of the statins, several primary and secondary prevention trials followed and are being continued. The West of Scotland Coronary Prevention Study Group (WOSCOPS) clearly demonstrated the efficacy of pravastatin in decreasing the risk of a fatal coronary events by 31% and the all-cause death rate by 22% (19) in men without known coronary artery disease. In another primary prevention trial, the Air Force/Texas Coronary Atherosclerosis Prevention Study (AFCAPS/TexCAPS) (20), lowering cholesterol concentrations with lovastatin decreased the relative risk of first major coronary events, myocardial infarctions, episodes of unstable angina, and coronary revascularization procedures in both men and women with mildly elevated serum total and LDL cholesterol levels.

The secondary prevention trials with the statins have been equally compelling. The Scandinavian Simvastatin Survival Study (4S) demonstrated a relative risk reduction in nonfatal coronary events, fatal coronary events, and all-cause mortality (21). The Cholesterol and Recurrent Events (CARE) study specifically examined subjects with known coronary artery disease and average lipid levels (22). This study demonstrated that the administration of pravastatin induced a 24% risk reduction for nonfatal and fatal coronary events in subjects with a total cholesterol of less than 240 mg/dL with a mean LDL-C of 139 mg/dL. More recently, the Long-Term Intervention with Pravastatin in Ischemic Disease (LIPID) study group has shown a reduction in mortality from both coronary heart disease (24%) and all causes (22%) in subjects with known coronary artery disease (23). Most recently, the Myocardial Ischemia Reduction with Aggressive Cholesterol Lowering (MIRACL) study demonstrated that high-dose atorvastatin, initiated within several hours of an acute coronary syndrome, significantly reduced the risk of death, nonfatal myocardial infarction, cardiac arrest, and worsening angina as well as the incidence of both fatal and nonfatal strokes (24). Thus, in the final analysis, treatment with lipid-lowering agents clearly and unquestionably appears to improve both primary and secondary prevention of coronary artery disease in subjects with hyperlipidemia.

Table 5
Low-Density Lipoprotein (LDL) Cholesterol Goals

Risk category	LDL goal (mg/dL)	LDL requiring dietary therapy	LDL requiring drug therapy
Highest risk— coronary artery disease or equivalents	<100	≥100	≥130; may consider at 100–129
Intermediate risk—two risk factors and 10-yr risk <20%	<130	≥130	≥130 for a 10-yr risk of 10–20% ≥160 for a 10-yr risk of <10%
Lowest risk— none to one risk factors	<160	≥160	≥190, may consider at 160–189

Data from ref. 15.

Guidelines for the Treatment of Dyslipidemia

With the recent knowledge regarding the efficacy of therapy with statins, the new NCEP recommendations evolved (Table 5). In the highest risk category, the NCEP recommends that both lifestyle modifications and drug therapy be initiated at diagnosis if the baseline LDL-C exceeds130 mg/dL. However, LDL-C levels between 100 and 129 mg/dL may necessitate either intensification of lifestyle modification and/or initiation of drug therapy at the discretion of the provider. Subjects in the intermediate-risk category are divided into two further subgroups, one with the 10-yr risk of 10–20% and the other with a 10-yr risk of less than 10% according to the Framingham risk stratification criteria. In the first subgroup, the NCEP recommends lifestyle modification for the initial 3 mo and later adjunctive drug therapy if the LDL-C level remains above 130 mg/dL. In the other subgroup, lifestyle changes should be instituted with a later addition of drug therapy if LDL-C of less than 160 mg/dL is not attained. However, many providers consider this goal less than adequate and use drugs to lower LDL below 130 mg/dL. Finally, the same recommendations were suggested by the NCEP for subjects in the low-risk category. Nevertheless, for most health care providers the LDL goal remains at less than 130 mg/dL in this group as well (Table 6). In addition, the decision to initiate drug therapy at diagnosis may be based on the presence of a single severe risk factor, multiple life-habit risk factors, or a 10-yr risk approaching 10%. Finally, if the LDL-C is greater than 190 mg/dL, drug

Table 6
Absolute Risk (%) of Developing Coronary Artery Disease
over 10 Years Based on Risk Factors

Risk factor	Absolute risk (%) with LDL of 130 mg/dL
Age 50 yr in men	6%
Hypertension: BP145/95 mmHg or on antihypertensive medications	10%
Smoking	20%

Data from ref. *15*.

treatment may be initiated with simultaneous emphasis on lifestyle modifications *(15)*.

Management Options

The tools that are available for disorders of lipid metabolism include therapeutic lifestyle changes and drugs. Weight loss, increased physical activity, and attention to diet form the first-line options (Table 7). The Mediterranean diet has been distinctly effective in achieving improvements in lipid profiles. However, it may not be appropriate for all ethnic populations to incorporate this diet because of differing cultural eating habits. Unfortunately, lifestyle changes are inherently difficult to maintain, and therefore patients frequently fail to attain the lipid goals, necessitating pharmacologic interventions. The appropriate choice of drugs should be focused on the type of the predominantly elevated lipid, namely, elevation of triglycerides, LDL, or both as well as the level of HDL-C.

For the lowering of total and LDL cholesterol levels, the most common agents presently used are the statins. These drugs are competitive inhibitors of HMG CoA reductase because they are similar in structure to HMG-CoA. Their inhibitory activity leads to the upregulation of LDL receptors and a decrease in release of LDL into the circulation. All statins primarily lower LDL-C, with variable reductions in triglycerides and increases in HDL. The most cost-effective of these appears to be atorvastatin *(25)*. The most common side effects are gastrointestinal upset, myalgias, and hepatic dysfunction. Rare side effects described are insomnia, vivid dreams, neuropathies, and rashes. The myositis, rhabdomyolysis, and hepatic dysfunction seem to occur more frequently in subjects simultaneously receiving other drugs metabolized by the cytochrome P450 system because of the occurrence of undesirable circulating levels of statins. Therefore, transaminases must be checked within the first 12 wk of treatment and periodically thereafter to avoid hepatotoxicity. The combination of any statin with niacin or fibrates has been reported to cause a myositis and rhabdomyolysis with a significant prevalence in the elderly with impaired renal function *(26)*.

Table 7
Dietary Modifications for Cholesterol-Lowering

Component	Modification
Total calories	Enough to maintain or lose desired weight
Protein	15% of total calories
Carbohydrate	50–60% of total calories
Total fat	25–35% of total calories
Saturated fat	<7% of total calories
Polyunsaturated fat	Up to 10% of total calories
Monounsaturated fat	Up to 20% of total calories
Fiber	20–30 g
Cholesterol	<200 mg/d

The resins such as cholestyramine and colestipol bind bile acids in the intestine, inducing interruption of their circulation to the liver via the portal vein and therefore enhancing excretion. This process promotes greater synthesis of bile acids by the liver using circulating cholesterol. However, the resins also promote VLDL synthesis by the liver and may cause a worsening of hypertriglyceridemia. The most common side effects of the resins include abdominal bloating, borborygmi, and constipation. In addition, these drugs tend to bind to other compounds besides bile acids and to inhibit their absorption. Therefore, they should not be administered with other medications (26). Finally, resins also inhibit the absorption of fat because of the unavailability of bile acids and may induce a deficiency of fat-soluble vitamins in the long term.

Niacin, the oldest of the lipid-lowering agents, is documented to have various effects on lipid metabolism. Mobilization of free fatty acids from peripheral tissues is inhibited by niacin, resulting in decreased synthesis of VLDL and therefore reduction in circulating triglycerides. Niacin also lowers Lp(a) levels, transforms phenotype B LDL to less atherogenic LDL, and increases serum HDL levels. Thus, niacin is the only agent that influences lipid metabolism toward a healthy outcome. However, few subjects tolerate niacin because of the frequent occurrence of side effects, the most frequent being cutaneous flushing. This side effect can be alleviated in some patients with administration of aspirin 1/2 h after each meal followed by a dose of niacin. Liver enzymes rise frequently with niacin administration. However, this does not pose a hazard and does not necessitate withdrawal unless these enzymes continue to rise instead of reaching a plateau. Hepatic dysfunction is more common with niacin at doses greater than 2 g compared with the statins. Unfortunately, the effective dose of niacin is usually 3–6 g/d. In addition, niacin may induce impaired glucose tolerance in susceptible populations and may worsen hyperglycemia in subjects with diabetes. Moreover, it may also raise uric acid levels with precipitation of gout in susceptible subjects. Another common side effect of niacin is gastrointestinal disturbances. Flushing is more common with short-acting preparations whereas gastrointestinal problems occur frequently with the sustained-release compound. Typically, niacin is used in combination with a statin or a resin *(26)*.

The fibrates, such as clofibrate, gemfibrozil, and fenofibrate, form the mainstay of therapy for lowering triglyceride levels. They facilitate the oxidation of free fatty acids by the liver and muscle, resulting in a decrease in release of VLDL into the circulation. They also tend to increase both LDL and HDL if the baseline concentrations are especially low. However, in the presence of both elevated triglyceride and LDL levels, the fibrates may lower the LDL. The most common side effects include gastrointestinal upset, increase in gallstone formation, and increased serum transaminases. Clofibrate can cause erectile dysfunction and the syndrome of inappropriate diuretic hormone (SIADH) and is rarely used at present because of the availability of safer, newer compunds. Finally, all the fibrates can cause myositis and rhabdomyolysis when used in patients with impaired renal function, especially when administered in combination with statins *(26)*.

Unfortunately, some subjects will not be able to tolerate the traditional lipid-lowering agents. Other therapies such as fiber in the form of oat bran or psyllium powder, orlistat, neomycin, and dextrothyroxine have been shown to be somewhat efficacious. In the past, intestinal bypass surgery had been used, but it led to significant morbidity. In children with a deficiency of the LDL receptor, a liver transplant has proved to be an effective therapy.

REFERENCES

1. Ginsberg, Henry N. Lipoprotein physiology. Endocrinol Metab Clin N Am 1998;27:503–520.
2. Malloy M, Kane J. Disorders of lipoprotein metabolism. In: Greenspan and Gardner, eds. Basic and Clinical Endocrinology, 6th ed., McGraw-Hill, New York, 2001, pp. 716–744.
3. Brown G, Stewart BF, Zhao XQ, Hinger LA, Poulin D, Albers JJ. What benefit can be derived from treating normocholesterolemic patients with coronary artery disease? Am J Cardiol 1995;76:93C–97C.
4. Frederickson D. An international classification of hyperlipidemias and hyperprotcinemias. Ann Int Med 1971;75:471.
5. Williams RR, Hopkins PN, Hunt SC, et al. Population based frequency of dyslipidemia syndromes in coronary-prone families in Utah. Arch Int Med 1990;150:582–588.
6. Stein J, Rosenson R. Lipoprotein Lp(a) excess and coronary heart disease. Arch Int Med 1997;157:1170–1176.
7. Slyper A. Low-density lipoprotein density and atherosclerosis. JAMA 1994;272:305–308.
8. Davignon J, Genest J Jr. Genetics of lipoprotein disorders. Endrocrinol Metab Clin N Am 1998;27:521–550.
9. Goldberg I. Diabetic dyslipidemia: causes and consequences. J Clin Endocrinol Metab 2001;86:965–971.
10. Pucci E, Chiovato L, Pinchera A. Thyroid and lipid metabolism. Int J Obes 2000;24:s109–s112.
11. Mujamdar A, Wheeler D. Lipid abnormalities in renal disease. J Roy Soc Med 2000;93:178–182.
12. Crippin J, Lindor KD, Jorgensen R, et al. Hypercholesterolemia and atherosclerosis in primary biliary cirrhosis: what is the risk? Hepatology 1992;15:858–862.

13. Donahoo W, Kosmiski L, Eckel R. Drugs causing dyslipoproteinemia. Endocrinol Metab Clin N Am 1998;27:677–698.
14. Manfredi R, Chiodo F. Disorders of lipid metabolism in patients with HIV disease treated with antiretroviral agents. J Infect 2001; 42:181–188.
15. Expert Panel. Executive summary of the third report of the National Cholesterol Education Program Expert Panel on Detection, Evaluation, and Treatment of High Blood Cholesteol in Adults. JAMA 2001;285:2486–2497.
16. Report of Committee of Prinicipal Investigators. WHO cooperative trial on primary prevention of ischaemic heart disease using clofibrate to lower serum cholesterol: mortality follow-up. Lancet 1980;2:379–385.
17. Lipid Research Clinics Program. The lipid research clinics coronary primary prevention trial results. JAMA 1984;251:351–364.
18. Frick M, Elo O, Haapa K, et al. Helsinki heart study: primary prevention tiral with gemfibrozil in middle-aged men with dyslipidemia. N Engl J Med 1987;317:1237–1245.
19. Sheperd J, Cobbe SM, Ford I, et al. Prevention of coronary heart disease with pravastatin in men with hypercholesterolemia. N Engl J Med 1995;333:1301–1307.
20. Downs J, Clearfield M, Wies S, et al. Primary prevention of acute coronary events with lovastatin in men and women with average cholesterol levels. Results of AFCAPS/TexCAPS. Air Force/Texas Coronary Atherosclerosis Prevention Study. JAMA 1998;279:1615–1622.
21. Scandinavian Simvastatin Survival Study Group. Randomised trial of cholesterol lowering in 4444 patients with coronary heart disease: the Scandinavian Simvastatin Survival Study (4S). Lancet 1994;344:1383–1389.
22. Sacks F, Pfeffer MA, Moye LA, et al. The effect of pravastatin on coronary events after myocardial infarction in patients with average cholesterol levels. N Engl J Med 1996;335:1001–1009.
23. The Long-Term Intervention with Pravastatin in Ischaemic Disease (LIPID) Study Group. Prevention of cardiovascular events and death with pravastatin in patients with coronary heart disease and a broad range of initial cholesterol levels. N Engl J Med 1998;339:1349–1357.
24. Schwartz GG, Olsson AG, Ezekowitz MD, et al. Effects of atorvastatin on early recurrent ischemic events in acute coronary syndromes. JAMA 2001;285:1711–1718.
25. Jones P, Kafonek S, Laapora I, Hunninghake D, et al. Comparative dose efficacy study of atorvastatin versus simvastatin, pravastatin, lovastatin, and fluvastatin in patients with hypercholesterolemia. Am J Cardiol 1998;81:582–587.
26. Knopp R. Drug treatment of lipid disorders. N Engl J Med 1999;341:498–511.

9

Polycystic Ovarian Syndrome

Anuja Dokras, MD, PhD, and William I. Sivitz, MD

CONTENTS

INTRODUCTION

Polycystic ovarian syndrome (PCOS) is the most common endocrine disorder in women of reproductive age. The clinical presentation commonly includes infertility, irregular menses, obesity, and hirsutism, and hence women may initially present to the gynecologist or reproductive endocrinologist. However, women with PCOS are also at an increased risk for a number of medical problems including diabetes, hypertension, coronary artery disease, and endometrial cancer and may first present to an internist, medical endocrinologist, gynecologic oncologist, or cardiologist. Thus, PCOS is a multifaceted endocrine and metabolic disorder, which needs early recognition and treatment to prevent long-term complications. In this chapter we present current views on diagnosis and therapy.

PCOS affects 5–10% of premenopausal women *(1)*. It is characterized by chronic anovulation and hyperandrogenism soon after puberty. Drs. Stein and Leventhal first described PCOS in 1935 in seven women with amenorrhea, hirsutism, and enlarged polycystic ovaries *(2)*. These ovaries are classically associated with multiple 2–8-mm cysts in a peripheral location, as well as a hypervascular, androgen-secreting ovarian stroma that is typically increased in

From: *Contemporary Endocrinology: Early Diagnosis and Treatment of Endocrine Disorders*
Edited by: R. S. Bar © Humana Press Inc., Totowa, NJ

Table 1
Frequency of Clinical and Laboratory Features Associated
with Polycystic Ovarian Syndrome

Feature	Frequency (%)
Chronic oligomenorrhea or anovulation	90
Hyperandrogenism - hirsutism, acne	70
Obesity	35–60
Polycystic ovaries on TVUS	70
Hyperinsulinemia	50–70

TVUS, transvaginal ultrasound.

volume. The clinical manifestations include hirsutism, acne, alopecia associated with androgen excess and obesity, menstrual irregularities (amenorrhea, oligomenorrhea), and infertility secondary to chronic anovulation *(3)*.

Given the variability in the clinical presentation, there is no strict definition for this syndrome. The 1990 National Institutes of Health-National Institute of Child Health and Development (NIH-NICHD) consensus conference stipulated that clinical symptoms including chronic oligo-ovulation or anovulation and hyperandrogenism should serve as the selection criteria for the syndrome, and hormonal results should be used to exclude related disorders of the pituitary, adrenals, and ovary *(4)*. The frequency with which women exhibit these features is shown in Table 1. Lean women may also exhibit features of PCOS and usually have elevated luteinizing hormone levels (LH) but normal insulin levels. Another subtype includes the HAIR-AN syndrome, characterized by hyperandrogenism, severe insulin resistance, acanthosis nigricans, and missense mutations in the insulin receptor *(5,6)*.

PATHOPHYSIOLOGY

The two-cell, two-gonadotropin system needs to be reviewed in order to understand the pathophysiology of PCOS. In preantral and antral ovarian follicles, LH receptors are present on theca cells, and LH plays a significant role in steroidogenesis by regulating the entry of cholesterol into the cell and further conversion of cholesterol to androgens *(7)*. The conversion of progesterone and 17-hydroxyprogesterone to androstenedione is catalyzed by the enzymes 17α-hydroxylase and 17,20 lyase. Both these steps are regulated by p450c17α and are under the influence of factors such as amplitude of LH secretion, insulinemia, and insulin-like growth factors (IGFs) (Fig. 1). During the menstrual cycle, androstenedione is used as a substrate by the granulosa cells and converted by the enzyme aromatase to estradiol. In women with polycystic ovaries, elevated levels of androgens within the theca cells inhibit aromatase activity, and androgens

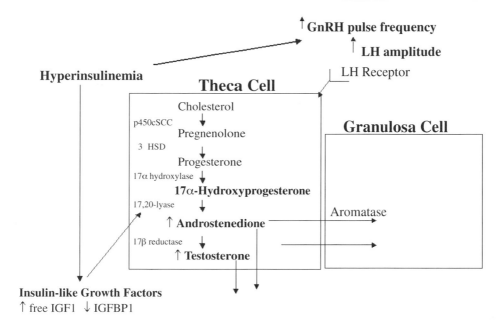

Fig. 1. Schematic depiction of factors regulating the production of androgens by the theca cell of the ovary. The conversion of cholesterol into androstenedione and testosterone within the theca cell is regulated by cytochrome p45017α enzymes (17α-hydroxylase and 17,20-lyase). These are further regulated by factors such as hyperinsulinemia and increased free insulin-like growth factor (IGF)-1. Elevated androgens within the theca cell inhibit the actions of aromatase and hence formation of estrogens in the granulosa cell. GnRH, gonadotropin-releasing hormone; IGFBP1, IGF binding protein 1; LH, luteinizing hormone.

are converted to their 5α metabolites *(8)*. Hence, the follicles are unable to change their microenvironment from androgen dominance to estrogen dominance. Although new follicular growth is continuously stimulated in the ovary in response to normal follicle-stimulating hormone (FSH) concentrations, the follicles fail to achieve complete maturation, contributing to the polycystic appearance. The increased estrogen levels in women with PCOS can be explained on the basis of peripheral conversion of androstenedione to estrone.

The underlying mechanisms that lead to the dysregulation of relationships among the hypothalamus, pituitary, and the ovary (resulting in elevated intracellular and peripheral androgens) still need investigation. Recently hyperinsulinemia and insulin resistance have been implicated as pivotal in the pathogenesis of PCOS through a number of mechanisms (Fig. 2), including direct action on the theca cells; increasing the amplitude of LH secreted by the pituitary; decreasing sex hormone binding globulin (SHBG) secretion by the

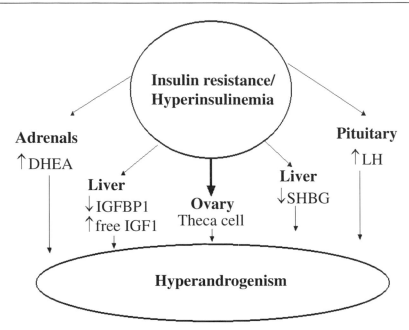

Fig. 2. The effects of hyperinsulinemia on a number of organs contribute to peripheral hyperandrogenism. Hyperinsulinemia directly or via luteinizing hormone (LH; pituitary) and the insulin-like growth factor (IGF) system (liver) increases ovarian androgen production. Elevated insulin levels can increase adrenal production of dehydroandrostenedione (DHEA), which may be reflected as elevated DHEA sulfate levels. A decrease in sex hormone binding globulin (SHBG) secondary to hyperinsulinemia results in elevated free androgen levels. IGFBP1, IGF binding protein 1.

liver; decreasing insulin-like growth factor binding protein 1 (IGFBP-1), thereby increasing free IGF-1; and possibly increasing dehydroandrostenedione (DHEA) secretion from the adrenals. The theca-interstitial compartment of the ovary contains an intact IGF system, with both ligands and receptors supporting its role in ovarian androgen production. Both insulin and IGFs have been shown to synergize with LH in vitro to modulate steroidogenesis and especially androgen production *(9–12)*. Furthermore, insulin may also act via the IGF-1 receptor to increase androgen production in thecal cells *(13)*. In many women, both the pulse amplitude and the frequency of LH are abnormally increased, resulting in chronically increased circulating LH concentrations. This may be an insulin effect or may reflect an increase in gonadotropin-releasing hormone (GnRH) pulsatile secretion *(14)*.

    To summarize, a number of aberrations develop in women with PCOS that (alone or in combination) lead to anovulation. The characteristic polycystic ovary develops when the state of anovulation persists for a long time.

Polycystic Ovarian Syndrome and Insulin Resistance

The association between insulin resistance and PCOS has been well recognized for almost two decades. Insulin resistance refers to an impairment of insulin-stimulated glucose uptake largely in skeletal muscle and an impairment in insulin-mediated inhibition of hepatic glucose output. In skeletal muscle and fat, insulin initiates several intracellular signals culminating in GLUT 4-mediated glucose uptake. Insulin also has a vasodilator effect on the normal skeletal muscle vasculature mediated by stimulation of endothelium-derived nitric oxide (NO). In endothelial cells in vitro, insulin-stimulated NO production shares signaling pathways similar to those mediating glucose uptake in muscle and fat (15–17).

The presence of insulin resistance leads to increased β-cell insulin secretion with compensatory hyperinsulinemia. Type 2 diabetes mellitus (DM) develops when insulin resistance is accompanied by β-cell dysfunction (15). Although a controlled randomized study has not been performed to determine the exact incidence, insulin resistance is present in approximately 50–75% of women with PCOS (18). Many women with PCOS also have insulin resistance independent of obesity (19). In 50% of women with PCOS, insulin resistance appears to be related to excessive insulin-independent serine phosphorylation of the β-subunit of the insulin receptor, which probably modulates the activity of the key regulatory enzyme of androgen biosynthesis, cytochrome P450c17α (20).

Hyperinsulinemia and insulin resistance are thought to play a critical role in the pathogenesis of PCOS and are associated with a high risk for type 2 DM, hypertension, hyperlipidemia, and atherogenesis (Fig. 3). Obese, premenopausal women with PCOS have a 31% incidence of impaired glucose tolerance, and 7.5% develop overt diabetes (6,21). Hypertension is uncommon in young women with PCOS, but its prevalence increases to 40% in the perimenopausal period (22). Although hypertension is common in patients with insulin resistance, it is unclear whether this is secondary to direct sympathetic activation by insulin or to insulin resistance to insulin-mediated vasodilation (23). Approximately 50–60% of women with PCOS have android obesity, with increased waist-hip ratio and an associated abnormal lipid profile—high triglyceride and low-density lipoprotein (LDL) cholesterol and low high-density lipoprotein (HDL) and apolipoprotein A-I levels (24). Also, impaired fibrinolytic activity reflected by increased plasminogen activator inhibitor-1 (PAI-1) levels have been found in women with PCOS (25,26).

Hence women with PCOS have a cluster of potent cardiovascular risk factors. Hyperinsulinemia and insulin resistance are often associated with central obesity, hypertension, dyslipidemia, atherosclerosis, and a predisposition to type 2 DM (Fig. 4). This constellation of features is known as the insulin resistance syndrome or metabolic syndrome X (27). The Quebec Cardiovascular Study demonstrated that hyperinsulinemia is an independent risk factor for develop-

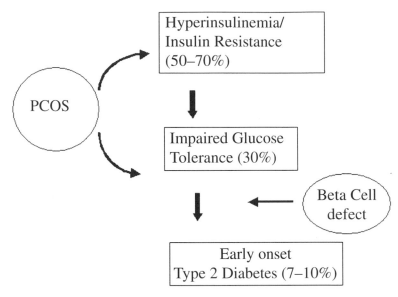

Fig. 3. Frequency of progression from hyperinsulinemia to type 2 DM in women with polycystic ovarian syndrome (PCOS). Approximately 50–70% of women with PCOS have hyperinsulinemia or insulin resistance, 30% have impaired glucose tolerance, and 7–10% have early-onset type 2 DM. It is not clear whether the earliest defect in the progression from normal glucose tolerance to diabetes is insulin resistance or a subtle defect in insulin secretion. However, insulin resistance is substantial early in the course, and diabetes appears to develop when insulin secretion can no longer keep up with the increased demand imparted by the resistance.

ment of coronary artery disease (28). The Insulin Resistance and Atherosclerosis Study (IRAS) was the first large epidemiologic study to report a direct relationship between insulin resistance and carotid artery thickness (an indicator of atherosclerosis) in Hispanic and non-Hispanic white subjects (29). Several studies have estimated that women with PCOS are at an increased risk for development of complications of coronary and cerebrovascular atherosclerosis, up to even four- to fivefold (31–34). Subclinical atherosclerosis has been demonstrated by carotid ultrasonography to be prevalent in premenopausal women with a history of anovulation and PCOS (30). In women undergoing coronary angiography, women with PCOS have been observed to have more extensive coronary artery disease (32). Therefore, it is not surprising that PCOS patients have a sevenfold increased risk for myocardial infarction (22). It is also of interest that hyperinsulinemia correlates significantly with a higher cardiovascular risk profile in these women independent of obesity (35).

The endothelium is the target organ for a variety of cardiovascular risk factors. Several studies have shown a correlation between endothelial dysfunction and

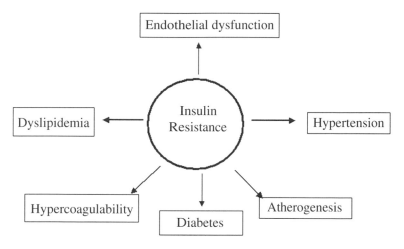

Fig. 4. Potential effects of insulin resistance on known cardiovascular risk factors.

smoking, hypercholesterolemia, hypertension, poorly controlled type 1 and type 2 diabetes, and the obesity/insulin-resistant state *(15,36)*. A recent study reported a significant association between endothelial dysfunction and insulin resistance in young first-degree relatives of patients with type 2 diabetes independent of the traditional cardiovascular risk factors *(37)*. One study has evaluated the effects of PCOS on endothelial function and reported no change in endothelial function in the conduit vessels. However, a major limitation of this study was the failure to evaluate the resistance vasculature. Another study recently showed evidence of endothelial dysfunction in women with PCOS *(38)*. A recent observation that may have important clinical implications is that metformin selectively improves endothelium-dependent dilation by acetylcholine in patients with type 2 DM *(39)*. However, the potential for these drugs to ameliorate endothelial dysfunction and the elevated cardiovascular risk in women with PCOS has not been systematically evaluated.

DIAGNOSIS

The clinical diagnosis of PCOS is usually made based on the history of oligomenorrhea or amenorrhea and hirsutism with or without obesity. The menstrual abnormalities of PCOS could also present as intermittent breakthrough bleeding, dysfunctional uterine bleeding, or menometrorrhagia. Some women may have regular cycles after puberty and then develop oligomenorrhea associated with weight gain. Hirsutism is excess terminal hair in a male distribution and is commonly noted on the upper lip, as sideburns, around the nipples, and as a linea alba on the lower abdomen and inner thighs.

Table 2
Recommended Laboratory Tests To Evaluate
Women with Features Suggestive of Polycystic
Ovarian Syndrome (Irregular Periods and Hirsutism)[a]

TSH, prolactin
Total testosterone
17-Hydroxy progesterone, DHEAS
Fasting glucose, fasting insulin
2-h GTT (if fasting glucose $\geq$ 110 mg/100 mL)
Fasting lipid panel

DHEAS, dehydroandrostenedione sulfate; GTT, glucose tolerance test; TSH, thyroid-stimulating hormone.

[a]Total testosterone levels are usually measured in women with worsening hirsutism.

The current laboratory tests suggested in the evaluation of women with PCOS are summarized in Table 2. Traditionally, the LH/follicle-stimulating hormone (FSH) ratio was determined and found to be elevated at least twofold in about 40–50% of these women. In addition, peripheral androgens (androstenedione, testosterone, and free testosterone) are elevated and SHBG levels reduced in many of these patients. Of these tests, we recommend only the testosterone level, which is useful to rule out a testosterone-producing tumor in patients with severe or rapidly progressing hirsutism (total testosterone > 200 ng/mL).

Other endocrine disorders to be considered in the differential diagnosis include hypothyroidism, hyperprolactinemia, adult-onset adrenal hyperplasia, and an adrenal source of androgens. To exclude these conditions, we check thyroid-stimulating hormone (TSH), 17-hydroxyprogesterone, and dehydroepiandro-stenedione sulfate (DHEA-S) levels. (The sulfated form of DHEA is measured in serum.)

Because of the strong association of diabetes with PCOS, we now recommend a test for insulin resistance. However, the more specific and sensitive tests for insulin resistance, such as glycemic clamp studies or the frequently sampled intravenous glucose tolerance test (GTT), are invasive and expensive. Surrogate tests that are used to predict insulin resistance include fasting insulin, fasting glucose/insulin ratio, or glucose and insulin response to a 3-h GTT. A fasting glucose/insulin ratio of less than 4.5 is used by some authors as a screening test for insulin resistance in obese white women with PCOS and shows a good correlation ($r = 0.73$) with the insulin sensitivity index and fasting insulin level (40). We routinely check a fasting glucose and insulin level in all women with PCOS and when indicated obtain a 2-h GTT. Clinical findings suggestive of insulin resistance in women with PCOS include body mass index (BMI) more than 27 kg/m^2, waist to hip ratio more than 0.85, waist more than 100 cm, acanthosis nigricans (grey-brown velvety discoloration of the skin in the neck, groin, or axilla or under the breasts), and numerous skin tags *(41)*.

Ultrasound of the ovaries is not routinely obtained, as the findings are not essential for the diagnosis. Approximately 75% of anovulatory women will have polycystic ovaries *(42)*, with 8–10 preantral and antral follicles less than 10 mm in size seen along the periphery of the ovaries, which also have increased volumes. In addition, 8–25% of normal women will have ultrasound features suggestive of polycystic ovaries *(43–45)*, and hence this finding alone is insufficient to make the diagnosis in women with regular menses and no signs of hyperandrogenism.

TREATMENT

The choice of treatment for PCOS is determined by the woman's desire to become pregnant. Therefore we will discuss treatment options in two categories: (1) women not interested in fertility, and (2) women interested in fertility.

Women Not Interested in Fertility

The medical treatment for menstrual regulation and hirsutism is summarized in Table 3.

MENSTRUAL REGULATION

The lack of menstrual regularity predisposes women with PCOS to a threefold risk of endometrial cancer *(46)*. Data from the Cancer and Steroid Hormone study found a fivefold increased risk of endometrial cancer in women with PCOS [Odds ratio (OR) 5.4; 95% confidence interval (CI) 2.4–12.3] *(47)*. This increased risk is attributed to prolonged periods of unopposed estrogens, resulting in mitogenic stimulation of the endometrium. Peripheral aromatization into estrone and low circulating SHBG levels, resulting in increased free estradiol concentrations, further contributes to the chronic estrogen action on the endometrium. Fortunately, most cases of endometrial cancer are detected at an early stage with well-differentiated histology and good prognosis *(48)*. Nonetheless, women with PCOS who are not interested in fertility should be treated with oral contraceptive pills (OCPs) or a 14-d course of cyclic progestin each month to induce regular withdrawal bleed and prevent endometrial hyperplasia *(49)*.

A newer alternative is metformin, which is a dimethyl biguanide and an antihyperglycemic agent. It has been in clinical use since 1957 but was only recently approved by the Food and Drug Administration for the treatment of type 2 DM. Metformin decreases hepatic gluconeogenesis, increases peripheral glucose uptake, and decreases free fatty acid oxidation *(50,51)*. The first study describing its use in women with PCOS showed a 29% decrease in total testosterone, 39% decrease in free testosterone, 50% increase in SHBG, and menstrual regulation with evidence of ovulation *(52)*.

Table 3
Drugs Used for Menstrual Regulation and Hirsutism in PCOS

Drug	Indication	Dose	Adverse effects	Efficacy[a]
Oral contraceptives	Menstrual regulation	Low-dose, third-generation OCPs	Weight gain, nausea, vomiting, gallbladder disease, migraine	+++
	Hirsutism			+/++
Progestins (medroxy-progesterone acetate)	Menstrual regulation	10 mg qd × 12–14 d each month	Bloating, depression	+++
Glucophage	Menstrual regulation	500 mg tid	Abdominal discomfort, nausea, diarrhea	++
	Hirsutism			+/−
Spironolactone	Hirsutism	50–200 mg qd	Hyperkalemia, irregular bleeding, light-headedness, gynecomastia	++
Flutamide	Hirsutism	250 mg tid	Diarrhea, cystitis, rectal bleeding, liver injury	++
Finasteride	Hirsutism	1 mg qd	Sexual dysfunction, breast tenderness	++
Eflornithine HCl 13.9%	Hirsutism	Apply thin layer to face bid	Redness, rash, burning, tingling	++

OCP, oral contraceptive pill.
[a]−, no efficacy; +, low; ++, moderate; +++, high; +/−, unkown.

There are few randomized studies comparing the long-term outcomes in women treated with OCPs versus metformin. In one study, women randomized to metformin showed a decrease in BMI, fasting glucose, and testosterone levels compared with the ethinyl estradiol-cyproterone acetate group *(53)*. Although an improvement in menstrual cyclicity was noted in six of eight subjects on metformin, the efficacy of this treatment in preventing endometrial hyperplasia and cancer needs to be evaluated.

HIRSUTISM

Because the response to medical treatment is slow (owing to the long hair growth cycle), therapy needs to be continued for 1–2 yr and combined with mechanical methods of hair removal such as plucking, waxing, laser photo-therapy, and electrolysis. Medical treatment of hirsutism includes ovarian suppression with OCPs, progestins, or GnRH analogs or antiandrogen compounds such as spironolactone, flutamide, and finasteride. In addition to decreasing LH-dependent ovarian androgen production, the estrogenic component of OCPs also acts directly on the liver to increase SHBG. Furthermore, the progestins in OCPs can directly inhibit 5α-reductase, which converts testosterone to dihydro-testosterone. The response to low dose OCPs is comparable to that observed with higher doses in patients with hirsutism *(54)*. Similarly, progestational agents including third-generation preparations such as desogestrel, gestodene, and norgestimate when used alone have effects similar to those of low-dose OCPs.

Spironolactone, an aldosterone antagonist and antidiuretic, is the next most commonly used drug. It competes for androgen receptors in the hair follicle, inhibits the enzyme 5α-reductase, and may have a direct effect on inhibiting ovarian steroid synthesis. The recommended doses are 50–200 mg daily, but the response to this agent is also slow (6 mo). Spironolactone can cause irregular menses and is teratogenic; hence it is usually prescribed in combination with OCPs, although this may not significantly improve the outcome *(55)*.

Flutamide inhibits the androgen receptor directly but has limited use because of the severe hepatotoxicity reported in a small number of cases *(56)*. Finasteride inhibits 5α-reductase activity, hence decreasing the conversion of testosterone to dihydrotestosterone, and has fewer side effects. A prospective randomized trial compared the efficacy of flutamide, finasteride, ketoconazole, and ethinyl-estra-diol-cyproterone acetate over a period of 360 d. Although an improvement in a modified Ferriman-Gallwey score was noted in all four groups, there was no statistically significant difference between groups *(57)*. Another randomized prospective trial compared the efficacy of spironolactone, flutamide, and finasteride and showed similar effectiveness at 6 mo *(58)*.

Eflornithine hydrochloride (HCl) cream (VANIQA(r)) is a topical medication that can irreversibly block ornithine decarboxylase (ODC), an enzyme responsible for regulating hair growth. This results in a decrease in the rate of hair growth as well as thinning of the hair. In a 24-wk randomized clinical trial, women using eflornithine cream showed significant improvement in a four-point physician global assessment with minimal side effects *(59)*. In an 8-wk follow-up study, it was found that the benefits diminished with discontinuation of the cream. The long-term efficacy and side effects from this drug, as well as its concomitant use with some of the above-mentioned agents, need to be examined.

METABOLIC SYNDROME

The metabolic syndrome seen in women with PCOS is associated with hyper-lipidemia, early-onset diabetes, and hypertension and macrovascular coronary artery syndrome. This underscores the importance of early intervention and treatment. Lifestyle modifications including weight loss and nutritional and exercise counseling remain the mainstay of therapy. In a recent multicenter, randomized, prospective trial sponsored by the NIH, intensive lifestyle modifi-cations in individuals with impaired glucose tolerance reduced the risk of pro-gressing to diabetes by 58%, and metformin reduced the risk of diabetes by 31% over a follow-up period of 3 yr *(60; see also* Chapter 5). Similar results for lifestyle changes were reported in the recent Finnish Diabetes Prevention Study *(61)*. How-ever, it is still unclear whether and how this applies to specific populations of women with PCOS.

The treatment of women with PCOS diagnosed with diabetes during the pre-liminary workup is clear; however, the treatment of women who have hyper-insulinemia or a glucose/insulin ratio less than 4.5 remains controversial. In a randomized control trial of 29 adolescents with hyperinsulinemia and obesity, treatment with metformin resulted in an improvement in the fasting glucose and insulin levels and a decrease in BMI *(62)*. These authors concluded that metformin may complement dietary and exercise counseling in selected patients with increased risk for diabetes.

In summary, women with PCOS who are not interested in fertility should be prescribed steroid hormones to regulate their menstrual cycles. If they present with a prolonged duration of amenorrhea, an endometrial biopsy should be per-formed prior to starting medical therapy. Periodic screening tests should include blood pressure checks, fasting lipids, glucose, and insulin. If they are obese or hyperinsulinemic, they should be aggressively counseled regarding weight loss and the use of insulin-sensitizing agents.

Women Interested in Fertility

MEDICAL TREATMENT

Most women with PCOS ovulate intermittently and can present with infertil-ity. However, only a subset have infertility secondary to anovulation, and most respond to ovulation-inducing agents. The current medical treatment strategy for PCOS patients to regulate menstruation and treat infertility includes use of an estrogen receptor agonist/antagonist such as clomiphene citrate. Clomiphene is typically administered in the follicular phase of the cycle, starting on d 3–5 for a total of 5 d. The starting dose is 50 mg/d, and this may be increased in an incremental manner until ovulation is detected, usually by measuring the midluteal progesterone level. Women are asked to time intercourse every other day for 1 wk starting 5 d after the last dose of clomiphene or to use an ovulation prediction kit. This ovulatory dose is then maintained for three to six cycles. It has been reported that 70% of women will ovulate at the 100-mg dose (63). Furthermore, most clomiphene-initiated conceptions will occur within the first six cycles. The common side effects associated with clomiphene include hot flashes, mood changes, abdominal discomfort, visual symptoms, and a multiple pregnancy rate of 5–8%. If there is no other cause for infertility, the pregnancy rates in this population approach that of the normal population (63). Approximately 20% of women with PCOS fail to ovulate on maximum doses of clomiphene (150–200 mg/d) and are then candidates for combination therapy with metformin or gonadotropins. Also, women who fail to become pregnant after three to six cycles of clomiphene are then treated with combination therapy.

Weight loss counseling is also important. It has been reported that weight loss of 5–7% of body weight will improve menstrual function (64–66). In a randomized trial, weight loss was associated with decrease in total testosterone and insulin levels, and four of six women had documented ovulation (67). In contrast, none of the five women in the control group ovulated. In another study, women with PCOS were placed on a low-calorie diet and randomized to placebo versus metformin (65). After 6 mo, the women in the metformin arm of the study had greater reduction of body weight (mean 9.7 kg) and abdominal fat and a decrease in serum fasting insulin (40%), testosterone (35%), and leptin levels. In addition, they had a significant improvement in menstrual irregularity.

Insulin sensitizers may also have a role in the treatment of infertility in PCOS. Approximately 80% of women with PCOS will respond to clomiphene, but only 50% will become pregnant. Although several studies have examined the role of insulin-sensitizing agents in women with PCOS (68–70), the appropriateness of administering insulin-lowering agents to women with normal fasting insulin remains to be validated (71). Obese PCOS women treated with metformin have a reduction in cytochrome P450c17α activity and a decrease in serum free testosterone (72). Metformin therapy for only 5 wk improves both the spontaneous ovulatory rate (34%) and clomiphene-induced ovulatory response (90%) compared with 4 and 8%, respectively, in controls (69). Laboratory data in the same study showed an improvement in the free testosterone and SHBG levels as well as the insulin area under the curve. A randomized controlled trial conducted over a 6-mo period showed similar improvements in biochemical profiles of women with PCOS administered metformin compared with placebo (n = 23) (58). In the metformin arm of the study, the authors noted an increase in menstrual frequency in 54.8% of women, and ovulation was detected in 74% of these women.

The use of metformin in conjunction with clomiphene will reduce the number of patients who will require gonadotropins for ovulation induction. This has potential benefits owing to the side effects associated with gonadotropin therapy, which include ovarian hyperstimulation syndrome (OHSS) and multiple gestation, as well as the lower cost and decreased patient monitoring requirements. Women who fail to ovulate with clomiphene/metformin combinations can then be treated with low-dose gonadotropins. In a review of 14 randomized controlled trials, it was noted that ovulation induction with FSH compared with human menopausal gonadotropin (HMG) resulted in a lower incidence of OHSS (OR 0.2; 95% CI 0.08–0.46) *(73)* but no significant improvement in pregnancy rate. On the other hand, addition of GnRH analogs to gonadotropin therapy showed a trend toward improved pregnancy rates, but there was a higher risk of overstimulation (OR 3.15; 95% CI 1.48–6.7). The addition of metformin to gonadotropin stimulation has been associated with an orderly growth of follicles and a lower risk of hyperstimulation *(74)*.

The use of metformin in women with PCOS undergoing in vitro fertilization has been recently examined. Women in the metformin arm had fewer follicles ($p < 0.005$) and lower estradiol levels ($p < 0.05$) compared with the group that did not receive metformin *(75)*. In addition, the number of mature oocytes and more than 4-cell-stage embryos was higher in the metformin group, suggesting a beneficial effect of metformin on follicular and oocyte development. Troglitazone, a member of the thiazolidinedione class of drugs, is another insulin-sensitizing agent that has been shown to have similar beneficial effects on biochemical parameters and menstrual function. However, troglitazone has been withdrawn for sale in the United States because of potentially fatal hepatotoxicity. The two available thiazolidinediones (rosiglitazone and pioglitazone) may have the same favorable effects on menstrual function as troglitazone.

SURGICAL TREATMENT

Modern surgical treatment for PCOS consists of laparoscopic ovarian "drilling." Ovarian wedge resection was the first established treatment for anovulatory PCOS women but was abandoned because of the increased risk of postoperative adhesions *(76)*. As previously mentioned, some women fail to respond to ovulatory agents such as clomiphene and have an exaggerated response to gonadotropins. Hence, there has been an ongoing effort to develop laparoscopic ovarian drilling as a relatively less invasive alternative to wedge resection. Several observational trials have reported an improvement in both the spontaneous ovulatory rate and the response to ovulation-inducing agents. A review of six randomized controlled trials comparing ovarian drilling with gonadotropins failed to show a statistically significant difference between the two treatment groups *(77)*. However, multiple pregnancy rates were significantly reduced in the ovarian drilling arm (OR 0.61; 95% CI 0.17–2.16) This treatment remains an option for women who fail to respond to oral ovulation-inducing agents and cannot afford expensive treatments including gonadotropins and assisted reproductive technologies.

OBSTETRIC COMPLICATIONS

Women with PCOS have an increased risk of miscarriages of unclear etiology *(78,79)*. This has led several authors to recommend (for patients achieving pregnancy on metformin) that the drug be continued at least through the first trimester *(80)*. This is based on the hypothesis that metformin will lower the miscarriage rate by decreasing insulin and PAI-1 levels *(81)* and increasing glycodelin and IGFBP-1 *(81)*. Women with PCOS also have an increased risk of other obstetric complications including diabetes and risks associated with multiple gestations. In one study *(82)*, the multiple pregnancy rate was 9.1% in women with PCOS compared with 1.1% in controls, and the risk of developing gestational diabetes was 20% in women with PCOS compared with 8.9% in controls. Interestingly, PCOS was an independent predictor of gestational diabetes. In contrast, PCOS was not a predictor of preeclampsia, as had been reported previously *(83,84)*.

In summary, most women with PCOS will achieve a successful pregnancy. However, a subset of these patients may fail to respond to oral ovulation-inducing agents and will hyperrespond when administered gonadotropins. Newer regimens including metformin and letrozole will decrease the number of women with PCOS that will require assisted reproductive technologies.

SUMMARY

PCOS is a heterogenous disorder with an appreciable increase in risk of diabetes and cardiovascular complications by the perimenopausal period. Although the short-term benefits of insulin-sensitizing agents are now being defined, it is crucial to determine the long-term effects of these agents on delaying or decreasing the risks of developing diabetes and hypertension.

REFERENCES

1. Knochenhauser ES, Key TJ, Kahser-Miller M, Waggoner W, Boots LR, Aziz R. Prevalence of polycystic ovary syndrome in unselected black and white women of the southeastern United States: a prospective study. J Clin Endocrinol Metab 1998;83:3078–3082
2. Stein IF, Leventhal ML. Amenorrhea associated with bilateral polycystic ovaries. Am J Obstet Gynecol 1935;29:181–191.
3. Rogerio AL, Enrico C. The importance of diagnosing the polycystic ovary syndrome Ann Intern Med. 2000;132:989–993.
4. Dunaif A, Givens JR, Haseltine FP, Merriam GR, eds. Current Issues in Endocrinology and Metabolism: Polycystic Ovary Syndrome. Blackwell Scientific Publications, Boston, 1992.
5. Barbieri RL, Ryan KJ. Hyperandrogenism, insulin resistance and acanthosis nigricans syndrome. A common endocrinopathy with distinct pathophysiologic features. Am J Obstet Gynecol 1983;147:90–101.

6. Barbieri RL. Some genetic syndromes associated with hyperandrogenism. Contemp OB Gyn 1994;39:35–48.
7. Magoffin DA. Regulation of differentiated functions in ovarian theca cells. Semin Reprod Endocrinol 1991;9:321–331.
8. Agarwal SK, Judd HL, Magoffin DA. A mechanism for the suppression of estrogen production in polycystic ovary syndrome. J Clin Endocrinol Metab 1996;81:3686–3691.
9. Barbieri RL, Makris A, Ryan KJ. Insulin stimulates androgen accumulation in incubations of human ovarian stroma and theca. Obstet Gynecol 1984;64(suppl 3):73S–80S.
10. Barbieri RL, Makris A. Randall RW. Daniels G. Kistner RW. Ryan KJ. Insulin stimulates androgen accumulation in incubations of ovarian stroma obtained from women with hyperandrogenism. J Clin Endocrinol Metab 1986;62:904–910.
11. Cara LF, Rosenfield RL. Insulin-like growth factor-I and insulin potentiate luteinizing hormone-induced androgen synthesis by rat ovarian thecal-interstitial cells. Endocrinology 1998;123:733–739.
12. Hernandez ER, Resnick CE, Svoboda ME, Van Wyk JJ, Payne SW, Adashi EY. Somatomedin-C insulin-like growth factor-I as an enhancer of androgen biosynthesis by cultured rat ovarian cells. Endocrinology 1988;122:1603–1612.
13. Bergh C, Carlsson B, Olsson J-H, Selleskog U, Hillensjo T. Regulation of androgen production in cultured human thecal cells by insulin-like growth factor I and insulin. Fertil Steril 1993;59:323–331.
14. Waldstreicher J, Santoro NF, Hall JE, Filicori M, Crowley WE. Hyperfunction of the hypothalamic-pituitary axis in women with polycystic ovary disease: indirect evidence of partial gonadotroph desensitization. J Clin Endocrinol Metab 1999;66:165–172.
15. Steinberg HO, Chaker H, Leaming R, Johnson A, Brechtel G, Baron AD. Obesity/ insulin resistance is associated with endothelial dysfunction—implications for the development of insulin resistance. J Clin Invest 1996;97:2601–2610.
16. Saltiel A. Series introduction: the molecular and physiological basis of insulin resistance: emerging implications for metabolic and cardiovascular diseases J Clin Invest 2000;106:163–164.
17. Garvey TW, Maianu L, Zhu JH, Brechtel-Hook G, Wallace P, Baron AD. Evidence for defects in the trafficking and translocation of GLUT4 glucose transporters in skeletal muscle as a cause of human insulin resistance. J Clin Invest 1998;101:2377–2386.
18. Dunaif A. Insulin resistance and the polycystic ovary syndrome: mechanism and implications for pathogenesis. Endocr Rev 1997;18:774–800.
19. Dunaif A, Segal KR, Futterweit W, Dobrjansky A. Profound peripheral insulin resistance, independent of obesity, in the polycystic ovary syndrome. Diabetes 1989;38:1165–1174.
20. Dunaif A, Xia J, Book CB, Schenker E, Tang Z. Excessive insulin receptor serine phosphorylation in cultured fibroblasts and in skeletal muscle. A potential mechanism for insulin resistance in polycystic ovary syndrome. J Clin Invest 1985;96:801–810.
21. Legro RS, Kunselman AR, Dodson WC, Dunaif A. Prevalence and predictors of the risk for type 2 diabetes mellitus and impaired glucose tolerance in polycystic ovary syndrome: a prospective, controlled study in 254 affected women J Clin Endocrinol Metab 1999;84:165–169
22. Dahlgren E, Johansson S, Lindstedt G, et al. Women with polycystic syndrome wedge resected in 1956 to 1965: a long term follow-up focusing on natural history and circulating hormones. Fertil Steril 1992;57:505–513
23. Scherrer U, Sartori C. Insulin as a vascular and sympathoexcitatory hormone Circulation 1997;96:4104–4113.
24. Wild S, Pierpoint T, McKeigue P, Jacobs H. Cardiovascular disease in women with polycystic ovary syndrome at long-term follow-up: a retrospective cohort study. Clin Endocrinol 2000; 52:595–600.
25. Sampson M, Kong C, Patel A, Unwin R, Jacobs HS. Ambulatory blood pressure profiles and plasminogen activator inhibitor (PAI-1) activity in lean women with and without polycystic ovary syndrome, Clin Endocrinol 1996;45:623–629.

26. Schneider DJ, Sobel BE. Synergistic augmentation of expression of PAI-1 induced by insulin, VLDL, and fatty acids, Coronary Artery Dis 1996;7:813–817.
27. Reaven GM, Lithell H, Landsberg L. Hypertension and associated metabolic abnormalities—the role of insulin resistance and sympathoadrenal system. N Engl J Med 1996;334:374.
28. Despres JP, Lamarche B, Mauriege P, et al. Hyperinsulinemia as an independent risk factor for ischemic heart disease. N Engl J Med 1996; 334:952–957.
29. Howard G, O'Leary DH, Zaccaro D, et al. Insulin sensitivity and atherosclerosis Circulation 1996;93:1809–1817.
30. Guzick DS, Talbott EO, Sutton-Tyrrell K, Herzog HC, Kuller LH, Wolfson SK Jr. Carotid atherosclerosis in women with polycystic ovary syndrome: initial results from a case-control study. Am J Obstet Gynecol 1996;174:1224–1232.
31. Talbott EO, Guzick DS, Sutton-Tyrrell K, et al. Evidence for association between polycystic ovary syndrome and premature carotid atherosclerosis in middle-aged women. Arterioscler Thromb Vasc Biol 2000;20:2414–2421.
32. Birdsall MA, Farquhar CM, White HD. Association between polycystic ovaries and extent of coronary artery disease in women having cardiac catheterization. Ann Intern Med 1997;126:32–35.
33. Pierpoint T, McKeigue PM, Isaacs AJ, Wild SH, Jacobs HS. Mortality of women with polycystic ovary syndrome at long-term follow-up. J Clin Epidemiol 1998;51:581–586.
34. Dahlgren E, Janson PO, Johansson S, Lapidus L, Oden A. Polycystic ovary syndrome and risk for myocardial infarction—evaluated from a risk factor model based on a prospective study of women. Acta Obstet Gynecol Scand 1992;71:599–604.
35. Mather KJ, Verma S, Corenblum B, Anderson TJ. Normal endothelial function despite insulin resistance in healthy women with the polycystic ovary syndrome J Clin Endocrinol Metab 2000;85:1851–1856.
36. Zeiher AM, Drexler H, Saurbier B, Just H. Endothelium-mediated coronary blood flow modulation in humans: effects of age, atherosclerosis, hypercholesterolemia, and hypertension. J Clin Invest 1993;92:652–662.
37. Balletshofer BM, Rittig K, Enderle MD, et al. Endothelial dysfunction is detectable in young normotensive first-degree relatives of subjects with type 2 diabetes in association with insulin resistance. Circulation 2000;101:1780–1784.
38. Paradisi G, Steinberg HO, Hempfling A, et al. Polycystic ovary syndrome is associated with endothelial dysfunction. Circulation 2001;103:1410–1415.
39. Haynes WG, Sinkcy CA, Wayson SM, Bar RS, Sivitz WI. Endothelial effects of sulfonylurea and biguanide therapy in type 2 diabetes mellitus. In: Proceedings of the American Diabetes Association Meeting, 2000, abstract #564.
40. Legro RS, Finegood D, Dunaif A. Fasting glucose to insulin ratio is a useful measure of insulin sensitivity in women with polycystic ovary syndrome. J Clin Endocrinol Metab 1998;83:2964–2968.
41. Barbieri RL. Induction of ovulation in infertile women with hyperandrogenism and insulin resistance. Am J Obstet Gynecol 2000;183:1412–1418.
42. Franks S. Polycystic ovary syndrome. N Engl J Med 1995;333:853–861.
43. Polson DW, Wadsworth J, Adams J, Franks S. Polycystic ovaries: a common finding in normal women. Lancet 1988;ii:870–872.
44. Clayton RN, Ogden V, Hodgkinson J, et al. How common are polycystic ovaries in normal women and what is their significance for the infertility of the population? Clin Endocrinol 1992;37:127–134.
45. Farquhar CM, Birdsall M, Manning P, Mitchell JM, France JT. The prevalence of polycystic ovaries on ultrasound scanning in a population of randomly selected women. Aust NZ Obstet Gynaecol 1994;34:67–72.
46. Coulam CG, Annegers FH, Krantz JS. Chronic anovulation syndrome and associated neoplasia. Obstet Gynecol 1983;61:403–407.

47. Escobedo LG, Lee NC, Peterson HB, Wingo PA. Infertility-associated endometrial cancer risk may be limited to specific subgroups of infertile women. Obstet Gynecol 1991;77:124–128.
48. McDonald TW, Malkasian GD, Gaffey TA. Endometrial cancer associated with feminizing ovarian tumor and polycystic ovarian disease. Obstet Gynecol 1976;49:654–658.
49. Greenbalt RG, Gambrell Js RD, Stoddard LD. The protective role of progesterone in the prevention of endometrial cancer. Pathol Res Pract 1982;174:297–318.
50. Patane G, Piro S, Rabuazzo A, Anello M, Vigneri R, Purrello F. Metformin restores insulin secretion altered by chronic exposure to free fatty acids or high glucose. Diabetes 2000;49:735–740.
51. Perriello G, Misericordia P, Volpi E, et al. Acute antihyperglycemic mechanisms of metformin in NIDDM. Evidence for suppression of lipid oxidation and hepatic glucose production. Diabetes 1994;43:920–928.
52. Velazquez EM, Menodza S. Hamer T, Sosa F, Glueck CJ. Metformin therapy in polycystic ovary syndrome reduces hyperinsulinemia, insulin resistance, hyperandrogenemia and systolic blood pressure, while facilitating normal menses and pregnancy. Metab Clin Exp 1994;43:647–654.
53. Morin-Papunin LC, Vauhkonen I, Koivunen R, Ruokonen A, Martikianen H, Tapanainen J. Endocrine and metabolic effects of metformin versus ethinyl estradiol-cyproterone acetate in obese women with polycystic ovary syndrome: a randomized study. J Clin Endocrinol Metabol 2000;85:3161-3168.
54. Palatsi R, Hirvensalo E, Liukko P, et al. Serum total and unbound testosterone and sex hormone binding globulin (SHBG) in female acne patients treated with two different oral contraceptives. Acta Derm Venereol 1984;64:517–523.
55. Pittaway DE, Maxson WS, Wentz AD. Spironolactone in combination drug therapy for unresponsive hirsutism. Fertil Steril 1985;43:878–882.
56. Andrade RJ, Lucena MI, Fernandez MC, et al. Fulminant liver failure associated with flutamide therapy for hirsutism. Lancet 1999;353:362–983.
57. Venturoli S, Marescalchi O, Colombo FM, et al. A prospective randomized trial comparing low dose flutamide, finasteride, ketoconazole and cyproterone acetate-estrogen regimens in the treatment of hirsutism. J Clin Endocrinol Metab 1999;84:1304–1310.
58. Moghetti P, Castello R, Negri C, et al. Metformin effects on clinical features, endocrine and metabolic profiles and insulin sensitivity in polycystic ovary syndrome: a randomized double-blind, placebo-controlled 6-months trial, followed by open, long-term clinical evaluation. J Clin Endocrinol Metab 2000;85:139–146.
59. Schrode K, Huber F, Staszak J, et al. Randomized, double-blind, vehicle-controlled safety and efficacy evaluation of eflornithine 15% cream in the treatment of women with excessive facial hair. Poster presented at the American Academy of Dermatology Annual Meeting, March 11–14, 2000, San Francisco, CA.
60. Knowler WC, Barrett-Connor E, Fowler SE, et al. Reduction in the incidence of type 2 diabetes with lifestyle intervention or metformin. N Engl J Med 2002;346:393–403.
61. Tuomilehto J, Lindstrom J, Eriksson JG, et al. Prevention of type 2 diabetes mellitus by changes in lifestyle among subjects with impaired glucose tolerance. N Engl J Med 2001;344:1343–1350.
62. Freemark M, Bursey D. The effects of metformin on body mass index and glucose tolerance in obese adolescents with fasting hyperinsulinemia and a family history of type 2 diabetes. Pediatrics 2001;107:E55.
63. Gorlitsky GA, Kase NG, Speroff L. Ovulation and pregnancy rates with clomiphene citrate. Obstet Gynecol 1978;51:265–269.
64. Pasquali R, Casimirri F, Vicennati V. Weight control and its beneficial effect on fertility in women with obesity and PCOS. Hum Reprod 1997;12:82–87.
65. Pasquali R, Gambineri A, Biscotti D, et al. Effect of long-term treatment of metformin added to hypocaloric diet on body composition, fat distribution, and androgen and insulin levels in

abdominally obese women with and without the polycystic ovary syndrome. J Clin Endocrinol Metab 2000;85:2767–2774.

66. Jakubowicz DJ, Nestler JE. 17 Alpha-hydroxyprogesterone response to leuprolide and serum androgens in obese women with and without PCOS after dietary weight loss. J Clin Endocrinol 1997;82:556–560.

67. Guzik DS, Wing R, Smith D, Berga SL, Winters SJ. Endocrine consequences of weight loss in obese, hyperandrogenic, anovulatory women. Fertil Steril 1994;61:589–604.

68. Velázquez E, Acosta A, Mendoza SG. Menstrual cyclicity and metformin therapy in PCOS. Obstet Gynecol 1997;90:392–395.

69. Nestler JE, Jakubowicz DJ, Evans WS, Pasquali R. Effects of metformin on spontaneous and clomiphene-induced ovulation in the polycystic ovary syndrome. N Engl J Med 1998;338:1876–1880

70. Glueck CJ, Wang P, Fontaine R, Tracy T, Sieve-Smith L. Metformin-induced resumption of normal menses in 39 of 43 (91%) previously amenorrheic women with PCOS. Metabolism 1999;48:511–519.

71. Sills ES, Perloe M, Palermo GD. Correction of hyperinsulinemia in oligoovulatory women with clomiphene-resistant PCOS: a review of therapeutic rationale and reproductive outcomes. Eur J Obstet Gynecol Reprod Biol 2000;91:135–141.

72. Nestler JE, Jakubowicz DJ. Decreases in ovarian cytochrome p450c17α activity and serum free testosterone after reduction of insulin secretion in polycystic ovary syndrome. N Engl J Med 1996;335:617–623.

73. Nugent D, Vandekerckhove P, Hughes E, Arnot M, Lilford R. Gonadotrophin therapy for ovulation induction in subfertility associated with polycystic ovary syndrome. Cochrane Database Systematic Rev 2000;(4):CD000410.

74. De Leo V, la Marca A, Ditto A, Morgante G, Cianci A. Effects of metformin on gonadotropin induced ovulation in women with PCOS. Fertil Steril 1999;72:282–286.

75. Stadmauer LA, Toma SK, Riehl RM, Talbert LM. Metformin treatment of patients with polycystic ovary syndrome undergoing in vitro fertilization improves outcomes and is associated with modulation of the insulin like growth factors. Fertil Steril 2001;75:505–509.

76. Portuondo JA, Melchor JC, Neyro JL, Alegre A. Periovarian adhesions following ovarian wedge resection or laparoscopic biopsy. Endoscopy 1984;16:143.

77. Farquhar C, Vandekerckhove P, Lilford R. Laparoscopic "drilling" by diathermy or laser for ovulation induction in anovulatory polycystic ovary syndrome. Cochrane Database of Systematic Rev 2001;(4):CD001122.

78. Sagle M, Bishop K, Ridley N, et al. Recurrent early miscarriage and polycystic ovaries. BMJ 1988;287:1027–1028.

79. Balen AH, Braat DD, West C, Patel A, Jacobs HS. Cumulative conception and live birth rates after treatment of anovulatory infertility: safety and efficacy of ovulation induction in 200 patients. Hum Reprod 1994;9:1563–1570.

80. Glueck CJ, Phillips H, Cameron D, Sieve-Smith L, Wang P. Continuing metformin throughout pregnancy in women with polycystic ovary syndrome appears to safely reduce first-trimester spontaneous abortion: a pilot study. Fertil Steril 2001;75:46–52.

81. Mikola M, Hiilesmaa V, Halttunen M, Suhonen L, Tiitinen A. Obstetric outcome in women with polycystic ovarian syndrome. Hum Reprod 2001;16:226–229.

82. Jakubowicz DJ, Seppala M, Jakubowicz S, et al. Insulin reduction with metformin increases luteal phase serum glycodelin and insulin-like growth factor-binding protein 1 concentrations and enhances uterine vascularity and blood flow in the polycystic ovary syndrome. J Clin Endocrinol Metab 2001;86:1126–1133.

83. De Vries MJ, Dekker GA, Schoemaker J. Higher risk of pre-eclampsia in the polycystic ovary syndrome. A case control study. Eur J Obstet Gynecol Reprod Biol 1998;14:91–95.

84. Radon PA, McMahon MJ, Meyer WR. Impaired glucose tolerance in pregnancy women with polycystic ovary syndrome. Obstet Gynecol 1999;94:194–197.

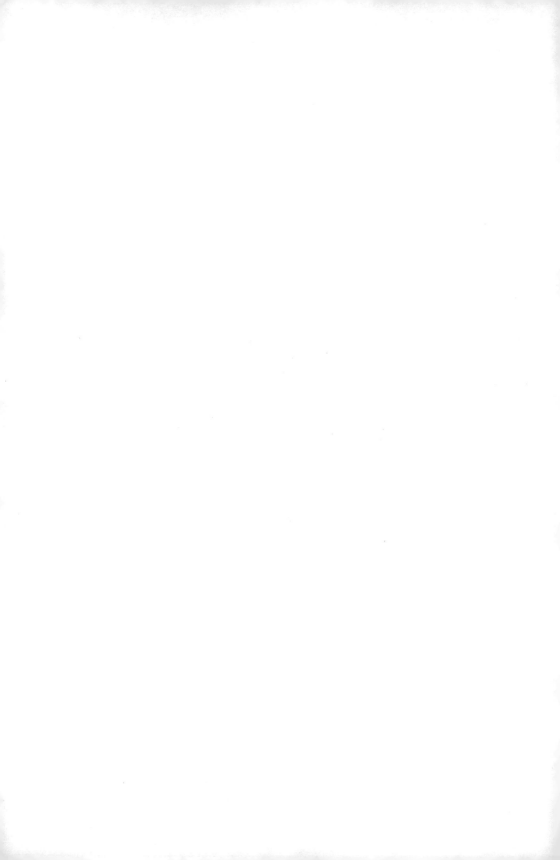

10   Acromegaly

Vivien Bonert, MD, and Shlomo Melmed, MD

INTRODUCTION

Acromegaly is a chronic, insidious, disfiguring disorder of adulthood caused by excess circulating growth hormone (GH) secretion occurring after epiphyseal closure with protean clinical manifestations affecting almost every major organ system. GH hypersecretion stimulates increased hepatic insulin-like growth factor (IGF-1) production, and both GH and IGF-1 contribute to the clinical features of hypersomatotrophism.

Acromegaly is rare, with a prevalence that varies from 38 to 69 cases/million depending on the community being studied (1–3) and an annual incidence of 3–4 new cases/million people. It is estimated that in the United States approximately 1000 new cases of acromegaly are diagnosed annually.

More than 95% of cases of acromegaly are caused by GH secreting pituitary adenomas, with nonpituitary disease rarely causing the syndrome. Acromegaly is characterized by elevated circulating GH levels, which stimulate increased hepatic IGF-1 secretion (4), (Fig. 1) both of which contribute to the clinical and pathologic features of hypersomatotrophism (5). GH-secreting pituitary adenomas are usually benign and may be slowly growing (densely granulated) or rapidly growing (sparsely granulated), pure somatotropinomas (6), or mixed

From: *Contemporary Endocrinology: Early Diagnosis and Treatment of Endocrine Disorders*
Edited by: R. S. Bar © Humana Press Inc., Totowa, NJ

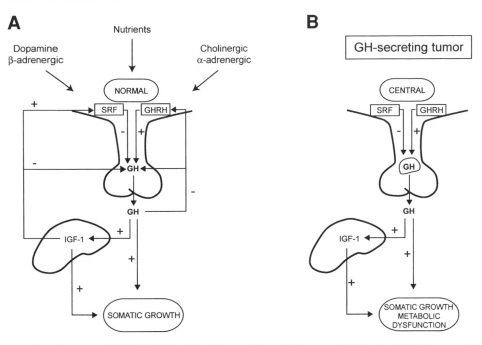

Fig. 1. (A) Normal GH/IGF-1 feedback loop. Growth hormone (GH), insulin-like growth factor-I (IGF-1), growth hormone-releasing hormone (GHRH), and somatostatin (SRF) feedback loop in the control of somatic growth. A stimulatory effect of GHRH and inhibitory effect of SRF interact to result in GH secretion from the anterior pituitary. GH stimulates IGF-1 production from the liver. This, in turn, has a negative feedback effect on pituitary GH secretion and a positive feedback effect on hypothalmic SRF release. Pituitary GH secretion has a negative autoregulatory feedback effect on pituitary GH secretion as well as a negative feedback effect on hypothalmic GHRH secretion. GH exerts an effect on somatic growth by direct action as well as indirectly via IGF-1. **(B)** GH-secreting pituitary adenoma. Development of a GH-secreting pituitary adenoma results in unrestrained pituitary GH hypersecretion with loss of the negative feedback regulation from peripheral GH and IGF-1. (Adapted from ref. *4.*)

GH-cell and prolactin (PRL)-cell adenomas, composed of two distinct cell types, somatotrophs expressing GH and lactotrophs expressing PRL *(7,8)*; or plurihormonal tumors secreting any combination of PRL, thyroid-stimulating hormone, adrenocorticotrophic hormone, or α-subunit *(9)* (Table 1). GH cell carcinomas with distant metastases are very rare *(10)* and must be distinguished from benign, rapidly growing, locally invasive somatotropinomas, which do not metastasize. Ectopic GH-secreting tumors can rarely occur in the sphenoid sinus, pancreas, lung, ovary, and breast or can manifest as carcinoid tumors.

Nonpituitary tumors secreting growth hormone-releasing hormone (GHRH) cause acromegaly by stimulating GH cell hyperplasia in the pituitary gland. Hyperplasia is difficult to distinguish from a GH cell adenoma *(11)*, but silver

Table 1
Causes of Acromegaly

	Prevalence (%)
Excess growth hormone secretion	
Pituitary	
Densely or sparsely granulated GH cell adenoma	98
Mixed GH-cell PRL-cell adenoma	60
Mammosomatotroph cell adenoma	25
Plurihormonal adenoma	10
GH-cell carcinoma or metastases	
Multiple endocrine neoplasia-1 (GH-cell adenoma)	
McCune-Albright syndrome (rarely; adenoma)	
Ectopic sphenoid or parapharyngeal sinus pituitary adenoma	
Extrapituitary tumor	
Pancreatic islet cell tumor	<1
Excess growth hormone-releasing hormone secretion	
Central	<1
Hypothalamic hamartoma, choristoma, ganglioneuroma	<1
Peripheral	1
Bronchial carcinoid, pancreatic islet cell tumor, small cell lung cancer, adrenal adenoma, medullary thyroid carcinoma, pheochromocytoma	

GH, growth hormone; PRL, prolactin.
Adapted from ref. 4.

staining may reveal an intact reticulin network without a surrounding pseudo-capsule. Excess GHRH may be eutopic (derived from a hypothalmic hamartoma) or ectopic (from a carcinoid tumor, pancreatic cell tumor, pheochromocytoma, adrenal adenoma, or small cell carcinoma of the lung).

Elevated circulating levels of GHRH or GH in the absence of a pituitary adenoma, with a significant arteriovenous hormone gradient across the ectopic tumor source, confirm a diagnosis of ectopic acromegaly. Clinical and biochemical diagnosis of ectopic acromegaly is important, as a different therapeutic approach is employed in that the ectopic GHRH-secreting tumor is surgically resected if possible, reversing the GH hypersecretion, and pituitary surgery is not performed. Somatostatin analogs suppress both ectopic GHRH tumor secretion as well as pituitary GH secretion in patients with recurrent carcinoid tumor or nonresectable or disseminated disease.

Acromegaloidism is a condition in which the soft tissue, skin changes, and bony features of acromegaly occur in patients in the absence of a pituitary or extrapituitary tumor. GH and IGF-1 levels are normal in these "acromegaloid" patients, with some evidence of insulin resistance and defective IGF-1 binding (12) and possibly a novel growth factor (13).

Acromegaly is also associated with a number of genetic familial syndromes *(14),* including McCune-Albright syndrome (polyostotic fibrous dysplasia, café-au-lait pigmentation, sexual precocity, hyperthyroidism, hypercortisolism, hyperprolactinemia, acromegaly), multiple endocrine neoplasia type 1 (MEN-1; tumors of the endocrine pancreas, parathyroid, and anterior pituitary), Carney's syndrome (skin and cardiac myxomas, Cushing's syndrome, and GH-secreting adenomas), and familial acromegaly (familial GH-secreting adenomas). The specific chromosomal localizations of the genes associated with these syndromes have been identified.

CLINICAL FEATURES

The characteristic clinical manifestations of acromegaly are caused by peripheral actions of excess GH and IGF-1 (Table 2). Presenting clinical complaints vary, with most cases being diagnosed by chance (Tables 3 and 4). However, as 70% of GH-secreting adenomas are macroadenomas (>10 mm), *(15)* the central features of an expanding pituitary mass are common. As with all pituitary masses, suprasellar extension results in visual field defects caused by optic chiasmal compression; lateral cavernous sinus extension impinges on cranial nerves III, IV, V, and VI, causing diplopia or facial pain, and inferior extension may be associated with cerebrospinal fluid rhinorrhea and nasopharyngeal sinus invasion. Central pressure effects from the expanding pituitary mass are often associated with headache and rarely hypothalamic and frontal lobe dysfunction.

Long-standing effects of GH hypersecretion on acral and soft tissues, as well as on several vital organ systems and metabolic function, result in the characteristic clinical manifestations of acromegaly (Fig. 2). The slow insidious change in appearance results in a mean delay from time of onset of symptoms to diagnosis of 9 yr *(1,16).* Acromegaly is frequently diagnosed incidentally when patients seek care for dental, rheumatologic, or orthopedic disorders *(17).* Acral enlargement results in the physical features of acromegaly including coarsening of facial features, bulbous nose, fleshy lips, frontal bossing, spade-like hands, and widened feet. Mandibular overgrowth causes widening of the maxilla, with prognathism, teeth separation, jaw malocclusion and overbite (Fig. 3). These slowly progressive subtle physical changes can often be appreciated by serial review of old photographs. Patients volunteer or admit to increase in shoe, ring or hat size on direct questioning. GH excess also results in generalized visceromegaly with enlargement of tongue, salivary glands, thyroid, and heart.

Arthropathy

Mono- or polyarticular arthropathy with joint swelling, hypermobility, and cartilaginous thickening *(18)* is common in acromegaly, affecting 70% of patients, up to half of whom are impaired in the performance of daily activities

Table 2
Clinical Features of Acromegaly

Local tumor effects
   Pituitary enlargement
   Visual field defects
   Cranial nerve palsy
   Headache
Somatic
   Acral enlargement
      Thickening of soft tissue of hands and feet
   Musculoskeletal
      Prognathism
      Malocclusion
      Arthralgias
      Carpal tunnel syndrome
      Acroparesthesia
      Proximal myopathy
      Hypertrophy of frontal bones
Skin
   Hyperhidrosis
   Oily
   Skin tags
Colon
   Polyps
Cardiovascular
   Left-ventricular hypertrophy
   Asymmetric septal hypertrophy
   Hypertension
   Congestive heart failure
   Sleep disturbances
   Sleep apnea
   Narcolepsy
Visceromegaly
   Tongue
   Thyroid
   Salivary gland
   Liver
   Spleen
   Kidney
Endocrine-metabolic
   Reproduction
      Menstrual abnormalities
      Galactorrhea
      Decreased libido, impotence, low sex hormone-binding globulin

(continued)

Table 2 *(continued)*

Multiple endocrine neoplasia (1)
    Hyperparathyroidism
    Pancreatic islet cell tumors
Carbohydrate
    Impaired glucose tolerance
    Insulin resistance and hyerinsulinemia
    Diabetes mellitus
Lipids
    Hypertriglyceridemia
Mineral
    Hypercalciuria, increased $1,25(OH)_2$ vitamin D3
    Urinary hydroxproline
Electrolyte
    Low renin
    Increased aldosterone
Thyroid
    Low thyroxine-binding globulin

Adapted from ref. *121.*

Table 3
Presentation of Acromegaly

Chief presenting complaint	*Frequency (%)*
Menstrual disturbance	13
Change in appearance/acral growth	11
Headaches	8
Paresthesias/ carpal tunnel syndrome	6
Diabetes mellitus/impaired glucose tolerance	5
Heart disease	3
Visual impairment	3
Decreased libido/impotence	3
Arthropathy	3
Thyroid disorder	2
Hypertension	1
Gigantism	1
Fatigue	0.3
Hyperhidrosis	0.3
Somnolence	0.3
Other	5
Chance (detected by unrelated physical or dental examination or x-ray)	40

Adapted from ref. *17.*

Table 4
Signs and Symptoms of Acromegaly

Sign/symptom	Screening test
↑Sweating (hyperhidrosis) with pungent odor	IGF-1
Prognathism, mandible overgrowth	
Carpal tunnel, especially bilateral	
Visual field defect with diplopia	
Widely spaced teeth, thickened tissue, persistent headache, sleep apnea/snoring, amenorrhea/impotence, colon polyps, unexplained ↑ prolactin	

IGF-1, insulin-like growth factor-1.

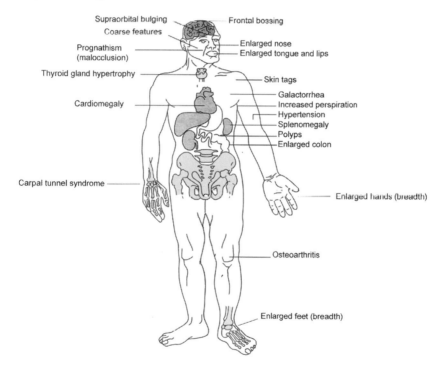

Fig. 2. Clinical features in acromegaly. Schematic representation of clinical signs in advanced acromegaly. (Adapted from ref. *123*.)

(19–21). Knees, hips, shoulders, lumbosacral joints, elbows, and ankles are commonly affected. Crepitus, stiffness, and tenderness commonly occur, with severe joint pain signifying irreversible joint degeneration. Carpal tunnel syndrome, (a painful entrapment median nerve neuropathy), occurs in up to 50% of patients and resolves early in the course of treatment. Dorsal spine kyphosis may result from osteophytosis, disc space widening, and increased anteroposterior verte-

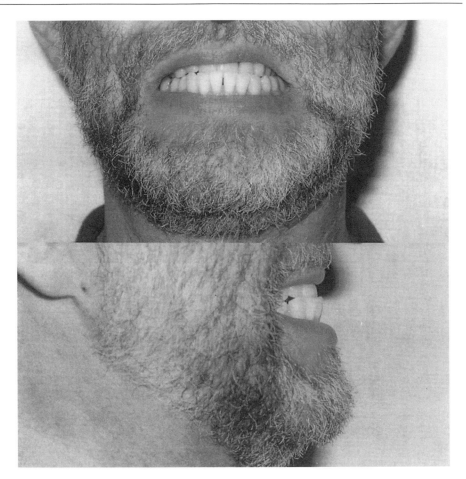

Fig. 3. Jaw overbite due to mandibular overgrowth in acromegaly.

bral length *(21)*. Severity of joint changes correlates with duration of excessive GH secretion *(21)*. Reversibility of joint symptoms with therapy depends on the degree of cartilage degeneration present.

Skin Changes

Hyperhidrosis with an unpleasant odor and oily skin occur early in the course of acromegaly in up to 70% of patients. Skin thickening caused by glycosaminoglycan deposition *(22)*, and increased collagen production, result in facial wrinkles, increased nasolabial fold, and heel pad thickness *(23)*. Skin tags are very common and are frequently associated with the presence of colonic polyps *(24)*.

Cardiovascular Disease

Cardiovascular disease accounts for approximately 60% of deaths in acromegaly *(25)* and is the most significant predictor of mortality. Coexisting hypertension and coronary artery disease occur *(25–29)*, in addition to a specific GH/IGF-1-mediated cardiomyopathy *(25)*.

Twenty percent of patients have symptomatic heart disease, expanded extracellular fluid volume owing to sodium and fluid retention, arterial hypertension, accelerated atherosclerosis, and cardiac arrhythmias. Fifty percent of patients have hypertension, with evidence of left-ventricular dysfunction in half *(29)*.

Fifty percent of normotensive patients have left-ventricular hypertrophy and asymmetric septal hypertrophy with subclinical left-ventricular diastolic dysfunction. Myocardial hypertrophy and interstitial fibrosis with lymphocytic myocardial infiltrates have been demonstrated. Fifty percent of patients have abnormal electrocardiograms, with ST-segment, T-wave abnormalities and arrythmias. The presence of cardiac disease at diagnosis worsens prognosis, and aggressive control of GH/IGF-1 improves cardiac function *(30)*.

Respiratory Disease

Respiratory complications contribute significantly to morbidity and mortality in acromegaly, accounting for 25% of deaths *(25)*. Both upper airway obstruction as well as central respiratory depression contribute to respiratory complication. Prognathism, macroglossia, hypertrophied nasal structures, tracheal calcification, and cricoarytenoid joint arthopathy contribute to significant upper airway obstruction *(31–33)*. Laryngeal mucosal and cartilaginous hypertrophy leads to vocal cord fixation and laryngeal stenosis with accompanying voice change *(31)*. These factors contribute to the difficulty in tracheal intubation often encountered in patients undergoing anesthesia. Central respiratory center depression, as well as upper airway obstruction, can result in sleep apnea and excessive snoring and also contribute to paroxysmal daytime sleepiness (narcolepsy) *(31)*.

Neuromuscular Disease

Carpal tunnel syndrome may occur, owing to increased edema *(34)*. Proximal myopathy may manifest as myalgia and proximal muscle weakness caused by hypertrophy and necrosis of skeletal muscle fiber *(35)*. A symmetric sensorimotor peripheral neuropathy, distinct from diabetic neuropathy, may rarely occur in patients who have had long-standing poorly controlled diabetes mellitus.

Endocrine Complications

Thirty percent of acromegalic patients have concomitant elevated serum PRL levels, with or without galactorrhea *(15)* owing to functional pituitary stalk compression by the adenoma, with interruption of tonic hypothalamic dopamine inhibition *(36)* or concomitant GH and PRL hypersecretion from mixed GH-cell and PRL-cell plurihormonal adenomas, monomorphous, mammosomatotroph adenomas, and acidophilic stem cell adenomas *(9)*.

Because most patients harbor macroadenomas, hypopituitarism develops from compression of normal surrounding pituitary tissue by the expanding tumor mass causing amenorrhea and impotence in half of acromegalic patients *(15,37)*, with secondary hypothyroidism and hypoadrenalism in approximately 20%.

Carbohydrate intolerance is caused by the direct antiinsulin effects of GH, and patients may develop insulin-requiring diabetes mellitus *(38)*, both of which improve with lowering of the elevated GH levels. Hypertriglyceridemia, hypercalciuria, and hypercalcemia are well described in acromegaly *(39)*. Acromegaly may be associated with MEN-1 syndrome, and thus hyperparathyroidism resulting in hypercalcemia can occur, as well as pancreatic tumors causing hypoglycemia.

Psychological Changes

There is no clear evidence for an increased incidence of psychological disorders in acromegaly *(40,41)*. However, decreased self-esteem could result from disfigurement, and depression and apathy may occur as part of any chronic disorder.

Colonic Polyps

Forty-five percent of patients with acromegaly have been reported to harbor colonic polyps *(38)*, which are potentially premalignant. However, a recent controlled study did not confirm an increased incidence of polyps in acromegaly *(42)*. Skin tags are present in most patients harboring colonic polyps *(24,43)*. Colonoscopy is recommended for diagnosis of colonic polyps with resection of these premalignant lesions.

DIAGNOSIS

Serum GH Levels

GH is secreted in a pulsatile manner, and normal serum levels fluctuate from undetectable up to 30 µg/L *(44)*. Thus evaluation of a random GH sample can be misleading. In the clinical setting of suspected acromegaly, GH estimation after an oral glucose load confirms the diagnosis. Serum GH levels that do not suppress to less than 1 µg/L 2 h after an oral glucose (75-g) load are diagnostic; paradoxically, glucose may actually stimulate GH secretion in about 10% of patients *(45)*. Using newer, highly sensitive GH assays *(46)*, random GH levels in acromegalic patients may be less than 1.0 µg/L, and even as low as 0.37 µg/ L when IGF-1 levels are still elevated postoperatively *(47)*. Thus biochemical exclusion criteria for acromegaly mandate a random GH of less than 0.4 µg/L or a GH nadir of less than 1 µg/L during oral glucose tolerance testing (OGTT), both with normal IGF-1 levels *(45)*.

Serum IGF-1 Levels

Elevated serum IGF-1 levels are a reliable screening test for acromegaly *(48)*, and the degree of elevation correlates well with the log of serum GH determinations *(49)*. IGF-1 levels must be matched for age and sex. Pregnancy and puberty also elevate serum IGF-1 levels. IGFbinding protein (BP)-3 levels are usually elevated in acromegaly but provide no diagnostic advantage over IGF-1 *(48)*.

Differential Diagnosis

IGF-1 levels are elevated in acromegaly, and GH levels fail to suppress to less than 1 µg/L after an oral glucose load *(49)*. More than 95% of patients harbor a GH cell pituitary adenoma *(4)*. However, it is important to confirm the rare diagnosis of extrapituitary acromegaly to plan appropriate treatment. After the biochemical diagnosis of acromegaly has been confirmed, anatomic localization of a pituitary tumor is confirmed using pituitary magnetic resonance imaging (MRI) with and without contrast. In rare patients who have a normal pituitary MRI, a strong suspicion of extrapituitary tumor should be entertained, and abdominal and chest computed tomography (CT) performed in an attempt to localize the ectopic source preoperatively. Elevated circulating GHRH levels, *(50)* normal pituitary MRI, and clinical and biochemical features of other tumors known to be associated with extrapituitary acromegaly are indicators for extrapituitary imaging. However, pituitary hyperplasia occurs in patients with ectopic GHRH-secreting tumors, resulting in an enlarged pituitary on MRI, which may be difficult to differentiate from a pituitary adenoma.

TREATMENT

Goals of Therapy

Successful therapy for acromegaly involves tumor mass control and normalization of GH/IGF-1 levels, while preserving normal anterior pituitary function, to prevent long-term clinical consequences of GH hypersecretion *(45,51)*. Mortality associated with poorly controlled acromegaly is two to three times *(24)* that of age- and sex-matched healthy controls (Fig. 4), and it is therefore important to reverse the mortality rate by aiming for tight control of GH with normalization of the GH/IGF-1 axis *(51)*. Clinical assessment of "cure" requires serum GH levels to be suppressed to less than 1 ng/mL after an oral glucose load with a normal age- and sex-matched serum IGF-1 level. Metabolic, acral, and soft tissue effects of GH hypersecretion, including glucose intolerance, hypertension, arthritis, and nerve entrapment syndromes, should also be reversed *(51)*. Current therapies for acromegaly include surgery, radiation therapy, and medical management.

Surgery

The success of surgery is largely dependent on the expertise of the neurosurgeon. Selective transsphenoidal surgery is the treatment of choice for somatotroph

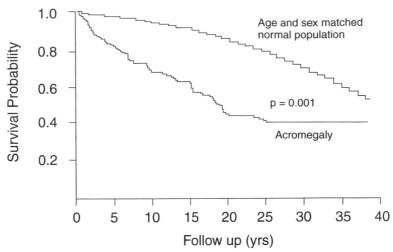

Fig. 4. Mortality in acromegaly. Mortality in patients with acromegaly (lower solid line) is two to three times that of matched normal controls (upper solid line). (Reproduced from Rajasoorya et al. Determinants of clinical outcome and survival in acromegaly. Clin Endocrinol 1994;41:95–102.

cell adenomas confined to the sella *(52–55)*. Fifty to 90% of patients with microadenomas achieved postoperative GH levels of less than 2.5 ng/mL, whereas less than 50% of patients with macroadenomas had postoperative GH levels of less than 2 ng/mL after glucose *(53)* (Table 5). Using normalized IGF-1 as a criterion for cure in 17 studies of 1284 patients, 82% of patients with microadenomas had normal IGF-1 levels, whereas 47% of patients with macroadenomas had normalized IGF-1 levels. A less invasive, endoscopic transnasal surgical approach has been developed. Long-term results of this procedure are being evaluated.

Surgical complications occur in approximately 10% of patients, including permanent diabetes insipidus, cerebrospinal fluid leaks, hemorrhage, secondary empty sella syndrome, meningitis, and sinusitis (Table 6). Approximately 20% of patients develop new hypopituitarism postoperatively, owing to surgical damage of the surrounding normal pituitary tissue *(56)*, which may require life-long hormone replacement therapy. The incidence of complications is related to the experience of the neurosurgeon as well as the tumor size. Approximately 7% of patients experience tumor recurrence, as shown by 10-yr postoperative follow-up.

Radiation Treatment

Radiation therapy (conventional external deep x-ray therapy and proton beam or heavy particle radiation therapy) has been used as primary or adjuvant therapy for acromegaly *(51)*, as it stops tumor growth and shrinks pituitary adenomas *(57)*. The major disadvantage of radiation therapy is the slow rate of cure, with

Table 5
Percentage of Patients with Acromegaly Achieving GH Levels of Less
Than 2.5 µg/L after Transsphenoidal Surgery in Selected Series

Patients (no.)	Microadenomas in remission (no.)	Macroadenomas in remission (no.)	Year	Reference
224	72	49	1992	53
76	84	73	1994	126
78	54	30	1950	127
100	61	30	1996	128
72	59	14	1998	129
162	91	48	1998	47
139	91	46	1999	130
66	86	52	1999	131

Adapted from ref. 52.

the National Institutes of Health (NIH) reporting that it takes up to 20 yr after radiation for 90% of patients to exhibit GH levels of less than 5 ng/mL (58). Pretreatment GH levels directly affect the biochemical response. In patients with GH levels of more than 100 ng/mL prior to radiation therapy, only 60% have a GH of less than 5 ng/mL after 18 yr (59). During the first 7 yr after radiation, less than 5% of patients normalize their IGF-1 levels (60), whereas only 70% normalize IGF-1 levels during longer follow-up (61). Thus a very high percentage of patients is exposed to continuing elevated GH levels in the initial years after radiation.

The recent advent of stereotactic radiation, using the γ-knife, has the potential to control tumor mass and normalize GH/IGF-1 levels more rapidly with a lower incidence of hypopituitarism (62,63). Long-term follow-up of this therapy is required (64).

SIDE EFFECTS OF RADIATION THERAPY

Of patients who undergo conventional radiation therapy, 1–2% experience hair loss, cranial nerve palsies, tumor necrosis with hemorrhage, and optic nerve damage or pituitary apoplexy with visual loss (65–69). Lethargy, memory loss, and altered personality are also reported (70). Half of patients treated with radiation therapy develop hypopituitarism within 10 yr of receiving radiation treatment (58,71), with an increased incidence annually thereafter (65), requiring permanent replacement with gonadal steroids, thyroid hormone, and cortisone. Secondary brain neoplasms arising in the radiation field have been rarely reported (72,73). Radiation therapy is highly effective in shrinking GH-secreting adenomas, but it takes 15–20 yr to control GH/IGF-1 levels in 90% of patients. Radiation therapy is recommended for patients not cured by surgical or medical

Table 6
Complications of Transsphenoidal
Pituitary Surgery

Transient
    Diabetes insipidus
    Cerebrospinal fluid leak and rhinorrhea
    Inappropriate ADH secretion
    Arachnoiditis
    Meningitis
    Postoperative psychosis
    Local hematoma
    Arterial wall damage
    Epistaxis
    Local abscess
    Pulmonary embolism
    Narcolepsy
Permanent (up to 10%)
    Diabetes insipidus
    Total or partial hypopituitarism
    Visual loss
    Inappropriate ADH secretion
    Vascular occlusion
    Central nervous system damage
        Oculomotor palsy
        Hemiparesis
        Encephalopathy
    Nasal septum perforation
Surgery-related mortality (up to 1%)
    Brain, hypothalamic injury
    Vascular damage
    Postoperative meningitis
    Cerebrospinal leak
    Pneumocephalus
    Acute cardiopulmonary disease
    Seizure

ADH, antidiuretic hormone.
Adapted from ref. *122.*

therapy, in view of the slow onset of action and high incidence of hypopituitarism.

Medical Therapy

Several different medical therapies have been used in acromegaly, either alone or in combination, to control GH secretion (Table 7). These drugs act at different sites in the GH/IGF-1 pathway (Fig. 5).

Table 7
Medical Therapy for Acromegaly

Dopamine agonist therapy
    Short-acting: oral administration bid or tid
        Bromocriptine (Parlodel®)
    Long-acting oral administration biw
        Cabergoline (Dostinex®)
Somatostatin analog therapy
    Short-acting: subcutaneous administration tid or bid
        Octreotide
    Long-acting: intramuscular administration monthly or q 7, 10, or 14 d
        Sandostatin LAR® depot
        Lanreotide®
Growth hormone receptor antagonist therapy
    Pegvisomant: subcutaneous daily administration

The hypothalamic peptides, somostatin (SRIF) and GHRH act together to inhibit and stimulate, respectively, pituitary GH secretion. GH in turn stimulates hepatic IGF-1 production. IGF-1 has a negative feedback on pituitary GH secretion and a positive feedback effect on hypothalamic SRIF release. GH acts both indirectly via IGF-1 and directly. Several medical therapies have been developed that mimic or block physiologic actions of the different components of this complex GH/IGF-1 feedback pathway, ultimately suppressing GH/IGF-1 action.

Dopamine Agonists

Dopamine inhibits GH secretion in about one-third of patients, suggesting the use of dopamine agonists as a potential therapy for GH hypersecretion. High doses of bromocriptine, a short-acting dopamine agonist administered orally two to three times daily or cabergoline, administered orally biweekly, are used as primary or adjuvant therapy for acromegaly *(74)*.

Higher doses of dopamine agonist than those used to suppress hyperprolactinemia in patients with prolactinomas are required to suppress GH hypersecretion in acromegaly. Bromocriptine doses of up to 20 mg/d or more may be required to suppress GH in acromegaly *(75)*. Although 75% of patients experience amelioration of symptoms including reduced perspiration, fatigue, headache, and soft tissue swelling, in only 15% of acromegalic patients are GH levels suppressed to less than 5 ng/mL, with 15% of patients experiencing minimal tumor shrinkage.

Experience with cabergoline, a long-acting dopamine agonist, is more limited, suggesting that up to one-third of acromegalic patients suppress GH levels to less than 2 ng/mL *(76–78)*. Side effects of dopamine agonists (especially the high doses of bromocriptine that are required) include gastrointestinal upset,

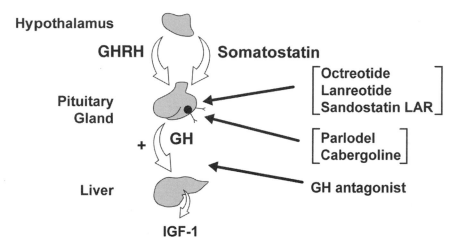

Fig. 5. Site of action of different medical therapies for acromegaly in the growth hormone/insulin-like growth factor-1 (GH/IGF-1) pathway. Dopamine agonists and somatostatin analogs bind to specific pituitary tumor receptors and inhibit pituitary GH secretion. The GH receptor antagonists bind to hepatic GH receptors, preventing receptor dimerization, thereby blocking the peripheral GH action, resulting in decreased IGF-1 generation. GHRH, growth hormone-releasing hormone.

nasal stuffiness, nausea, vomiting, headache, and postural hypotension resulting in dizziness and (rarely) peripheral vasospasm.

Somatostatin Analogs

Five somatostatin receptor subtypes (SSTR1–5), are widely expressed and mediate several physiologic functions including inhibition of pituitary GH hypersecretion, attenuation of insulin secretion, and regulation of gastrointestinal secretion and motility *(79)*.

Hypothalamic somatostatin (SRIF) inhibits pituitary GH secretion. SSTR2 and SSTR5 are preferentially expressed on somatotroph and thyrotroph cell surfaces *(80)*. Several somatostatin analogs, which mimic the physiologic actions of native somatostatin, have been developed for treating acromegaly (Fig. 6).

Octreotide

Octreotide, an octapeptide, was the first somatostatin analog developed. Octreotide is 45 times more potent than native somatostatin in suppressing GH secretion and has a prolonged half-life of up to 2 h in the circulation *(81)* as opposed to the 2-h circulating half-life of native SRIF. Octreotide weakly inhibits insulin secretion compared with native SRIF, whereas effects on gastrointes-

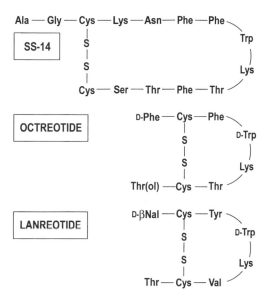

Fig. 6. Amino acid sequences of the three available somatostatin analogs, compared with endogenous somatostatin-14 (SS-14). (Reproduced from van der Lely AJ, Lamberts SWJ. Medical therapy for acromegaly. In Wass J, ed. Handbook of Acromegaly. BioScientifica, Bristol, UK, 2001, p. 52.

tinal motility are more pronounced, resulting in some of the gastrointestinal side effects of octreotide.

Octreotide binds to SSTR2 and SSTR5. The increased potency and prolonged suppression of GH hypersecretion *(82,83)* and lack of rebound GH hypersecretion on withdrawal contribute to the development of octreotide as a useful therapy in acromegaly *(84–87)*.

In a double-blind, placebo-controlled trial, octreotide administered subcutaneously significantly suppressed GH and IGF-1 levels in 90% of patients, with integrated GH levels of less than 2 ng/mL in 25% of patients and IGF-1 normalization in about 70% of patients *(87)* (Fig. 7).

An average daily dose of 150–200 µg tid or qid offers optimal responses; maximum doses of 1500 mg/d can be used *(88)*. Elderly male patients and patients with lower pretreatment GH levels and smaller tumors exhibit greater sensitivity to octreotide *(89)*. Tolerance to the suppressive effects of GH hypersecretion does not develop during long-term treatment with octreotide *(90–92)*.

Long-Acting Somatostatin Analogs

Sandostatin LAR depot is a sustained release intramuscular depot preparation of octreotide *(93–96)*. A single, intramuscular, 10-, 20-, or 30-mg injection results

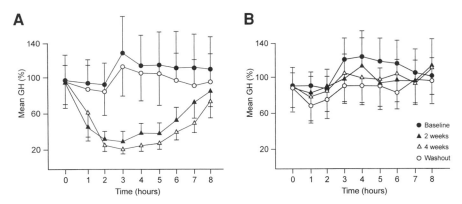

Fig. 7. Effect of octreotide or placebo on hourly growth hormone (GH) levels in acromegaly. Mean percentage changes (± SE of basal values) of serum GH concentrations in patients with acromegaly treated with either 100 μg octreotide subcutaneously every 8 h ($n = 52$; **a**) or placebo ($n = 47$; **b**) subcutaneously every 8 h. Blood was sampled before an injection and every hour for 8 subsequent h before treatment (baseline), at the end of wk 2 and 4 of treatment, and 4 wk after discontinuation of treatment (washout). Octreotide or placebo was administered just after the 0-h sampling. (Reproduced from Ezzat S, Snyder PJ, Young WF, et al. Octreotide treatment of acromegaly: a randomized multicenter study. Ann Intern Med 1992;117:711–718.)

in peak drug levels at 28 d with sustained suppression of integrated GH levels for up to 49 d (Fig. 8). GH is suppressed after monthly injections for up to 18 mo *(97)*. IGF-1 levels are suppressed in 60–70% of patients receiving Sandostatin LAR depot.

Lanreotide, a 30-mg slow release intramuscular preparation injectable every 7, 10, or 14 d *(98–100)*, suppresses integrated GH to less than 2.5 ng/mL in 60% of patients and normalizes IGF-1 in 60–70% of patients *(100)*. It is not yet approved in the United States.

CLINICAL RESPONSE TO SOMATOSTATIN ANALOGS

Octreotide reduces tumor size by 20–80% possibly in a dose-related fashion in about a third of patients *(87,101,102)*, usually within the first 4 mo of initiating therapy. Preoperative octreotide for 3–6 mo may improve postoperative biochemical control *(103,104)*.

Clinical features of acromegaly improve as GH/IGF-1 levels decrease during chronic administration of octreotide *(103,105)*. Headache frequently resolves rapidly, within minutes of injection *(106)*. Soft tissue swelling, caused by sodium and water retention in acromegaly, resolves rapidly with treatment in more than 70% of patients *(87)* and is accomplished by decreased swelling of face, feet, and hands, and reduced parasthesias and numbness caused by nerve entrapment.

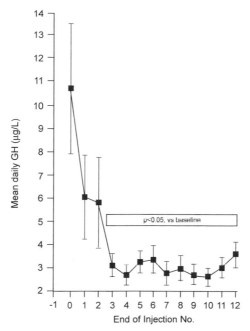

Fig. 8. Long-term serum growth hormone (GH) responses to monthly LAR injections. Results are expressed as mean (SE of either 12-h or 8-h daily GH profiles. The dose of Sandostatin LAR was 10 mg (*n* = 3), 20 mg (*n* = 2), or 30 mg (*n* = 3) every 60 d for injections 1 and 2 and 20 mg (*n* = 2), 30 mg (*n* = 5), or 40 mg (*n* = 1) every 28 (*n* = 4) or 42 d (*n* = 4) thereafter. GH profiles were taken at baseline (no treatment) and on the last day of each injection. (Adapted from ref. *95*.)

Improved control is associated with decreased blood pressure, heart rate, and left-ventricular wall thickness *(29, 107)* in patients without cardiac, renal, or liver disease. Octreotide improves left-ventricular ejection fraction and reduces systemic arterial resistance, oxygen consumption, and fluid volume in patients with cardiac failure. Joint function improves in those patients with bone and cartilage involvement, which can be reversed with chronic therapy *(108)*. Sleep apnea improves after several months *(109)*.

SIDE EFFECTS

The side effects of somatostatin analogs, usually transient, are caused by the inhibitory effects of somatostatin on gastrointestinal hormones, motility, and secretion *(84)*. Loose stools, flatulence, and nausea occur in approximately one-third of patients.

Patients with diabetes mellitus have lowered insulin requirements, although neither hypoglycemia nor hyperglyemia occur commonly. Reduced gallbladder contractility and delayed emptying occur in up to 25% of patients on octreotide, with subsequent development of gallbladder sludge *(110,111)*. Clinically apparent cholelithiasis is uncommon. The incidence of gallbladder sludge or stones occurs most frequently in China *(111)*, Australia *(112)*, and the United Kingdom *(104)*. In the United States, serial ultrasound suggests that one-third of patients experience echogenic gallbladder deposits, usually within 18 mo of initiating therapy *(113)*, with no further episodes.

GH Receptor Antagonist Therapy

GH binds to its hepatic receptors, inducing dimerization, which signals a cascade of molecular events culminating in IGF-1 generation *(114)*. Pegvisomant, a genetically engineered GH analog, binds to the GH receptor (Fig. 9) and prevents functional GH receptor dimerization, thereby preventing GH signal transduction and subsequent IGF-1 generation *(115–117)*. This novel mechanism of action inhibits peripheral GH action, rather than decreasing GH secretion. Pegvisomant administered by daily subcutaneous injection normalizes IGF-1 levels in more than 90% of patients, with decreased fatigue, soft tissue swelling and perspiration *(117)*. Pegvisomant has not yet been approved by the Food and Drug Administration.

APPROACH TO THERAPY

Several different treatment modalities are available to attain tight control of GH hypersecretion in order to improve morbidity and mortality in patients with acromegaly. Multiple treatment options may be required, and an individualized therapeutic approach is recommended for each patient (Fig. 10).

In assessing the role of surgery as primary therapy, the likelihood of cure must be seriously considered. Surgery is the primary treatment for pituitary microadenomas or macroadenomas that have not spread beyond the sella. However, 70% of acromegalic patients have macroadenomas at the time of presentation, which have spread beyond the sella turcica and are not amendable to curative resection. There are no conclusive trials confirming that preoperative treatment with somatostatin analog therapy improves the surgical outcome. Postoperatively, patients who are not "cured" require medical therapy. Dopamine agonist therapy has a low efficacy but is inexpensive, with mild side effects, and can be used initially. Subsequently somatostatin analog therapy can be instituted, initially by a subcutaneous injection of 50–100 µg with measurement of GH and IGF-1 after 2 h *(118)* to assess efficacy. Tolerability and efficacy are assessed by administering octreotide subcutaneously three to four times a day, for 3–4 d. If GH levels are suppressed by more than 50% *(97)* and patients do not experience intolerable gastrointestinal side effects, therapy with Sandostatin LAR is initiated.

Patients treated with somatostatin analogs require assessment of postprandial glucose levels every 3 mo. Gallbladder ultrasound is performed only if symp-

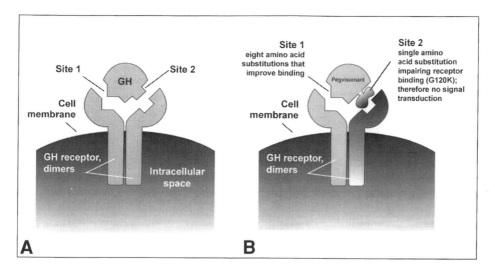

Fig. 9. Action of growth hormone (GH) receptor antagonist. (**A**) Normally a single molecule of GH binds two GH receptors through sites 1 and 2, and the GH signal transduction pathway is activated. (**B**) Pegvisomant increases binding of the GH receptor to site 1 and blocks binding at site 2 to prevent functional GH receptor dimerization, initiation of GH action, and induction of IGF-1 synthesis and secretion. The peripheral effects of excess GH are antagonized at the cellular level, independent of the presence of somatostatin or dopamine receptors on the pituitary tumor. (Adapted from ref. *124.*)

toms of cholelithiasis occur. The development of asymptomatic gallbladder sludge does not require monitoring by serial ultrasound.

Primary medical therapy is recommended in patients who are at high risk for surgery or anesthesia or those who refuse surgery. There is also a role for primary medical therapy in patients with invasive macroadenomas not amenable to curative surgical resection, with a high likelihood of persistently elevated postoperative GH levels, who will require somatostatin analog therapy postoperatively despite surgery *(119).*

In patients whose pituitary lesions abut the optic chiasm with visual field defects, surgical resection is indicated. A second surgical resection is recommended for patients with tumor recurrence.

Radiation therapy is indicated in patients who are intolerant to medical therapy or fail to respond. However, medication may still be required for several years after radiation, until GH levels are lowered.

The criteria for "cure" of acromegaly include a GH suppressed to less than 1 ng/mL after an OGTT and normal age- and sex-matched IGF-1 levels. Patients should be followed quarterly with titration of the dose of medication until biochemical control is achieved. In patients with no residual tumor tissue

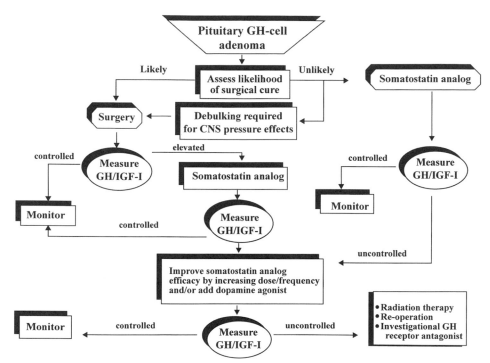

Fig. 10. Algorithm for decision making in the treatment of acromegaly. GH, growth hormone; IGF-1, insulin-like growth factor-1. (Adapted from ref. *125*.)

remnant and biochemical cure, IGF-1 levels should be assayed annually with a pituitary MRI repeated every 1–2 yr *(121)*.

In patients with residual tumor tissue or those with hypopituitarism requiring hormone replacement medical treatment, as well as patients who have received pituitary radiation, testing of adrenal, gonadal, and thyroid reserve should be performed semiannually and pituitary MRI annually. Mammogram and colonoscopy should be performed annually in patients over the age of 50 yr, especially if skin tags are present.

REFERENCES

1. Alexander L, Appleton D, Hall R, Ross WM, Wilkinson R. Epidemiology of acromegaly in the Newcastle region. Clin Endocrinol 1980;12:71–79.
2. Bengtsson B-A, Eden S, Ernest I, Oden A, Sjogren B. Epidemiology and long-term survival in acromegaly. Acta Med Scand 1988;223:27–35.
3. Ritchie CM, Atkinson AB, Kennedy Al, et al. Ascertainment and natural history of treated acromegaly in Northern Ireland. Ulster Med 1990;59:55–62.

4. Melmed S. Acromegaly. N Engl J Med 1990;322:966–977.
5. Lindah A, Isgaard J, Carlsson L, Isaksson OGP. Differential effects of growth hormone and insulin-like growth factor 1 on colony formation of epiphysial chondrocytes in suspension culture in rats of different ages. Endocrinology 1987;121:1061–1019.
6. Asa SL, Kovacs K. Pituitary pathology in acromegaly. Endocrinol Metab Clin 1992;21:553–574.
7. Lloyd RV, Cano M, Chandler WF, Barkan AL, Horvath E, Kovacs K. Human growth hormone and prolactin secreting pituitary adenomas by in situ hybridization. Am J Pathol 1989;134:605–613.
8. Halmi NS. Occurrence of both growth hormone and prolactin immunoreactive materials in the cells of human somatotropic pituitary adenomas contain in mammotropic elements. Virchows Arch [A] 1982;398:19–31.
9. Kovacs K, Horvath E, Asa SL, et al. Pituitary cells producing more than one hormone. Trends Endocrinol Metab 1989;1:104–108.
10. Stewart PM, Carey MP, Graham CT, Wright AD, London DR. Growth hormone secreting pituitary carcinoma: a case report and literature review. Clin Endocrinol 1992;37:189–195.
11. Thorner MO, Perryman RL, Cronin MJ, et al. Somatotroph hyperplasia: successful treatment of acromegaly by removal of pancreatic islet tumor secreting a growth hormone-secreting factor. J Clin Invest 1982;70:965–972.
12. Low L, Chernausek SD, Sperling MA. Acromegaloid patietns with type A insulin resistance: parallel defects in insulin and insulin-like growth factor-I receptors and biological responses in cultured fibroblasts. J Clin Endocrinol Metab 1988;69:329–337.
13. Ashcroft MW, Hartzband PI, Van Herle A, et al. A unique growth factor in patients with acromegaloidism. J Clin Endocrinol Metab 1983;57:272–276.
14. Prezant T, Melmed S. Pathogenesis of pituitary tumors. In Besser GM, Thomas M, eds. Comprehensive Clinical Endocrinology, 3rd ed. Harcourt, London, 2001.
15. Drange MR, Fram NR, Bonert VH, Melmed S. Pituitary tumor registry: a novel clinical resource. J Clin Endocrinol Metab 2000;85:168–174,.
16. Melmed S, Braunstein GD, Chang RJ, Becker DP. Pituitary tumors secreting growth hormone and prolactin [clinical conference]. Ann Intern Med 1986;105:238–253.
17. Molitch ME. Clinical manifestations of acromegaly. Clin Endocrinol Metab 1992;21:597–614.
18. Lieberman SA, Bjorkengren AG, Hoffman AR. Rheumatologic and skeletal changes in acromegaly. Endocrinol Metab Clin 1992;21:615–631.
19. Ibbertson HK, Manning PJ, Holdaway IM, et al. The acromegalic rosary. Lancet 1991;337:154–156.
20. Layton MW, Fudman EJ, Barkan A, et al. Acromegalic arthopathy. Characteristics and response to therapy. Arthritis Rheum 1988;31:1022–1028.
21. Dons RF, Roseelet P, Pastakia B, et al. Arthropathy in acromegalic patients before and after treatment; a long-term follow-up study. Clin Endocrinol 1988;28:515–524.
22. Matsuoka LY, Wortsman J, Kupchella CE, et al. Histochemical characterization of the cutaneous involvement of acromegaly. Arch Intern Med 1932;142:1820–1833.
23. MacSweeny JE, Baxter MA, Joplin GF. Heel pad thickness is an insensitive index of biochemical remission in acromegaly. Clin Radiol 1990;42:348–350.
24. Leavitt J, Klein I, Kendricks F, Gavaler J, Vanthiel DH. Skin tags: a cutaneous marker for colonic polyps. Ann Intern Med 1983;98:928–930.
25. Rajasoorya C, Holdaway IM, Wrightson P, et al. Determinants of clinical outcome and survival in acromegaly. Clin Endocrinol 1994;41:95–107.
26. Bates AS, Van't Hoff W, Jones JM, et al. An audit of outcome of treatment in acromegaly. Q J Med 1993;86:293–299.
27. Lombardi G, Colao A, Marzullo P, et al. Is growth hormone bad for your heart? Cardiovascular impact of GH deficiency and of acromegaly. J Endocrinol 1997;155:S33–S39.

28. Colao A, Cuocolo A, Marzullo P, et al. Impact of patient's age and disease duration on cardiac performance in acromegaly: a radionuclide angiography atudy. J Clin Endocrinol Metab 1999;84:1518–1523.

29. Luboshitzki R, Hammerman H, Barzilai D, et al. The heart in acromegaly: correlation of echocardiographic and clinical findings. Isr J Med Sci 1980;16:378–383.

30. Colao A, Cuocolo A, Marzullo P, et al. Effects of 1-year treatment with octreotide on cardiac performance in patients with acromegaly. J Clin Endocrinol Metab 1999;84:17–23.

31. Trtoman-Dickenson B, Weetman AP, Hughes JMB. Upper airflow obstruction and pulmonary function in acromegaly: relationship to disease activity. Q J Med 1991;79:527–533.

32. Barnes AJ, Pallis C, Joplin GF. Acromegaly and narcolepsy. Lancet 1979;ii:332–333.

33. Pekkarinen T, Partinen M, Pelkonen R, et al. Sleep apnoea and daytime sleepiness in acromegaly: relationship to endocrinological factors. Clin Endocrinol 1987;27:649–54.

34. Jenkins JP, Sohaib SA, Akker S, et al. The pathology of median neuropathy in acromegaly. Ann Intern Med 2000;133:197–201,.

35. O'Duffy JD, Randall RV, MacCarty CS. Median neuropathy (carpal-tunnel syndrome) in acromegaly. A sign of endocrine overactivity. Ann Intern Med 1973;78:379–383.

36. Barkan AL. Acromegaly diagnosis and therapy. Endocrinol Metab Clin 1989;18:277–310.

37. Kaltsas GA, Mukherjee JJ, Jenkins PJ, et al Menstral irregularity in women with acromegaly. J Clin Endocrinol Metab 1999;84:2731–2735.

38. Melmed S. Acromegaly and cancer: not a problem? J Clin Endocrinol Metab 2001;86:2929–2934.

39. James RA, Moller N, Chatterjee S, et al. Carbohydrate tolerance and serum lipids in acromegaly before and during treatment with high dose octreotide. Diabetic Med 1991;8:517–523.

40. Abed RT, Clark J, Elbadawy MHF, et al. Psychiatric morbidity in acromegaly. Acta Psychiatric Scand 1987;75:635–639.

41. Furman K, Ezzat S. Psychological features of acromegaly. Psychother Psychosom 1998;67:147–153.

42. Renehan AG, Bhaskar P, Painter JE, et al. The prevalence and characteristics of colorectal neoplasia in acromegaly. J Clin Endocrinol Metab 2000;85:3417–3424.

43. Ezzat S, Strom C, Melmed S. Colon polyps in acromegaly. Ann Intern Med 1991;114:754–758.

44. Hartman ML, Veldhuis JD, Vance ML, et al. Evidence of an endrogenous digitalis-like factor in the plasma of patients with acromegaly reduced by successful therapy. J Clin Endocrinol Metab 1990;70:1375–1384.

45. Giustina A, Barkan A, Casanueva F, et al. Criteria for cure of acromegaly: a consensus statement. J Clin Endocrinol Metab 2000;85:526–529.

46. Veldhuis JD, Liem AY, South S, et al. Differential impact of age, sex steroid hormones, and obesity on basal versus pulsatile growth hormone secretion in men as assessed in an ultrasensitive chemiluminescence assay. J Clin Endocrinol Metab 1995;80:3209–3222.

47. Freda PU, Post KD, Powell JS, Wardlaw SL. Evaluation of disease status with sensitive measures of growth hormone secretion in 60 postoperative patients with acromegaly. J Clin Endocrinol Metab 1998;83:3808–3816.

48. Clemmons DR, Van Wyk JJ, Ridgway E, et al. Evaluation of acromegaly by radioimmunoassay somatomedin C. N Engl J Med 1979;301:1138–1142.

49. Melmed S, Ho K, Klibanski A, Reichlin S, Thorner M. Recent advances in pathogenesis, diagnosis and management of acromegaly. J Clin Endocrinol Metab 1995;80:3395–3302.

50. Frohman LA. Ectopic hormone production by tumors. Clin Neuroendocr Perspect 1984;3:201–224.

51. Melmed S, Jackson I, Kleinberg D, Klibanski A. Current treatment guidelines for acromegaly. J Clin Endocrinol Metab 1998;83:2646–2652.

52. Stewart PM. Current therapy for acromegaly. Trends Endocrinol Metab 2000;11:128–132.

53. Fahlbusch R, Honegger J, Buchfelder M. Surgical management of acromegaly. Endocrinol Metab Clin North Am 1992;21:669–692.
54. Ross DA, Wilson CB. Results of transsphenoidal microsurgery for growth hormone secreting pituitary adenomas in a series of 214 patients. J Neurosurg 1988;68:854–867.
55. Jho HD, Carrau RL. Endoscopic endonasal transsphenoidal surgery: experience with 50 patients. J Neurosurg 1997;87:44–51.
56. Ciric I, Ragin A, Baumgartner C, et al. Complications of transsphenoidal surgery: results of a national survey, review of the literature, and personal experience. Neurosurgery 1997;40:225–236.
57. Biermasz NR, van Dulken H, Roelfsema F. Long-term follow-up results of postoperative radiotherapy in 36 patients with acromegaly. J Clin Endocrinol Metab 2000;85:2476–2482.
58. Eastman RC, Gorden P, Glatstein E, Roth J. Radiation therapy of acromegaly. Endocrinol Metab Clin North Am 1992;21:693–712.
59. Feek CM, McLellan J, Seth J, et al. How effective is external pituitary irradiation for growth hormone-secreting pituitary tumors? Clin Endocrinol 1984;20:401 408.
60. Barkan AI, Halasz I, Dornfeld KJ, et al. Pituitary irradiation is ineffective in normalizing plasma insulin-like growth factor I in patients with acromegaly. J Clin Endocrinol Metab 1997;82:3187–3191.
61. Powell JS, Wardlaw SL, Post KD, Freda PU. Outcome of radiotherapy for acromegaly using normalization of insulin-like growth factor I to define cure. J Clin Endocrinol Metab 2000;85:2068–2071.
62. Laws JE, Vance ML. Radiosurgery for pituitary tumors and craniopharyngiomas. Neurosurg Clin North Am 1999;10:327–336.
63. Landolt AM, Haller D, Lomax N, et al. Stereotactic radiosurgery for recurrent surgically treated acromegaly: comparison with fractionated radiotherapy. J Neurosurg 1998;88:1002–1008.
64. Pan L, Zhang N, Wang E, Wang B, Xu W. Pituitary adenomas: the effect of gamma knife radiosurgery on tumor growth and endocrinopathies. Stereotact Funct Neurosurg 1998;70:119–126.
65. Van der Lely AJ, Herder WW, Lamberts SWJ. Editorial: the role of radiotherapy in acromegaly. J Clin Endocrinol Metab 1997;82:3185–3186.
66. Millar JL, Spry NA, Lamb DS, Delahunt J. Blindness in patients after external beam irradiation for pituitary adenomas: two cases occurring after small daily fractional doses. Clin Oncol 1991;3:291–294.
67. Alexander MJ, DeSalles AA, Tomiyasu U. Multiple radiation-induced intracranial lesions after treatment for pituitary adenoma. Case report. J Neurosurg 1998;88:111–115.
68. Ahmed M, Kanaan I, Rifai A, et al. An unusual treatment-related complication in a patient with growth hormone-secreting pituitary tumor. J Clin Endocrinol Metab 1997;82:2816–2820.
69. Al-Mefty O, Kersh JE, Routh A, et al. The long-term side effects of radiation therapy for benign brain tumors in adults. J Neurosurg 1990;73:502–512.
70. Crossen JR, Garwo D, Glatstein E, et al. Neurobehavioral sequelae of cranial irradiation in adults: a review of radiation-induced encephalopathy. J Clin Oncol 1994;12:627–642.
71. Eastman RC, Gordon P, Roth J. Conventional supervoltage irradiaiton is an effective treatment for acromegaly. J Clin Endocrinol Metab 1979;48:931–940.
72. Brada M, Ford D, Ashley S, et al. Risk of second brain tumor after conservative surgery and radiotherapy for pituitary adenoma. BMJ 1992;304:1343–1346.
73. Tsang RW, Laperriere NJ, Simpson WJ, et al. Giloma arising after radiation therapy for pituitary adenoma. A report of four patients and estimation of risk [published erratum appears in Cancer 1994;73:492]. Cancer 1993;72:2227–2233.
74. Vance ML, Evans WS, Thorner MO. Bromocriptine. Ann Intern Med 1984;100:78–91.

75. Jaffe CA, Barkan AL. Treatment of acromegaly with dopamine agonists. Endocrinol Metab Clin 1992;3:713–735.
76. Jackson SN, Fowler J, Howlett TA. Cabergoline treatment of acromegaly: a preliminary dose finding study. Clin Endocrinol (Oxf) 1997;46:745–749.
77. Muratori M, Arosio M, Gambino G, et al. Use of cabergoline in the long-term treatment of hyperprolactinemia and acromegalic patients. J Endocrinol Invest 1997;20:537–546.
78. Abs R, Verhelst, Maiter D, et al. Cabergoline in the treatment of acromegaly : a study in 64 patients. J Clin Endocrinol Metab. 1998;83:374–378.
79. Reichlin S. Somatostatin. N Engl J Med 1983;309:1495–1501.
80. Shimon I, Taylor JE, Dong JZ, et al. Somatostatin receptor subtype specificity in human fetal pituitary cultures. Differential role of SSTR2 and SSTR5 for growth hormone, thyroid-stimulating hormone, and prolactin regulation. J Clin Invest 1997;99:789–798.
81. Wass JAH. Octreotide treatment of acromegaly. Horm Res 1990;1(suppl):1–5.
82. Plewe C, Beyer J, Krauve U, Neufeld M, del Pozo E. Long-acting and selective suppression of growth hormone secretion by somatostatin analogue SMS 201-995 in acromegaly. Lancet 1984;i:782–784.
83. Lamberts SWJ. The role of somatostatin in the regulation of anterior pituitary hormone secretion and the use of its analogs in the treatment of human pituitary tumors. Endocr Rev 1988;9:417–436.
84. Lamberts SWJ, van der Lely AJ, de Herder WW, et al. Octreotide. N Engl J Med 1996;334:246–254.
85. Lamberts SWJ, Uitterlinden P, Verschoor L, et al. Long-term treatment of acromegaly with the somatostatin analogue SMS 201-995. N Engl J Med 1985;313:1576–1580.
86. Sassolas G, Harris AG, James-Deidier, et al. Long-term effect of incremental doses of the somatostatin analog SMS 201-995 in 58 acromegalic patients. J Clin Endocrinol Metab 1990;71:391–397.
87. Ezzat S, Snyder PJ, Young WE, et al. Octreotide treatment of acromegaly: a randomized, multicenter study. Ann Intern Med 1992;117:711–718.
88. Quabbe HJ, Plockinger U. Dose response study and long-term effect of the somatostatin analog octreotide in patients with therapy resistant acromegaly. J Clin Endocrinol Metab 1989;68:873–881.
89. Van der Lely AJ, Harris AG, Lamberts SWJ. The sensitivity of growth hormone secretion to medical treatment in acromegalic patients: influence of age and sex. Clin Endocrinol 1992;37:181–185.
90. Newman CB, Melmed S, Snyder PJ, et al. Safety and efficacy of long-term octreotide therapy of acromegaly: results of a multicenter trial in 103 patients—a clinical research center study. J Clin Endocrinol Metab 1995; 80: 2768–2775.
91. Wang C, Lam KSL, Arceo E, Chan FL. Comparison of the effectiveness of 2-hourly versus 8-hourly subcutaneous injections of a somatostatin analog (SMS 201-995) in the treatment of acromegaly. J Clin Endocrinol Metab 1989;69:670–677.
92. Tauber JP, Babin TH, Tauber MT, et al. Long-term effects of continuous subcutaneous infusion of the somatostatin analog octreotide in the treatment of acromegaly. J Clin Endocrinol Metab 1988;68:917–924.
93. Flogstad AK, Halse J, Haldorsen T, et al. Sandostatin LAR in acromegalic patients: a dose-range study. J Clin Endocrinol Metab 1995;80:3601–3607.
94. Gillis JC, Noble S, Goa KL. Octreotide long-acting release (LAR): a review of its pharmacological properties and therapeutic use in the management of acromegaly. Drugs 1997;53:618–699.
95. Stewart PM, Kane KF, Stewart SE, et al. Depot long-acting somatostatin analog (Sandostatin-LAR) is an effective treatment for acromegaly. J Clin Endocrinol Metab 1995;80:3267–3272.

96. Lancran I, Atkinson AB, and the Sandostatin LAR Group. Results of a European multicentre study with Sandostatin LAR in acromegalic patients. Pituitary 1999;1:105–114.
97. Flogstad AK, Halse J, Bakke S, et al. Sandostatin LAR in acromegalic patients: long term treatment. J Clin Endocrinol Metab 1997;82:23–28.
98. Giusti M, Gussoni G, Cuttica CM, et al. Effectiveness and tolerability of slow release lanreotide treatment in active acromegaly: Six-month report on an Italian Multicenter Study. Italian Multicenter Slow Release Lanreotide Study Group. J Clin Endocrinol Metab 1996;81:2089–2097.
99. Caron P, Morange-Ramos I, Cogne M, et al. Three-year follow-up of acromegalic patients treated with intramuscular slow-release lanreotide. J Clin Endocrinol Metab 1997;38:18–22.
100. Giusti M, Cicccarelli E, Dallabonzan D, et al. Clinical results of long-term slow-release lanreotide treatment of acromegaly. Eur J Clin Invest 1997;27:277–284.
101. Barakat S, Melmed S. Reversible shrinkage of a growth hormone secreting pituitary adenoma by a long-acting somatostatin analog octreotide. Arch Intern Med 1989;149:1443–1445.
102. Barkan AL, Lloyd RV, Chandler WE, et al. Preoperative treatment of acromegaly with long-acting somatostatin analog SMS 201-995. Shrinkage of invasive pituitary macroadenomas and improved surgical remission rate. J Clin Endocrinol Metab 1988;67:1040–1048.
103. Colao A, Ferone D, Cappabianca P, et al. Effect of octreotide pretreatment on surgical outcome in acromegaly. J Clin Endocrinol Metab 1997;82:3308–3314.
104. Biermaz NR, van Dulkin H, Roelfsema F. Direct postoperative and follow-up results of transsphenoidal surgery in untreated matched controls. J Clin Endocrinol Metab 1999;84:3551–3555.
105. Page MD, Millward ME, Taylor A, et al. Long-term treatment of acromegaly with long-acting analogue of somatostatin, octreotide. Q J Med 1990;274:189–201.
106. Pascual J, Freijanes J, Berciano J, Pesquera C. Analgesic effect of octreotide in headache associated with acromegaly is not mediated by opioid mechanisms. Pain 1991;47:341–344.
107. Chanson P, Timsit J, Masquet C, et al. Cardiovascular effects of the somatostatin analog octreotide in acromegaly. Ann Intern Med 1990;113:921–923.
108. Layton MW, Fudman EJ, Barkan A, et al. Acromegalic arthropathy: characteristics and response to therapy. Arthritis Rheum 1988;31:1022–1028.
109. Ip MM, Tan KB, Peh WG, Lam KL. Effect of Sandostatin LAR on sleep apnoea in acromegaly: correlation with computerized tomographic cephalometry and hormonal activity. 2001;55:477–483.
110. Melmed S, Dowling RH, Frohman L, et al. Consensus statement: benefits vs. risks of medical therapy for acromegaly. Ann J Med 1994;97:468–473.
111. Shi Y-F, Zhu XF, Harris AG, Zhang JX, Dai Q. Prospective study of long-term effects of somatostatin analog (octreotide) on gallbladder function and gallstone formation in Chinese acromegalic patients. J Clin Endocrinol Metab 1993;76:32–37.
112. Ho KY, Weissberger AJ, Marbach P, et al. Therapeutic efficacy of the somatostatin analog SMS 201-995. (octreotide) in acromegaly. Effects of dose and frequency and long-term safety. Ann Intern Med 1990;112:173–181.
113. Newman CB, Melmed S, Snyder PJ, et al. Safety and efficacy of long-term octreotide therapy of acromegaly: results of a multicenter trial in 103 patients—a clinical research center study. J Clin Endocrinol Metab 1995;80:2768–2775.
114. Chen, WY, Wight DC, Wagner TE, Kopchick JJ. Expression of a mutated bovine growth hormone gene suppresses growth of transgenic mice. Proc Natl Acad Sci USA 1990;87:5061–5065.
115. Fuh G, Cunnigham BC, Fukunaga R, Nagata S, Goeddel DV, Wells JA. Rational design of potent antagonist to the human growth hormone receptor. Science 1992;256:1677–1680.
116. Chen WY, Wight DC, Wagner TE, Kopchick JJ. In vitro and in vivo studies of antagonistic effects of human growth hormone analogs. J Biol Chem 1994;269:15,892–15,897.

117. Trainer PJ, Drake WM, Katznelson L, et al. Treatment of acromegaly with the growth hormone receptor antagonist pegvisomant. N Engl J Med 2000;342:1171–1177.
118. Lamberts SWJ, Uitterlinden P, Schuijff PC, Khjn JGM. Therapy of acromegaly with Sandostatin. The predictive value of an acute test, the value of serum somatomedin-C measurements in dose adjustment and the definition of a biochemical "cure." Clin Endocrinol 1988;29:411–420.
119. Newman C, Melmed S, George A, et al. Octreotide as primary therapy for acromegaly. J Clin Endocrinol Metab 1998;83:3034–3040,.
120. Shimon I, Melmed S. Management of pituitary tumors. Ann Intern Med 1998;129:472–483.
121. Melmed S, Fagin J. Acromegaly update. West J Med 1985;146:328–336.
122. Williams Textbook of Endocrinology, 10th. WB Saunders, Philadelphia, in press.
123. Harris AGH. Diagnosis of Acromegaly (Chap. 5) In: Acromegaly and Its Management. Lippincott Raven, New York, 1996, p. 36.
124. Van der Lely AJ, Lamberts SWJ. Medical gherapy for acromegaly. In: Wass J, ed. Handbook of Acromegaly. Bioscientifica, Bristol, UK 2001; p. 59.
125. Braunwald E, ed. Harrison's Principles of Internal Medicine, 10th ed, McGraw-Hill, New York, 2001;Chap. 328, p. 2046.
126. Osman IA. Factors determining the long-term outcome of surgery for acromegaly. Q J Med 1994;87:617–623.
127. Moon HD, Simpson ME, Li CH, Evans HM. Neoplasms in rat treated with pituitary growth hormone 1. Pulmonary and lymphatic tissues. Cancer Res 1950;10:297–308.
128. Sheaves R, Jenkins P, Blackburn P, et al. Outcome of transsphenoidal surgery for acromegaly using strict criteria for surgical care. Clin Endocrinol 1996;45:407–413.
129. Lissett CA, Peacy SR, Laing I, Tetlow L, Davis JR, Shalet SM. The outcome of surgery for acromegaly: the need for a specialist pituitary surgeon for all types of growth hormone (GH) secreting adenome. Clin Endocrinol 1998;49:653–657.
130. Ahmed S, Elsheikh M, Stratton I, Page RC, Adams CB, Wass JA. Outcome of transsphenoidal surgery for acromegaly and its realtionship to surgical experience. Q J Med 1999;50:561–567.
131. Gittoes NJL, Sheppard MC, Johnson AP, Stewart PM. Outcome of surgery for acromegaly—the experience of a dedicated pituitary surgeon. Q J Med 1999;92:741–745.

11 Pituitary Tumors Other Than Acromegaly

Nicholas Clarke, MD, and
Udaya M. Kabadi, MD, FRCP(C), FACP, FACE

CONTENTS

PROLACTINOMA

Prolactinoma, an adenoma, is the most common hormone-secreting pituitary tumor. Pituitary tumors arise from the functioning or hormone-producing cells as well as stromal cells. The prevalence of prolactinoma in the general population is unknown. However, autopsy results demonstrate that 23–27% of individuals have pituitary microadenomas without prior clinical evidence, and 40% of these stain positive for prolactin by immunocytochemical analysis *(1,2)*. Adenomas are frequently classified according to their size, with microadenomas being less than 10 mm in diameter and larger lesions labeled macroadenomas. Most prolactinomas are microadenomas and enlarge (if at all) extremely slowly over time. The risk of progression of untreated microadenomas to macroadenomas is approximately 7%, based on several longitudinal series of patients followed over long periods *(3–8)*. The pathogenesis of prolactinomas is unknown. Clonal analysis of tumor DNA indicates a monoclonal origin and thus a *de novo* formation *(9,10)*.

Prolactinoma is more common in women than in men. The clinical presentation of prolactinoma depends on the age and sex of the patient, the size of the tumor, and the duration of the hyperprolactinemia *(11)*. Premenopausal women

From: *Contemporary Endocrinology: Early Diagnosis and Treatment of Endocrine Disorders*
Edited by: R. S. Bar © Humana Press Inc., Totowa, NJ

may present with menstrual dysfunction and/or galactorrhea. Menstrual dysfunction includes amenorrhea, oligomenorrhea, menorrhagia, or normal periods with anovulation and thus infertility. Galactorrhea may be present in 30–80% of these women *(11)*. They may also experience symptoms of estrogen deficiency including vaginal dryness, decreased libido, and dysparunia. Finally, osteopenia/osteoporosis is also a concern owing to the lack of estrogen. Therefore, most of the premenopausal women manifest microadenoma, presenting with the classic symptoms of hyperprolactinemia early in the course of the disease. In contrast, postmenopausal women tend to manifest macroadenoma; the delay in diagnosis during the earlier stage of the disease is caused by a lack of galactorrhea in the absence of estrogenized breast tissue and the presence of amenorrhea, which is attributed to menopause itself.

Similarly, most men also present with macroadenoma. However, in some men, microadenoma may be detected if they express manifestations of hypogonadisim, i.e., erectile dysfunction, decreased libido and/or infertility problems, a decrease in testicular size, diminishing masculine hair pattern; clinical galactorrhea is reported in only 14–33% of men with marked hyperprolactinemia *(12,13)*.

Finally, postmenopausal women and men may also present initially with local symptoms related to the tumor size, i.e., headache and visual disturbances. Bitemporal hemianopsia, i.e., loss of temporal vision bilaterally owing to compression of the optic chiasm by the adenoma, is the classic but not the most common visual abnormality.

Hyperprolactinemia is a common clinical entity induced by disorders affecting the hypothalamic-pituitary lactotroph axis. Functional hyperprolactinemia in the absence of tumor is a reflection of increased production and/or decreased degradation or clearance. Hypothalamic disorders and medications cause hyperprolactinemia by inhibiting the action of dopamine on prolactin secretion. In actuality, the most common cause is psychiatric medications such as neuroleptics (dopamine receptor blockers), tricyclic antidepressants, and monoamine oxidase inhibitors *(14–16)* Moreover, the commonly used drugs verapamil and metoclopramide may also induce hyperprolatinemia, via the same mechanism *(17)*. Alternatively, hypothyroidism, primary as well as secondary (pituitary), may stimulate prolactin secretion by elevated thyrotropin-releasing hormone (TRH) levels. Finally, chronic renal failure and cirrhosis may cause elevated prolactin levels because of reduced clearance or degradation. The prolactin levels in these conditions (medications, hypothalamic disorders, and systemic disease) rarely exceed 200 ng/mL. However, occasionally, multiple causes in the same patient may induce very high levels i.e., a patient with gastroparesis from diabetes receiving melodopromidy who has chronic renal failure as well as hypothyroidism. Therefore knowledge of the degree of hyperprolactinemia is frequently helpful in the clinical assessment.

A macroadenoma is most likely to be a prolactinoma with a serum prolactin level more than 200 ng/mL *(18)*. Macroadenoma is mostly pituitary in the presence of a serum prolactin level less than 200 ng/mL, because of pituitary stalk compression interfering with dopamine transport from the hypothalamus to the anterior pituitary. Such macroadenomas are frequently classified as nonfunctional because of the lack of expression of clinical hormonal effects, although they may actively secrete follicle-stimulating hormone (FSH) and rarely luteinizing hormone (LH) or the α-subunit and are of gonadotroph origin *(19)*. When these tumors are either neurologic or large in size, symptons may be caused by mass- like effects; when they are of endocrine origin, symptoms may be caused by atrophy or suppression of functioning of pituitary cells, i.e., hypogonadism in men. The distinction between a macroprolactinoma and a nonfunctional macroadenoma is extremely important in terms of therapeutic management. In both situations, a dopamine agonist reduces serum prolactin, but tumor shrinkage is unlikely with the nonfunctional adenoma *(20)*. A nonfunctional adenoma must be suspected when the prolactin level declines without shrinkage of the tumor because most patients with nonfunctional macroadenoma require surgery. Patients with pituitary microadenomas usually manifest serum prolactin levels of 60–200 ng/mL.

Elevated prolactin levels between 20 and 200 ng/mL are difficult to interpret because of a distinct overlap between functional cancer and microadenoma. A thorough history and detailed physical examination must always be done. Prolactin is secreted episodically and therefore serum prolactin should be determined on several occasions to confirm elevation. The best time to assess a serum prolactin level is the early morning, as prolactin levels peak between 4:00 and 7:00 AM. If the prolactin level remains elevated, magnetic resonance image (MRI) with gadolinium enhancement should be obtained, especially in the absence of distinct functional etiologies. Other tests should be performed as appropriate, i.e., for testosterone (in men), insulin-like growth factor-1, prolactin, AM cortisol, α-subunit, and β-human chorionic gonadotropin. In patients with a suspected or confirmed pituitary tumor, the following laboratory tests are recommended to assess pituitary function: electrolytes, thyroid stimulating hormone (TSH), free T4, LH, and FSH. Patients with no identified cause for the hyperprolactinemia and a normal MRI are classified as having idiopathic hyperprolactinemia.

Management of prolactinoma consists of amelioration of the clinical effects of hyperprolactinemia and correction of mechanical effects caused by tumor size. Therapeutic options include observation, administration of depressive agonists, surgery, and radiation (Table 1). For patients with mild to absent microadenoma symptoms, observation may be appropriate if other forms of therapy are contraindicated, since 95% of microprolactinomas do not enlarge over a 4–6 yr period *(18)*. Similarly, many patients with asymptomatic microadenomas may be observed safely with serial prolactin levels, follow-up

Table 1
Management of Prolactinoma

Type	Early signs/symptoms	Test	Early treatment
Microadenoma	Galactorrhea, infertility, oligo-menorrhea	Prolactin level	Observe unless fertility desired, then dopamine agonist
Macroadenoma	Headache, visual field defect	Prolactin level →MRI	Dopamine agonist

MRIs, and periodic bone mineral density measurements. However, other definitive forms of treatment are indicated if MRI documents enlargement or if clinical manifestations ensue. Moreover, if prolactin levels rise significantly, repeat MRI imaging is necessary and specific medical therapy with a dopamine agonist should be initiated. Finally, macroadenomas require intervention, especially in patients who are symptomatic from the hyperprolactinemia, e.g., amenorrhea, hypogonadism, and other symptoms.

Since 1971, bromocriptine, an active dopamine agonist, has been used for the treatment of hyperprolactinemia with and without adenomas . Bromocriptine binds to and stimulates the dopamine receptors on normal and adenomatous lactotroph cells (21,22). It inhibits prolactin synthesis and secretion, decreases cellular DNA synthesis, and ultimately retards and reverses tumor growth (23,24). Numerous studies have documented the efficacy of dopamine agonists, including bromocriptine, in lowering serum prolactin levels, reducing tumor size, and improving neurologic abnormalities such as visual field and cranial nerve defects with restoration of gonadal function (11). In most patients, rapid shrinkage of the tumor occurs during the first 3 mo of therapy, followed by further gradual reduction (25). With treatment, 80–90% of women attain normal prolactin concentrations and regain normal ovulatory menstrual cycles and fertility (18).

Bromocriptine is well tolerated; nausea, dizziness, and othostatic hypotension occur in only 5–10% of patients. We recommend that bromocriptine be taken at a lower dose at night with a snack and that the dose be increased gradually over a 1–2-wk period. The usual dose of bromocriptine is 2.5 mg three times a day. Intravaginal bromocriptine is a therapeutic option for women who cannot tolerate oral bromocriptine. This method of administration provides better absorption with fewer side effects and therefore can provide excellent clinical results (26). Other available long-acting dopamine agonists include quinagolide and cabergoline (available in the United States). Cabergoline is administered once or twice weekly, is as efficacious as bromocriptine, and appears to be better tolerated by some patients *(27–31)*. As little as 0.25 mg of cabergoline weekly may be sufficient to lower the prolactin level and restore normal hypothalamic-pituitary-gonadal function.

Prior to the advent of medical therapy, or in the presence of intolerance to drugs, surgery is the effective therapy for prolactinoma. Transsphenoidal microsurgical resection remains the preferred approach because of minimal morbidity and the possibility of a cure. Complete resolution of hyperprolactinemia with resumption of cyclic menses occurs in 40% of patients with macroadenomas and 80% of patients with microadenomas *(32)*. Recurrence of tumor is a long-term risk with surgery and ranges from 10 to 15% in patients with microadenomas and from 0 to 90% for macroadenomas over 5 yr *(33–38)*. The best results are noted in patients who have a lesser degree of hyperprolactinemia (150–500 ng/mL) and a relatively smaller tumor size and who are in the early stage (11, 32). Surgery is also effective in debulking macroadenomas, but hyperprolactemia usually persists and requires adjuvant therapy *(39)*. The mortality risk with surgery is less than 1% in experienced hands. Potential operative and perioperative complications include cerebrospinal fluid rhinorrhea, diabetes insipidus, infection, and damage to the visual pathways *(11)*.

Primary radiation therapy may be an option of last resort if medical therapy is not tolerated and surgery is contraindicated. This therapy gradually reduces prolactin levels and prevents the further growth of the prolactinoma. Results of treatment are less than impressive, with only 2 of 28 patients normalizing their prolactin level 2–10 yr after treatment *(40)*. The recommended radiation dose is a total of 45 Gy administered as 1.8 Gy/d over 25 d *(11)*. Potential complications of therapy include hypothalamic insufficiency, hypopituitarism, optic chiasm or optic nerve injury, brain necrosis, development of malignant tumors, and loss of mental function.

Stereotactic radiosurgery with a γ-knife or a highly focused linear accelerator may produce less hypopituitarism by sparing the hypothalamus *(11)*. It is now available in many medical centers. Furthermore, pituitary tumors in general are an optimal target for such precise radiosurgery. However, medical therapy remains the most preferred option because of the efficacy, ease of administration, and convenience.

NONFUNCTIONING PITUITARY TUMORS

Clinically nonfunctioning pituitary adenomas make up a third of all pituitary tumors. They usually do not cause a hypersecretory syndrome and so are called nonsecreting. They also do not stain with hematoxylin-eosin and so have been called chromophobe adenomas *(41)*. These tumors present clinically only after they have grown large enough to cause symptoms secondary to local pressure on or invasion into nearby structures. Headache is a frequent symptom, because of the rise in intrasellar pressure and stretching of the dural membrane. If the tumor extends into the suprasellar region and encroaches on the optic chiasm or tracts, visual field defects ensue, with infrequent presentation of classic homonomous hemianopsia or other visual field defects. The tumor can also expand laterally, into the cavernous sinuses, leading to third, fourth, and sixth cranial nerve palsies, with resulting diplopia, ptosis, and opthalmoplegia. Rarely, tumors extend into the frontal lobes, causing seizures or erode through the sella floor, leading to cerebrospinal fluid rhinorrhea. Occasionally, these tumors bleed, with consequent pituitary apoplexy presenting with meningeal signs and acute onset of hypopituitarism, usually of a partial nature.

TSHOMA

TSH secreting pituitary tumors are rare, being less than 1% of all pituitary tumors. They present with symptoms of hyperthyroidism, a nonsuppressed TSH, and occasionally focal signs of compression of the local neurologic structures by the tumor because of its size *(42)*. Classically, they demonstrate a lack of TSH response to TRH stimulation, an elevated α-subunit and a high α-subunit/whole TSH molar ratio, and a pituitary lesion on MRI *(43)*. In patients with these symptoms, TSHoma is often misdiagnosed as a more common form of hyperthyroidism such as Graves' disease or toxic multinodular goiter; such patients may undergo unnecessary thyroidectomies or radioiodine ablations. These procedures are hazardous since they eliminate the negative feedback of thyroid hormone to the pituitary and hypothalamous and therefore enhance tumor growth. With this risk of misdiagnosis, a long duration usually elapses between the onset of symptoms and the accurate diagnosis, as documented in a large study in which this duration was almost 9 yr *(43)*. The delay in detection may be responsible for the presence of headaches and visual field defects.

Forty percent of the patients who had macroadenomas at the time of diagnosis manifested thyroid nodules at diagnosis, probably secondary to sustained stimulation by elevated TSH concentrations over a prolonged period. The disease is often difficult to diagnose, especially in the absence of microadenomas, and may be confused with functional TRH or TSH excess or the syndrome of thyroid hormone resistance (STHR) *(44)*. Classically, STHR demonstrates a robust response to TRH, whereas in 50% of cases a TSHoma does not respond to TRH with a significant rise in TSH. Measurement of the α-subunit, which is the same for FSH, LH, and hCG, is helpful in the diagnosis of TSHoma (Table 2). TSH-secreting pituitary tumors should be considered whenever a patient has persistently elevated free T4 and free T3 and increased TSH or inappropriately detectable TSH.

Table 2
Differential Diagnosis of TSHoma

	Early signs/ symptoms	Test	Early treatment
Clinically non-functioning adenomas	Headache, visual loss, cranial nerve palsies	MRI	Transsphenoidal surgery
TSHoma	Signs and symptoms of hyperthyroidism: weight loss, tremor, amenorrhea, sleep difficulties, ↑ free T4 with nonsuppressed TSH	Lack of TSH response to TRH, elevated α-subunit, ↑ α-subunit/ TSH ratio	Transsphenoidal surgery, somatostatin analogs in the 2/3 of cases in which surgery does not cure the patient
Gonadatrophinoma	Usually clinically silent	Elevated LH, FSH	Transsphenoidal surgery

FSH, follicle-stimulating hormone; LH, luteinizing hormone; TRH, thyrotropin-releasing hormone; TSH, thyroid-stimulating hormone.

Transsphenoidal surgery is the preferred treatment. Unfortunately, these tumors are unusually hard and fibrous and have often progressed to macro-adenomas at diagnosis, making surgery curative in only about a third of patients *(45)*. In many patients, surgery provides incomplete remission and therefore radiotherapy is recommended. Unfortunately, with external radiation, it takes months to years to attain complete remission, and hypopituitarism, impaired cognitive function, and infertility can often result.

Fortunately, both dopamine and somatostatin receptors have been located on these tumors, leading to bromocriptine and octreotide being used in their management. Octreotide normalized thyroid hormone levels in 73% of patients in a recent study *(46)*. Octreotide may be superior to bromocriptine since octreotide may affect glycoisomer distribution, leading to a decrease in TSH secretion and bioactivity (Table 2) *(43)*.

The differential diagnosis includes generalized thyroid hormone resistance and selective pituitary resistance to thyroid hormone. All these conditions are rarely seen. The physician confronted with a patient who has elevated thyroxine with an inappropriately elevated TSH has a difficult problem. Defining the correct etiology is important because different diagnostic tests and treatment methods are required, and dangerous (but unfortunately common) mistreatment must be avoided *(41–49)*.

FSH- AND LHOMAS:
PITUITARY TUMORS SECRETING FSH OR LH

FSH- and LH-secreting tumors are usually clinically silent. Rare cases of tumors presenting with clinical features have been reported. A 28-yr-old Finnish woman presented with oligoamenorrhea and pelvic pain. A detailed assessment revealed elevated FSH and estradiol with an appropriately suppressed LH; enlarged ovaries with multiple cysts were seen on pelvic ultrasound examination. Both gonadotropins and the α-subunit exhibited a paradoxic response to TRH, and MRI revealed a pituitary macroadenoma. After removal of the pituitary tumor, all hormone values normalized, and the patient resumed normal menstrual cycles. In another report, transsphenoidal tumor resection was found in a girl who presented with precocious puberty. LH hypersecretion from a pituitary adenoma was also documented in two cases. Thus, varying degrees of hypopituitarism may occur in these patients, with decreased libido and erectile dysfunction in men and oligo- or amenorrhea in women. Alternatively, central hypothyroidism and secondary adrenal insufficiency have also been described. Mild hyperprolactinemia, with levels of 100 ng/mL or less, is often seen and is attributed to stalk compression by the tumor.

REFERENCES

1. Costello RT. Subclinical adenoma of the pituitary gland. Am J Pathol 1936;12:205–216.
2. Burrow GN, Wortzman G, Rewcastle NB, et al. Microadenomas of the pituitary gland and abnormal sellar tomograms in an unselected autopsy series. N Engl J Med 1980;304:156–158.
3. Schlechte J, Dolan K, Sherman B, et al. The natural history of untreated hyperprolactinemia: a prospective analysis. J Clin Endocrinol Metab 1989;68:412–418.
4. Koppelman MCS, Jaffe MJ, Rieth KG, et al. Hyperprolactinemia, amenorrhea, and galactorrhea. Ann Intern Med 1984;100:115–121.
5. March CM, Kletzky OA, Davajan V, et al. Longitudinal evaluation of patients with untreated prolactin-secreting pituitary adenomas. Am J Obstet Gynecol 1981;139:835–844.
6. Sisam DA, Sheehan JP, Sheeler LR. The natural history of untreated microprolactinomas. Fertil Steril 1987;48:67–71.
7. Von Werder K, Eversmann T, Fahlbusch R, et al. Development of hyperprolactinemia in patients with adenomas with and without prior operative treatment. Excerpta Med Int Congr Ser 1982;584:175–188.
8. Weiss MH, Teal J, Gott P, et al. Natural history of microprolactinomas: six-year follow-up. Neurosurgery 1983;12:180–183.
9. Herman I, Gonsky R, Fagin J, et al. Clonal origin of secretory and non-secretory pituitary tumors. Clin Res 1990;38:296A (abstract).
10. Molitch ME. Pathogenesis of pituitary tumors. Endocrinol Metab Clin North Am 1987;16:503–527.
11. Wilson JD, Foster DW, Kronenberg HM, Larsen PR, eds. Williams Textbook of Endocrinology, 9th ed. WB Saunders, Philadelphia, 1998, pp. 288–340.
12. Thorner MO, Edwards CRW, Hanker JP, et al. Prolactin and gonadotropin interaction in the male. In: Troen P, Nankin H, eds. The Testis in Normal and Infertile Men. Raven, New York, 1977, pp. 351–366.
13. Carter JN, Tyson JE, Talis G, et al. Prolactin-secreting tumors and hypogonadism in 22 men. N Engl J Med 1978;299:847–852.

14. Langer G, Sachar EJ. Dopaminergic factors in human prolactin regulation: effects of neuroleptics and dopamine. Psychoneuroendocrinology 1977;2:373–378.
15. Meltzer HY, Fang VS, Tricou BJ, et al. Effect of antidepressants on neuroendocrine axis in humans. In Costa E, Racagni G, eds. Typical and Atypical Antidepressants: Clinical Practice. Raven, New York, 1982, pp. 303–316.
16. Slater SL, Lipper S, Shiling DJ, et al. Elevation of plasma-prolactin by monoamine oxidase inhibitors. Lancet 1977;2:275–276.
17. Gluskin LE, Strasberg B, Shah JH. Verapamil-induced hyperprolactinemia and galactorrhea. Ann Intern Med 1981;95:66–67.
18. Molitch ME. Advances in pituitary tumor therapy. Endocrinol Metab Clin 1999;28:143–168.
19. Katznelson L, Alexander JM, Bikkal HA. Clinically nonfunctioning pituitary adenomas. J Clin Endocrinol Metab 1993;76:1089–1094.
20. Boulanger CM, Mashchak CA, Chang RJ. Lack of tumor reduction in hyperprolactinemic women with extrasellar macroadenomas treated with bromocriptine. Fertil Steril 1985;44:532–535.
21. Foord SM, Peters JR, Dieguez C, et al. Dopamine receptors on intact anterior pituitary cells in culture: functional association with the inhibition of prolactin and thyrotropin. Endocrinology 1983;112:1567–1577.
22. Sibley DR, Creese I. Interactions of ergot alkaloids with anterior pituitary D-2 dopamine receptors. Mol Pharmacol 1983;23:585–593.
23. MacLeod RM, Lehmeyer JE. Suppression of pituitary tumor growth and function by ergot alkaloids. Cancer Res 1973;33:849–855.
24. Maurer RA. Dopaminergic inhibition of prolactin synthesis and prolactin messenger RNA accumulation in cultured pituitary cells. J Biol Chem 1980;255:8092–8097.
25. Mori H, Mori S, Saitoh Y, et al. Effects of bromocriptine on prolactin-secreting pituitary adenomas. Cancer 1985;56:230–238.
26. Ginsburg J, Hardiman P, Thomas M. Vaginal bromocriptine—clinical and biochemical effects. Gynecol Endocrinology 1992;6:119–125.
27. Biller BMK, Molitch ME, Vance ML, et al. Treatment of prolactin-secreting macroadenoms with the once-weekly dopamine agonist cabergoline. J Clin Endocrinol Metab 1996;81:2338–2343.
28. Ciccarelli E, Giusti M, Miola C, et al. Effectiveness and tolerability of long term treatment with cabergoline, a new long-lasting ergoline derivative, in hyperprolactinemic patients. J Clin Endocrinol Metab 1989;69:725–728.
29. Ferrari C, Mattei A, Melis GB, et al. Cabergoline: Long-acting oral treatment of hyperprolactinemic disorders. J Clin Endocrinol Metab 1989;68:1201–1206.
30. Ferrari C, Paracchi A, Mattei AM, et al. Cabergoline in the long-term therapy of hyperprolactinemic disorders. Acta Endocrinol 1992;126:489–494.
31. Webster J, Piscitelli G, Polli A, et al., for the Cabergoline Comparative Study Group. A comparison of cabergoline and bromocriptine in the treatment of hyperprolactinmeic amenorrhea. N Engl J Med 1994;331:904–909.
32. Speroff L, Glass RH, Kase NG. Amenorrhea. In: Speroff L, Glass RH, Kase NG, eds. Clinical Gynecologic Endocrinology and Infertility, 5th ed. Williams & Wilkins, Baltimore, 1994, pp. 401–456.
33. Nelson PB, Goodman M, Maroon JC, et al. Factors in predicting outcome from operation in patients with prolactin-secreting pituitary adenomas. Neurosurgery 1983;13:634–641.
34. Tucker HS, Grubb SR, Wigand JP, et al. Galactorrhea-amenorrhea syndrome: follow-up of forty-five patients after pituitary tumor removal. Ann Intern Med 1981;94:302–307.
35. Woosley RE, King JS, Talbert L. Prolactin-secreting pituitary adenomas: neurosurgical management of 37 patients. Fertil Steril 1982;37:52–60.
36. Rodman EF, Molitch ME, Post KD, et al. Long-term follow-up of transsphenoidal selective adenomectomy for prolactinoma. JAMA 1984;252:921–924.

37. Thomson JA, Teasdale GM, Gordon D, et al. Treatment of presumed prolactinoma by transsphenoidal operation: early and late results. BMJ 1985;291:1550–1553.
38. Parl FF, Cruz VE, Cobb CA, et al. Late recurrence of surgically removed prolactinomas. Cancer 1986;57:2422–2426.
39. Hubbard JL, Scheithauer BW, Abboud CF, et al. Prolactin-secreting adenomas: the preoperative response to bromocriptine treatment and surgical outcome. J Neurosurg 1987;67:816–821.
40. Sheline GE, Grossman A, Jones AE, et al. Radiation therapy for prolactinoma. In: Clack PMcL, Zervas NT, Ridgway EC, et al, eds. Secretory Tumors of the Pituitary Gland. Progress in Endocrine Reseach and Therapy, vol 1. Raven, New York, 1984, pp. 93–108.
41. Snyder PJ. Clinically nonfunctioning pituitary adenomas. Endocrinol Metab Clin North Am 1993;22:163–175.
42. Weiss D, Bar RS, Weidner N, Wener M, Lee F. Oncogenic osteomalacia: strange tumors in strange places. Postgrad Med J 1985;61:349–355.
43. Brucker-Davis F, Oldfield EH, Skarulis MC, Doppman JL, Weintraub BD. Thyrotropin-secreting pituitary tumors: diagnosis criteria, thyroid hormone sensitivity, and treatment outcome in 25 patients followed at the National Institutes of Health. J Clin Endocrinol Metab 1999;84:476–486.
44. Refetoff S, Weiss RE, Usala SJ. The syndromes of resistance to thyroid hormone. Endocr Rev 1993;14:348–399.
45. McCutcheon IE, Weintraub BD, Oldfield EH. Surgical treatment of thyrotropin-secreting pituitary adenomas. J Neurosurg 1990;73:674–683
46. Chanson P, Weintraub BD, Harris AG. Octreotide therapy for thyroid-stimulating hormone-secreting pituitary adenomas. A follow-up of 52 patients. Ann Intern Med 1993;119:236–240.
47. Samuels MH, Ridgway EC. Glycoprotein-secreting pituitary adenomas. Baillieres Clin Endocrinol 1995;9:337–358.
48. Greenman Y, Melmed S. Thyrotropin-secreting pituitary tumors. In: Melmed S, ed. The Pituitary. Blackwell, Boston, 1995, pp. 526–558.
49. Weintraub BD, Gershengorn MC, Kourides IA, Fein H. Inappropriate secretion of thyroid-stimulating hormone. Ann Intern Med 1981;95:339–351.

12 Multiple Endocrine Neoplasia Types 1, 2a, and 2b

Christina Orr, MD, and Thomas O'Dorisio, MD

CONTENTS

INTRODUCTION

The multiple endocrine neoplasia (MEN) syndromes form a rare distinct group of genetic tumor syndromes inherited in an autosomal dominant fashion. MEN is characterized by the occurrence of tumors involving two or more endocrine glands within an individual. The MEN syndromes consist of two major types based on their clinical characteristics, genetic inheritance, and biochemical features (Table 1). MEN-1 (Wermer's syndrome) is characterized by tumors of the parathyroid (mostly hyperplasia), neuroendocrine pancreaticoduodenal tumors, and tumors of the anterior pituitary gland. MEN-2 (Sipple's syndrome) consists of several subtypes, MEN-2a, MEN-2b, and familial medullary thyroid carcinoma (MTC). MEN-2a involves the association of MTC, pheochromocytomas, and parathyroid tumors (hyperplasia). The association of MTC and pheochromocytomas with a marfanoid habitus and mucosal neuromas describes MEN-2b. MTC is the sole manifestation of familial medullary thyroid cancer (FMTC). The recognition of an individual with a MEN syndrome has important implications for other family members, since first-degree relatives have a 50% risk of developing the disease *(3)*. Thus, biochemical and genetic screening of family members is important and is covered in this review.

From: *Contemporary Endocrinology: Early Diagnosis and Treatment of Endocrine Disorders*
Edited by: R. S. Bar © Humana Press Inc., Totowa, NJ

Table 1
Genetics and Clinical Manifestations of Multiple Endocrine Neoplasia (MEN)

MEN Type	Genetics	Tumors/clinical manifestations
MEN-1	Autosomal dominant MENIN gene	Primary hyperparathyroidism Pituitary adenomas Prolactinoma Growth hormone-secreting Pancreaticoduodenal tumors Gastrinoma, insulinoma
MEN-2a	Autosomal dominant *RET* protooncogene mutation (codons 609, 611, 618, 620, 634)	Medullary thyroid carcinoma Pheochromocytoma Parathyroid hyperplasia Cutaneous lichen amyloidosis
MEN-2b	Autosomal dominant *RET* protooncogene mutation (codon 918)	Medullary thyroid carcinoma Pheochromocytoma Mucosal neuroma Marfanoid habitus Intestinal ganglioneuromas
Familial medullary thyroid cancer (variant of MEN-2a)	Autosomal dominant	Medullary thyroid cancer only

Data from refs. *1* and *2*.

MEN-1 (3PS, PARATHYROID, PANCREAS, AND PITUITARY TUMORS)

MEN-1 is a rare disorder with an estimated prevalence of 2 in 100,000 persons *(4)*. It is defined by the presence of hypercalcemia secondary to parathyroid hyperplasia, gastrointestinal and pancreatic islet cell tumors, and anterior pituitary tumors. Primary hyperparathyroidism is the most common component of MEN-1; hypercalcemia is the most common initial presentation of the disorder, occurring in 80–100% of patients by age 40 *(5)*. Four-gland parathyroid hyperplasia and/or adenomatous tumors occur in 95% of patients. Approximately 1–2% of all cases of primary hyperparathyroidism are caused by MEN-1 *(6)*.

Primary hyperparathyroidism in the setting of MEN-1 differs from the common sporadic form of the disease. In MEN-1, the male-to-female ratio is 1:1, compared with 2–3:1 in sporadic primary hyperparathyroidism. Hyperparathyroidism presents earlier, usually in the second to fourth decade, about two decades earlier than the sporadic form. Multiple gland involvement is typical with hyperplasia of all four glands, whereas sporadic hyperparathyroidism is characterized by an adenoma within a single gland. Lastly, there is a high rate of recurrent hyperparathyroidism after subtotal parathyroidectomy in patients with MEN-1 owing to the strong proliferative drive in the parathyroid cells *(6)*.

Gastrointestinal and pancreatic islet cell tumors are the major cause of morbidity and mortality in patients with MEN-1 *(3)*. Approximately 30–40% of patients will develop clinical symptoms. Gastrinomas and insulinomas are the most common and the second most common type, respectively. Glucagonomas and vasoactive intestinal peptide-secreting tumors (VIPomas) are rare, whereas pancreatic polypeptidomas (PPomas) are more common but asymptomatic *(3)*.

Gastrinomas, leading to Zollinger-Ellison syndrome, account for most of the morbidity and mortality in patients with MEN-1 *(3)*. By age 50 yr, approximately 50% of affected patients with MEN-1 develop gastrinomas. They are often small, multifocal, and metastatic at diagnosis, with 15% progressing to an aggressive malignancy *(5)*, thus making surgical resection difficult. G-cells, the precursor cells of gastrinomas, are normally present in the fetal pancreas but gastrinomas in MEN-1 are ectopic tumors most often located in the duodenum. Excess gastrin secretion by the tumors causes prolific production of gastric acid, with patients developing multiple ulcers in the duodenum and jejunum *(7)*. Diarrhea also develops. Some patients remain asymptomatic despite an elevated gastrin level. Hypercalcemia (primary hyperparathyroidism) may cause an elevation of the serum gastrin level and exacerbate the symptoms of Zollinger-Ellison syndrome. Also, the hypergastrinemia seen in primary hyperparathyroidism may mimic the peptic ulcer disease normal hyperacid state of gastrinoma syndrome. Thus, addressing the primary hyperparathyroidism first is essential.

Insulinomas are the second most common pancreatic islet cell tumor with an incidence of 10–35% *(5)*. Insulinomas associated with MEN-1 are most often multifocal, small, and associated with the simultaneous expression of other islet cell tumors. Approximately 1–5% of all patients with an insulinoma have MEN-1, and in 10% of patients insulinoma may be the initial manifestation *(8)*. The clinical diagnosis is based on Whipple's triad, which consists of symptoms of hypoglycemia (tremor, diaphoresis, anxiety, confusion, seizure), documented hypoglycemia with symptoms, and improvement of symptoms soon after glucose ingestion or perfusion.

Anterior pituitary tumors associated with MEN-1 occur in approximately 30% of patients. Prolactinomas are the most common pituitary tumor, constituting approximately 60% of the total *(3)*. They are multicentric and large but usually respond well to dopamine agonists (e.g., bromocriptine or cabergiline). Growth hormone-producing tumors are the second most common pituitary tumor, affecting 10–25% of patients *(3)*. Overproduction of growth hormone results in acromegaly in adults and gigantism in children. Nonfunctional tumors and corticotrophinomas account for less than 15% of associated pituitary MEN-1 tumors *(3)*. In general, pituitary tumors are expressed much less frequently than neuroendocrine pancreatic tumors.

Other tumors associated with MEN-1 include foregut carcinoid tumors, adrenal cortical tumors, angiofibromas, and collagenomas. The foregut carcinoid tumors are located in the bronchus, thymus, or stomach. MEN-1 carcinoids rarely cause carcinoid syndrome or hypersecrete a hormone [serotonin or adrenocortiocotropin (ACTH) or calcitonin] *(5)*.

Genetics

The MEN-1 gene is believed to be a tumor suppressor gene *(9,10)* and has been localized to chromosome 11,11q13 *(9,11–16)*. It contains 10 exons, extends across 9 kb, and encodes a 610-amino- acid protein called menin. The cellular and biochemical function of menin is currently unknown. Tumor development in MEN-1 follows Knudson's two-hit hypothesis, that is, individuals with MEN-1 have been observed to harbor a germline inactivating mutation of the MEN-1 gene and a second hit with a somatic loss of heterozygosity on chromosome 11 *(3)*. Approximately 150 germline mutations distributed across the nine coding exons of the MEN-1 gene have been identified thus far *(1)*. Most result in premature protein truncation caused by frameshift mutations (deletions or insertions) and nonsense mutations, findings consistent with a loss of function of the tumor suppressor gene and thus tumor growth and expression *(1)*. Approximately 10% of the germline MEN-1 mutations arise *de novo*, and up to 10–30% are not currently detectable *(5)*.

Diagnosis and Management

Primary hyperparathyroidism is diagnosed by an elevated serum calcium with an inappropriately normal or elevated parathormone level. Primary hyperparathyroidism in MEN-1 is managed in the same manner as in individuals with sporadic primary hyperparathyroidism. In the symptomatic individual (*see* discussion in Chapter 15) or an asymptomatic individual younger than 50 yr, surgery is recommended. Surgery is recommended for the younger patient because of long life expectancy and risk of complications from prolonged hypercalcemia (osteoporosis, nephrolithiasis). Most patients have multiple parathyroid gland hyperplasia or adenomas. Preoperative localization is not necessary, except for recurrent hyperparathyroidism. Sestamibi scanning detects more than 90% of parathyroid adenomas preoperatively but detects only about 60% of enlarged glands in multiglandular parathyroid disease. There are two surgical options for patients, either total parathyroidectomy with autotransplantation in the forearm or 3 1/2 gland parathyroidectomy. Both are effective. Recurrent hyperparathyroidism is common in MEN-1 and usually occurs within 15 yr of initial surgery.

We recommend that treatment of the hyperparathyroid condition be addressed prior to further workup for a pancreatic neuroendocrine tumor, since the hypercalcemia of hyperparathyroidism may be a provocative stimulus for normal neuropeptides such as gastrin, glucagon, and insulin.

The pancreaticoduodenal tumors, gastrinoma and insulinoma, are diagnosed biochemically and then localized. Gastrinoma is diagnosed by finding an elevated fasting gastrin level usually greater than 1000 pg/mL or a moderately elevated gastrin level that increases by 200 pg/mL within 15 min after intravenous secretin. Secretin is no longer commercially available in the United States. Localization of a gastrinoma is imperfect and can be done by several imaging techniques including, computed tomography (CT), magnetic resonance imaging (MRI), ultrasonography, endoscopic ultrasonography, octreotide scanning (Octreoscan®), transhepatic portal venous sampling, or selective arterial secretin infusions. Somatostatin receptor scintigraphy has been recommended to be the most cost-efficient and sensitive imaging procedure for gastrinomas.

Most gastrinomas in MEN-1 are located in the duodenal wall. Despite localization, gastrinomas in MEN-1 are difficult to resect surgically because of multiple locations, frequent metastasis, and easily missed duodenal gastrinomas (17–20). Surgical resection does not decrease the mortality of the disease or the likelihood that metastasis will develop; thus medical therapy is warranted (21,22). The gastric acid overproduction is controlled medically by high-dose H2 receptor blockers or proton-pump inhibitors. A reexamination of the role of surgery has been explored with the recognition that most gastrinomas are small and located in the duodenum (17–20). Some surgeons now operate on individuals with MEN-1 who have Zollinger-Ellison syndrome that persists after correction of hyperparathyroidism. A duodenotomy (more sensitive than intraoperative ultrasound) is done to localize the duodenal gastrinoma with a subtotal pancreatectomy (23–25). Surgical debulking may offer some benefit to patients with hepatic metastases but is not routinely done.

Insulinomas are the most benign of all pancreatic neuroendocrine tumors and clinically present with fasting or exercise-induced hypoglycemia. Common symptoms of hypoglycemia include mental confusion, blurred vision, slurred speech, seizures, tremors, anxiety, hunger, diaphoresis, palpitations, and headaches. Hypoglycemia (glucose < 55 mg/dL in men or < 40 mg/dL in women) with simultaneous hyperinsulinemia (insulin > 5 µU/mL) occurring spontaneously or during a supervised 72-h fast confirms the diagnosis. Localization of an insulinoma can be difficult, especially with multiple small adenomatous insulinomas in MEN-1. Imaging studies include CT scan, ultrasonography, intraoperative ultrasonography, and transhepatic portal vein sampling, with intraoperative ultrasonography providing the best localization technique. Surgical resection is indicated for a single insulinoma and is usually successful. The multiple insulinomas in MEN-1 make surgical resection difficult, and some experienced surgeons recommend local excision of any tumors in the head of the pancreas plus a distal subtotal pancreatectomy (26).

Individuals with pituitary tumors in MEN-1, prolactinomas and growth hormone-secreting adenomas, present clinically and should be managed in the same manner as individuals with sporadic adenomas. MRI is highly sensitive for detecting pituitary adenomas, and plasma levels of prolactin and insulin-like growth factor-1 (IGF-1) are elevated in individuals with a prolactinoma and growth hormone-secreting adenomas, respectively. Medical management of prolactinoma and growth hormone-secreting tumors include bromocriptine and octreotide, respectively (discussed in the pituitary tumor Chapter 11).

Screening for Tumors

Despite the availability of genetic screening for MEN-1, it is currently not done in individuals or family members with MEN-1. Since primary hyperparathyroidism is the most common and initial presentation of MEN-1, screening family members with serum calcium should be done on an annual basis. Biochemical or radiologic screening for other tumors (pancreaticoduodenal and pituitary tumors) is usually not necessary unless patients are symptomatic.

MEN-2

MTC is the most common and serious manifestation of the MEN-2 syndromes. MEN-2 has three subtypes; MEN-2a, MEN-2b, and FMTC. MEN-2a describes the association of MTC, pheochromocytomas, and tumors of the parathyroid glands. MTC is usually the first manifestation of MEN-2a, has a high penetrance as it develops in approximately 95% of individuals, and results from the malignant transformation of C-cell (parafollicular thyroid cell) hyperplasia, the precursor of MTC (27). In comparison with sporadic MTC, MTC in MEN-2a develops at a younger age (as young as 2 yr) and is multifocal (affects the upper one-third of the gland) and bilateral. MTC may secrete calcitonin or other peptides (somatostatin, vasoactive intestinal peptide, carcinoembryonic antigen, neurotensin, and ACTH), and individuals may develop symptoms secondary to peptide cosecretion (28).

The second most common manifestation of MEN-2a is pheochromocytoma, which affects 40–50% of individuals (29). They progress from their precursor, adrenal medullary hyperplasia, and may also be multifocal and bilateral, but rarely extraadrenal. Pheochromocytomas in individuals with MEN-2a secrete greater amounts of epinephrine compared with sporadic pheochromocytomas; thus hypertension is less common. Primary hyperparathyroidism secondary to asymmetric multiglandular parathyroid hyperplasia/adenoma develops in 25–35% of individuals (29). In those who develop hyperparathyroidism, parathyroid hyperplasia occurs in approximately 84%, and a parathyroid adenoma is present in 16% of individuals (30). Cutaneous lichen amyloidosis has recently been described as a component of MEN-2a (2).

The combination of MTC, pheochromocytomas, marfanoid habitus, and mucosal neuromas describes MEN-2b. Primary hyperparathyroidism is not a manifestation of MEN-2b. As with all MTCs in MEN-2, they are multifocal and bilateral, although they tend to be more aggressive and occur at a younger age than MEN-2a and FMTC *(31)*. Forty to 50% of individuals develop pheochromocytomas. All individuals develop mucosal neuromas, located in the gastrointestinal tract, on the lips, tongue, and conjunctiva *(29)*. In some affected individuals a gastrointestinal neuroma may be a source of occult gastrointestinal bleeding. MEN-2b patients have a marfanoid habitus but lack ectopia lentis (ectopic lens) or aortic aneurysms associated with Marfan's syndrome *(32)*. Additional features include hypertrophic peripheral nerves and megacolon *(29,31)*. The former can be detected by silt lamp examination demonstrating myelinated nerve fibers at the corneal limbic junction.

MTC without any other endocrinopathies or clinical abnormalities of MEN-2a or 2b characterizes FMTC. It may be difficult to distinguish from MTC in MEN-2a prior to the diagnosis of hyperparathyroidism or pheochromocytoma. In general, it has a much more benign course than either MEN-2a or MEN-2b.

Genetics

MEN-2a, MEN-2b, and FMTC are all inherited in an autosomal dominant manner, mapped to chromosome 10q11.2, a region containing the *RET* (REarranged during Transfection) protooncogene. The *RET* protooncogene was discovered about 15 yr ago when a rearranged form of this gene was shown to transform NIH 3T3 cells. It encodes a transmembrane tyrosine kinase receptor with a large cysteine-rich extracellular domain, a ligand binding extracellular domain, and two intracellular tyrosine kinase domains. The *RET* protooncogene is expressed in many tissues, including neural crest derivatives (C-cells of the thyroid, adrenal medulla, parasympathetic and sympathetic ganglia) where its primary role involves the development and migration of neural crest tissue *(1)*.

Activating mutations located on exon 10 (codons 609, 611, 618, and 620) and exon 11 (codon 634) in the *RET* protooncogene on chromosome 10 are responsible for most of MEN-2 syndromes *(1,33)*. A single amino-acid change in the conserved cysteine extracellular domain is responsible for most of the mutations *(34)*. MEN-2a develops from mutations in codons 609, 611, 618, 620, and 634, with a mutation in codon 634 being the most common (80–90%) *(1,33)*. This mutation is located on the cysteine extracellular domain in exon 11 with individuals developing MTC, hyperparathyroidism, and pheochromocytomas. Once the mutation is identified in the index patient (MTC at surgery), all other family members who will develop MTC will have the same mutation *(34)*. Individuals who do not have the mutation will not develop MTC. This allows early detection and early treatment (thyroidectomy) before MTC develops. Individuals without the mutation do not have to be screened yearly *(30)*.

Mutations of codons 609, 611, and 618 account for less than 5% of all mutations, and individuals with codon 609 mutations do not develop pheochromocytomas *(1,33)*. Ninety-five percent of individuals with MEN-2b have a single Met to Thr mutation in codon 918 (exon 16) located in the intracellular tyrosine domain *(1)*. Other codon mutations in MEN-2b include 883 and 922 *(1)*. Identified mutations in FMTC include 609, 611, 618, 620, and 634, with a single family having a mutation in codon 768 (exon 13). Other codon mutations in FMTC described include 804 (exon 14) and 891 (exon 15), both found in the intracellular tyrosine kinase domain *(1)*. Why individuals develop only MTC is unclear since they harbor the same codon mutations as individuals with MEN-2a. Individuals with sporadic MTC have a 1–7% incidence of a *germline RET* protooncogene mutation and a 25–35% incidence of a *somatic RET* protooncogene mutation *(1,34)*.

Clinical Manifestations

Prior to the availability of genetic screening, patients with MEN-2 presented clinically with MTC as a thyroid nodule or cervical lymphadenopathy. Cervical lymph node involvement included the central and lateral compartments, with lung, liver, and bone as the primary sites of distant metastases *(29)*. Individuals also presented with a secretory diarrhea related to a humoral factor or symptoms of Cushing's syndrome (weight gain, abdominal striae, amenorrhea, and easy bruising) secondary to ACTH secretion by MTC (usually seen in sporadic MTC). MTC is the only thyroid cancer that may present with symptomatic diarrhea, especially sporadic MTC. Since genetic testing is now available, affected individuals with MEN-2 have surgery prior to clinically relevant MTC and rarely have lymph node or distant metastases. In individuals who are the index case (previous diagnosed family member), the serum calcitonin level correlates with tumor load and is almost always elevated in patients with a palpable tumor. Basal calcitonin and stimulated calcitonin levels (described later) and carcinoembryonic antigen (early dedifferentiation) are useful markers for following patients postsurgically *(28,34)*. Evidence of a pheochromocytoma usually presents about 10 yr after MTC *(35)*. Symptoms are similar to those of individuals with sporadic pheochromocytoma and include palpitations, anxiety, tachycardia, diaphoresis, and headaches; only about one-third of individuals have hypertension at the time of diagnosis *(36)*.

Prior to surgery for MTC, patients with MEN-2 should be evaluated for an unrecognized pheochromocytoma. If diagnosed, the pheochromocytoma should be surgically removed prior to the total thyroidectomy since there is a substantial risk to the surgical patient with an undiagnosed pheochromocytoma. Individuals with hyperparathyroidism in MEN-2a usually have an asymptomatic elevation of serum calcium (like hypercalcemia/hyperparathyroidism in MEN-1), but may present with symptoms of hypercalcemia (polyuria, polydipsia, constipation, nephrolithiasis, or abdominal pain).

Genetic Screening

A recent consensus statement in the *Journal of Clinical Endocrinology and metabolism (34)* provides a guide to individuals who should be genetically screened for *RET* protooncogene mutations. These include individuals who are the index case, those suspicious for MEN-2 based on expression of two or more MEN-2-related tumors, and symptomatic and asymptomatic family members to define the carrier state. Ninety-eight percent of MEN-2 index cases have an identifiable *RET* mutation. First-degree relatives have a 50% chance of inheriting the mutation and developing disease. Most MTCs in MEN-2 develop prior to age 20, with a 25% mortality rate if they are metastatic at the time of diagnosis. Screening is prudent, as an early total thyroidectomy can prevent disease development. Current techniques to detect mutations rely on polymerase chain reaction (PCR) amplification of genomic DNA followed by DNA sequencing. A limited number of MEN-2 mutations have been identified by the presence of *RET* on exons 10, 11, 13, 14, 15, and 16 and should be tested routinely. If these exons are negative, the remaining 15 exons should be sequenced. If a mutation is detected, family members should be tested for the same *RET* protooncogene mutation. Individuals with a mutation should then be considered for a prophylactic total thyroidectomy and further screening for pheochromocytoma and hyperparathyroidism (MEN-2a; *see* Management section below). Children of individuals with MEN-2b should be screened for the *RET* mutation as a neonate. There have been reported cases of MTC with metastases in children as young as 1 and 6 yr of age. Unaffected individuals do not need further biochemical screening, as they can be 95% reassured that they will not develop the disease.

Despite excellent screening with PCR, a negative *RET* analysis does not exclude hereditary disease with 100% certainty, since only 95% of recognized families have identifiable *RET* mutations. If an individual with a negative analysis desires complete certainty, biochemical screening for MTC, pheochromocytoma, and hyperparathyroidism can be implemented (*see* next subheading). Individuals with sporadic MTC should be genetically screened, as they may harbor a *de novo RET* protooncogene mutation.

Management

MTC should be managed surgically with a total thyroidectomy and central lymph node dissection for several reasons *(31,37)*. MTC is usually multicentric and bilateral. In contrast to differentiated thyroid carcinoma, MTC does not take up radioactive iodine. Chemotherapy and radiation are usually equally ineffective *(37,38)*. MTC is usually more aggressive than differentiated thyroid carcinoma. MTC in MEN-2b is more aggressive than in MEN-2a or FMTC, and surgery may not be curative *(34)*. Early total thyroidectomy with central lymph node dissection offers the best chance for cure. The timing of the total thyroidectomy is based on the *RET* protooncogene mutation identified *(34)*. Most experts recommend a prophylactic total thyroidectomy for children with *RET* codon mutations 611, 618, 620, or 634 between ages 5 to 7 yr old and classify these individuals as class 2 or high risk. The highest risk (class 3) children are those with MEN-2b and/or *RET* codon mutation 883, 918, or 920; these individuals should have a total thyroidectomy within the first 6 mo of life and preferably within the first year of life. Children with *RET* codon 609, 768, 790, 791, 804, and 891 mutations are classified as level 1 (least high risk), but they should still undergo a total thyroidectomy. The timing of the thyroidectomy is uncertain in this group but should probably occur between ages 5 and 10 yr.

Prior to surgery, patients with MEN-2 should be evaluated for a pheochromocytoma; if one is found, it should be removed prior to thyroidectomy. Currently unilateral surgery is recommended for a pheochromocytoma, with the understanding that one-third to one-half of patients will develop a pheochromocytoma of the other adrenal *(39)*. Removing only one adrenal gland allows patients to be free of life-long glucocorticoid and mineralcorticoid replacement. Most pheochromocytomas can be removed laparoscopically *(29)*. Parathyroid disease can be addressed at the same time as the total thyroidectomy. Bilateral neck dissection to identify all affected glands should be performed in individuals with known or suspected MEN-2a. There are two different surgical approaches to hyperparathyroidism: (1) a total parathyroidectomy with autotransplantation into the nondominant forearm performed at the time of the total thyroidectomy; and (2) a subtotal parathyroidectomy (three glands, often with cervical thymectomy). Both approaches are equally effective *(40,41)*.

Biochemical Diagnosis of Medullary Thyroid Cancer in MEN-2

Prior to genetic testing, MTC in MEN-2 was diagnosed with a provocative calcitonin stimulation test. This test could be done with either pentagastrin or calcium; pentagastrin-stimulated increase in calcitonin was the more sensitive test *(30)*. A stimulated increase in plasma calcitonin level was seen in C-cell hyperplasia and MTC. Currently pentagastrin is not commercially available. The role of the calcium stimulation test is detection of persistent or recurrent disease in patients with surgically treated MTC and in concerned unaffected individuals (negative genetic screen). Approximately one-third of patients with MTC have a normal baseline serum calcitonin level but an excessive rise after calcitonin stimulation by pentagastrin (in the past) or calcium *(29)*. Calcium is currently used as a stimulus for calcitonin secretion in the following protocol *(29)*: Infuse intravenous calcium gluconate (2 mg/kg over 1 min) and obtain blood samples at 0, 1, 2, 3, and 5 min after infusion. Plasma calcitonin levels usually peak at 1–2 min, but normal and abnormal stimulated levels have not been established to date. Erdogan et al. *(42)* noted that proton-pump inhibition (omeprazole) leads to endogenous elevation of gastrin and abnormal stimulation of calcitonin in

Table 2
Biochemical Screening for Multiple Endocrine Neoplasia (MEN)

Type	Hyperparathyroidism	Frequency	Pheochromocytoma
MEN-1	Serum calcium, PTH	Annually	
MEN-2a	Serum calcium, PTH	Annually in patients with codon 634 mutation	24-h urine: total fractionated catecholamines, VMA, and metanephrine
		Every 2–3 yr: codon mutation 609, 611, 618, 620, 790, 791	
MEN-2b			24-h urine: total fractionated catecholamines, VMA, and metanephrine

PTH, parathyroid hormone; VMA, vanillylmandelic acid.
Data from ref. *34*.

affected MTC individuals and thus could be used postoperatively in the follow-up of individuals with MTC.

Screening for Tumor Expression in MEN-2 Carriers

The timing of biochemical screening of MEN-2 carriers is based on the level of risk of *RET* codon mutations *(34)* (Table 2). Pheochromocytoma has been found in kindreds of all *RET* protooncogene mutations except those in codons 609, 768, val804met, and 891. Biochemical screening for pheochromocytoma should begin at the age that thyroidectomy would be considered or by the age of 5–7 yr, and it should be performed annually in individuals in the highest risk groups. In individuals with mutations of less high-risk codons (609, 768, val804met, and 891), screening may be initiated at a later age, and less frequent biochemical screening may be appropriate. Biochemical screening is done by measuring a 24-h urine collection for total fractionated catecholamines (epinephrine and norepinephrine), vanillylmandelic acid, and metanephrine. A recent report recommends measurement of plasma metanephrine and normetanephrine (plasma metabolites of epinephrine and norepinephrine, respectively) *(43)*. An elevated 24-h urine metanephrine is the most specific test for pheochromocytoma, and an elevated plasma metanephrine is the most sensitive test for diagnosis. After the biochemical diagnosis of a pheochromocytoma is established, the initial imaging study should be either an MRI or metaiodo benzylguanidine (MIBG) or CT scan depending on the radiology availability. MRI with T2-weighted images is the most sensitive for localization of extraadrenal pheochromocytomas; MRI and CT demonstrate equal sensitivity for localization of adrenal pheochromocytomas *(43)*. The possibility of bilateral pheochromocytomas should be kept in mind with MEN-2 individuals.

Screening for hyperparathyroidism should be done annually in individuals with a 634 codon mutation *(34)*. Mutations at codons 609, 611, 618, 620, 790, and 791 are less frequently associated with hyperparathyroidism *(34)*. Serum calcium and parathyroid hormone should be measured every 2–3 yr *(34)*. Technetium scanning should be done in recurrent hyperparathyroidism to help localize parathyroid tissue.

REFERENCES

1. Hoff A, Cote G, Gagel R. Multiple endocrine neoplasias. Annu Rev Physiol 2000;62:377–411.
2. Donovan D, Levy M, Furst E, et al. Familial cutaneous lichen amyloidosis in association with multiple endocrine neoplasia type 2A: a new variant. Henry Ford Hosp Med J 1989;37:147–150.
3. Thakker R. Multiple endocrine neoplasia syndromes of the twentieth century. J Clin Endocrinol Metab 1998;83:2617–2620.
4. Teh B, Mcardle J, Parameswaran V, et al. Sporadic primary hyperparathyroidism in the setting of multiple endocrine neoplasia type 1. Arch Surg 1996;131:1230–1232.
5. Schussheim D, Skarulis M, Agarwal S, et al. Multiple endocrine neoplasia type 1: new clinical and basic findings. Trends Endocrinol Metab 2001;12:173–178.
6. Fitzpatrick L. Hypercalcemia in the multiple endocrine neoplasia syndromes. Endo Metab Clin North Am 1989;18:741–752.
7. Cadiot G, Laurent-Piug P, Thuille B, et al. Is the multiple endocrine neoplasia type I gene a suppressor for fundic argyrophil tumors in Zollinger-Ellison syndrome? Gastroenterology 1993;105:579–582.
8. Metz D, Jensen R, Bale A, et al. Multiple endocrine neoplasia type 1: Clinical features and management. In: Bilezekian J, Levine M, Marcus R, eds. The Parathyroids. New York, Raven, 1994, p. 591.
9. Bystrom C, Larsson C, Blomberg C, et al. Localization of the MEN-1 gene to a small region within chromosome 11q13 deletion mapping in tumours. Proc Natl Acad Sci USA 1990;87:1968–1972.
10. Knudson AG. Mutation and cancer: statistical study of retinoblastoma. Proc Natl Acad Sci USA 1971;68:820–823.
11. Larsson C, Skogseid B, Oberg K, et al. Multiple endocrine neoplasia type I maps to chromosome 11 and is lost in insulinoma. Nature 1988;332:85–87.
12. Nakamura Y, Larsson C, Julier C, et al. Localization of the genetic defect in multiple endocrine neoplasia type I within a small region chromosome 11. Am J Hum Genet 1989;44:751–755.
13. Thakker, Rv, Bouloux P, Wooding C, et al. Association of parathyroid tumors in familial multiple endocrine neoplasia type I. N Engl J Med 1989;321:218–224.
14. Friedman E, Sakaguchi K, Bale AE, et al. Clonality of parathyroid tumors in familial multiple endocrine neoplasia type I. N Engl J Med 1989;321:213–218.
15. Radford DM, Ashley SW, Wells SA Jr, et al. Loss of heterozygosity of markers on chromosome 11 in tumors from patients with multiple endocrine neoplasia syndrome type I. Cancer Res 1990;50:6529–6533.
16. Bale AE, Norton JA, Wong EL, et al. Allelic loss on chromosome 11 in hereditary and sporadic tumors related to familial multiple endocrine neoplasia type I. Cancer Res 1991;51:1154–1157.
17. Pipeleers-Marichal M, Somers G, Willems G, et al. Gastrinomas in the duodenums of patients with multiple endocrine neoplasia type 1 and the Zollinger-Ellison syndrome. N Engl J Med 1990;322:723–727.

18. Donow C, Pipeleers-Marichal M, Stamm B, et al. Pathology of insulinoma and gastrinoma: site, size, multicentricity, association with multiple endocrine neoplasia type 1 and malignancy. Dtsch Med Wschr 1990;115:1386–1391.
19. Donow C, Pipeleers-Marichal M, Schroder S, et al. Surgical pathology of gastrinoma: site, size, multicentricity, association with multiple endocrine neoplasia type 1, and malignancy. Cancer 1991;68:1329–1334.
20. Lamers C. Gastrinoma in multiple endocrine neoplasia type 1. Acta Oncol 1991;30:489–492.
21. Jensen R, Gardner J. Gastrinoma. In: The Pancreas: Biology, Pathobiology and Diseases, 2nd ed. Raven, New York, 1993, p. 931.
22. Ruszniewski P, Podevin P, Cadiot G, et al. Clinical, anatomical, and evolutive features of patients with the Zollinger-Ellison syndrome combined with type 1 multiple endocrine neoplasia. Pancreas 1993;8:295–304.
23. Sugg S, Norton J, Fraker D, et al. A prospective study of intraoperative methods to diagnose and resect duodenal gastrinomas. Ann Surg 1993;218:138–144.
24. Thompson N, Pasieka J, Fukuuchi A. Duodenal gastrinomas, duodenotomy, and duodenal exploration in the surgical management of Zollinger-Ellison syndrome. World J Surg 1993;17:455–462.
25. Thompson N, The surgical management of hyperparathyroidism and endocrine disease of the pancreas in the multiple endocrine neoplasia type 1 patient. J Intern Med 1995;238:269–280.
26. Demeure M, Klonoff D, Karam J, et al. Insulinomas associated with multiple endocrine neoplasia type I: the need for a different surgical approach. Surgery 1991;110:998–1005.
27. Gagel R. Multiple endocrine neoplasia. In: Wilson JD, Foster DW, Larsen PR, Kronenberg H, eds. Williams' Textbook of Endocrinology. Saunders, Philadelphia, 1998, pp.1627–1649.
28. Moley J. Medullary thyroid cancer. Surg Clinics North Am 1995;75:405–420.
29. Phay J, Moley J, Lairmore T. Multiple Endocrine Neoplasias. Semin Surg Oncol 2000;18:324–332.
30. Ledger G, Khosla S, Lindor M, et al. Genetic testing in the diagnosis and management of multiple endocrine neoplasia type II. Ann Intern Med 1995;122:118–124.
31. Raue F, Frank-Raue K, Grauer A. Multiple endocrine neoplasia type 2: clinical features and screening. Endocrinol Metab Clin North Am 1994;23:137–156.
32. O'Riordain D, O'Brien T, Crotty T, et al. Multiple endocrine neoplasia type 2B: More than an endocrine disorder. Surgery 1995;118:936–942.
33. Eng C, Clayton D, Schuffenecker I, et al. The relationship between specific RET proto-oncogene mutations and disease phenotype in multiple endocrine neoplasia type 2. International RET mutation consortium analysis. JAMA 1996;276:1575–1579.
34. Brandi M, Gagle R, Angeli A, et al. Consensus Guidelines for Diagnosis and Therapy of MEN Type 1 and Type 2. J Clin Endocrinol Metab 2001;86:5658–5671.
35. Utiger R. Medullary thyroid carcinoma, genes, and the prevention of cancer. N Engl J Med 1994;331:870–871.
36. Pomares F, Canas R, Rodriguez J, et al. Differences between sporadic and multiple endocrine neoplasia type 2A phaeochromocytoma. Clin Endocrinol 1998;48:195–200.
37. Gagel R, Robinson M, Donovan D, et al. Clinical review 44: Medullary thyroid carcinoma: Recent progress. J Clin Endocrinol Metab 1993;76:809–814.
38. Snow K, Boyd A. Management of individual tumor syndromes: medullary thyroid carcinoma and hyperparathyroidism. Endocrinol Metab Clin North Am 1994;23:157–166.
39. Evans D, Lee J, Merrel R, et al. Adrenal medullary disease in multiple endocrine neoplasia type 2: appropriate management. Endocrinol Metab Clin North Am 1994;23:167–176.
40. O'Riordain D, O'Brien T, Grant C, et al. Surgical management of primary hyperparathyroidism in multiple endocrine neoplasia type 1 and 2. Surgery 1993;114:1031–1039.
41. Wells S, Donis-Keller H. Current perspectives on the diagnosis and management of patients with multiple endocrine neoplasia type 2 syndromes. Endocrinol Metab Clin North Am 1994;23:215–228.

42. Erdogan M, Gullu S, Baskal N, et al. Omeprazole: calcitonin stimulation test for the diagnosis follow-up and family screening in medullary thyroid carcinoma. J Clin Endocrinol Metab 1997;82:897–899.

43. Pacak K, Linehan W, Eisenhofer G, et al. Recent advances in genetics, diagnosis, localization, and treatment of pheochromocytoma. Ann Intern Med 2001;134:315–329.

13 Addison's Disease

Robert G. Spanheimer, MD

CONTENTS

INTRODUCTION

Although adrenal insufficiency is unusual, its recognition and treatment are life-saving. The prevalence of primary adrenal insufficiency (Addison's disease) is between 110 and 120 cases per million population (1), with a mean age of onset at 40 yr old. Advanced cases are usually easily diagnosed, but the recognition of early phases can be a challenge.

In 1855, Thomas Addison described "anemia, general languor, debility, remarkable feebleness of the heart's action, irritability in the stomach, and a peculiar change of color in the skin." These changes were associated with destruction of the adrenal glands as found on autopsy, but no therapy was known and patients inevitably died. In 1949 (2), the synthesis of cortisone and cortisol for treatment of inflammatory diseases led to their availability for adrenal insufficiency and thus changed the course of the disease in patients with Addison's disease.

Two famous historical figures (one fictional) have recently been reviewed in the literature with regard to their likely diagnosis of Addison's disease. The story of John F. Kennedy (3) illustrates the subtle but progressive changes early in the

From: *Contemporary Endocrinology: Early Diagnosis and Treatment of Endocrine Disorders*
Edited by: R. S. Bar © Humana Press Inc., Totowa, NJ

disease. In childhood he was diagnosed with asthma and remained very thin until adulthood. After one year at Princeton, he withdrew because of "ill health" and transferred to Harvard to be close to his home and doctors. In August of 1944 he had successful disc surgery following a back injury during the well-publicized PT-109 incident, but recovery was slow and he received a medical discharge from the United States Navy on December 6, 1944. Of interest, during his naval service, he was diagnosed with malaria solely on the basis of 8% eosinophilia yet had negative blood smears for parasites, which was likely attributable to his Addison's disease. In 1945 in London and 1951 in Japan, Kennedy became critically ill with fevers of 106°F, which probably represented adrenal crisis. The only medical note referring to Addison's disease was a letter dated March 20, 1953 from Dr. Vernon Dick to Dr. William Herbst, both urologists, stating that diagnosis and treatment for Addison's disease began in October 1947. Whether these early findings were missed by other physicians or covered up by the Kennedy family is still debated, but at autopsy no evidence of adrenal tissue was found, thus documenting his Addison's disease.

Weir and Fleming *(4)* presented an amusing case of microcardia "2 sizes too small" secondary to chronic adrenocortical insufficiency, to stump colleagues and students. Because of the absence of laboratory resources, the diagnosis of Addison's disease was made on the available clinical evidence of salt craving, hyperpigmentation, and microcardia in the Christmas Grinch.

ADRENAL PHYSIOLOGY

Each adrenal gland is composed of cortical and medullary areas. The cortex is divided histologically and functionally into three concentric zones: the zona glomerulosa, which secretes aldosterone, the fasiculata, which secretes cortisol, and the reticularis, which secretes adrenal androgens. The adrenal medulla secretes catecholamines, principally epinephrine.

Cortisol secretion is closely regulated by a negative feedback mechanism, as shown in Fig. 1. Pituitary adrenocorticotropic hormone (ACTH) directly stimulates cortisol release from the adrenal glands. ACTH release is stimulated by the hypothalmic hormone corticotropin-releasing hormone (CRH) and inhibited by cortisol at the level of the pituitary and hypothalmus by reducing CRH and ACTH release. Aldosterone secretion is directly stimulated by ACTH but also potassium (hyperkalemia) and renin (hypovolemia). Regulation of adrenal androgens is not well defined. Plasma cortisol concentration reaches its maximum a few hours before and lasts 1 h after awakening (Fig. 2). Plasma cortisol then declines during the day to reach its lowest point in the late evening. This diurnal variation can be changed by altered sleep-wake patterns, as seen in shift workers.

Acute stress also stimulates cortisol release through increased CRH and ACTH secretion. Surgery is one of the most potent stimuli, but so is severe trauma, fever, or infection. Failure to provide adrenally insufficient patients with stress levels

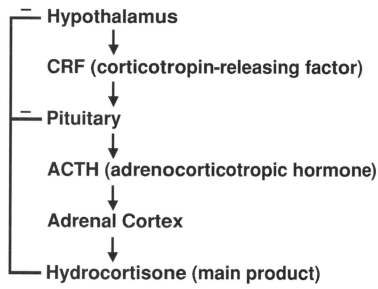

Fig. 1. Regulation of adrenal glucocorticoid production. The product of adrenal gluco-corticoid synthesis is hydrocortisone, which is closely regulated by a negative feedback mechanism. Hydrocortisone inhibits ACTH (adrenocortiotropic hormone) at the level of the corticotrophs of the pituitary and CRF (corticotropin-releasing factor) release from the hypothalamus.

of cortisol under these conditions will result in a rapidly worsening course, eventually resulting in death. Unexplained hypotension or fever during surgical procedure, or poor recovery post-op, may be the earliest signs of adrenal insufficiency.

ETIOLOGY

Primary Adrenal Insufficiency (Addison's Disease)

Primary adrenocorticol insufficiency results from any disease process (Table 1) that damages the entire adrenal cortex, thus resulting in deficiencies of cortisol, aldosterone, and adrenal androgens. Approximately 75–80% of cases are owing to autoimmune adrenalitis *(5)*, a shift from the predominant cause in 1928–1938, which was tuberculous adrenalitis (now only accounting for 10–20% worldwide). Although circulating antibodies to adrenal antigens, predominately 21-hydroxylase *(6)*, are found in 70% of patients, their role in the etiology is not clear, although they may be present years before the clinical diagnosis. It is recommended that adults and children with other organ-specific autoimmune disease (see below) particularly hypoparathyroidism and type 1 diabetes, be screened for the presence of 21-hydroxylase autoantibody; if this is positive, such patients should be screened for adrenal function every 6 mo *(7)*.

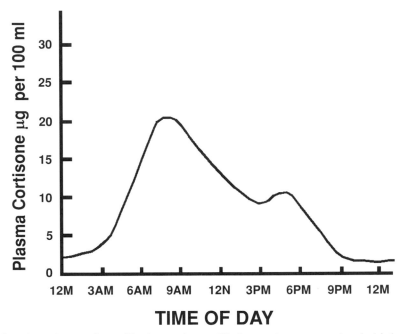

Fig. 2. Diurnal secretion of hydrocortisone. Hydrocortisone secretion is higher in the morning and gradually decreases throughout the day, with the lowest levels between 9 PM and midnight. This pattern may be disrupted by altered work shifts.

Table 1
Common Causes of Adrenal Insufficiency

Primary adrenal insufficiency
    1. Autoimmune adrenalitis (75%)
    2. Infectious adrenal destruction [tuberculosis (20%), fungal, AIDS with opportunistic infection]
    3. Metastatic carcinoma (lung, breast, lymphoma)
    4. Adrenal hemorrhage in patients on anticoagulation therapy
Secondary adrenal insufficiency
    1. Withdrawal from prolonged glucocorticoid therapy
    2. Pituitary or hypothalamic tumor, surgery, or irradiation
    3. Lymphocytic hypophysitis, sarcoidosis, or histocytosis

Autoimmune adrenocorticol insufficiency has a genetic predisposition and is associated with a high incidence of other endocrine gland failure. Although initially named after those who described the syndrome [Schmidt's syndrome (adrenal insufficiency and thyroiditis) or Carpenter's syndrome (hypoadrenalism, hypothyroidism, and type 1 diabetes mellitus)], these disorders are now grouped into polyglandular failure syndrome types I and II *(8).* Type I is inherited in an autosomal recessive pattern, with hypoparathyroidism, mucocutaneous candidiasis, and adrenal insufficiency being the most infamous triad of endocrine gland failures. Type II is familial half the time and is linked to HLA antigens B8 (DW3), DR3, and DR4. In type II patients, adrenal insufficiency is present in 100% of patients, with autoimmune thyroid disease, 70%, or insulin-dependent type 1 diabetes mellitus, 50%, in decreasing order of occurrence. Although these syndromes are uncommon, it is important to be aware that one autoimmune gland failure is associated with a higher risk of a second gland failure.

Other causes of primary adrenal insufficiency include adrenal hemorrhage in adults on anticoagulant therapy or in children because of meningococcal or *Pseudomonas* septicemia. Adrenomyeloneuropathy is an X-linked recessive disorder affecting 1 in 25,000 males, resulting in accumulation of long-chain fatty acids in central and peripheral nervous tissues as well as the adrenals and gonads; it is characterized by spastic paralysis and adrenal insufficiency (9). Although the adrenal insufficiency is clearly treatable, the cranial deficits are, unfortunately, progressive, with no known effective therapy. Through opportunistic infections, systemic fungal infections (histoplasmosis, cryptococcus, blastomycosis) and AIDS also result in adrenal insufficiency in 5% of patients. Primary adrenal insufficiency may also be iatrogenic owing to medications such as aminoglutethimide, metyrapon, and ketoconazole that reversibly inhibit steps in steroidogenesis. The anesthetic medication etomidate, as well as drugs that accelerate cortisol synthesis such as barbituates, refampin, and phenytoin, may precipitate adrenal insufficiency. Although metastic cancer (lung, breast, and kidney) and lymphoma often occur in the adrenal gland, adrenal insufficiency is infrequent; however, it may be overlooked in the terminal stages of the primary cancer because of overlapping symptoms.

Secondary Adrenal Insufficiency

The most common cause of secondary adrenocorticol insufficiency is iatrogenic, caused by withdrawal of therapy from patients who have been treated with pharmocologic doses of glucocorticoids (10). Clinical experience suggests that more than 30 d of supraphysiologic glucocorticoid treatment (e.g., prednisone at doses of >7.5 mg/d) may suppress CRH and ACTH for 3–6 mo; an additional 3–6 mo may then be required for cortisol to respond to ACTH since ACTH is trophic for the adrenal glands. Both topical and inhaled steroids (11) have now been reported to suppress the hypothalamic-pituitary adrenal axis, so withdrawal from prolonged use of these agents must be monitored for adrenal insufficiency.

The next most common causes of secondary adrenocortical insufficiency are tumors of the pituitary and/or hypothalmic region (most commonm after surgical and radiation treatment to the pituitary) as well as lymphocytic hypophysitis, sarcoidosis, and histocytosis. In these cases, ACTH is rarely the only pituitary hormone deficiency. Patients may present with either symptoms suggestive of a cranial mass, such as headache or visual field defects, or defects in other pituitary hormones such as gonadotropins, which usually are lost first (female: irregular or absent menses; male: erectile dysfunction), followed by hypothyroid symptoms, followed finally by loss of ACTH.

Causes of acute onset of secondary adrenal insufficiency are postpartum pituitary necrosis (Sheehan's syndrome) usually associated with heavy blood loss and the need for transfusions at delivery, head trauma with shearing of the pituitary stalk, or bleeding into pituitary macroadenomas.

CLINICAL FEATURES

In primary adrenal insufficiency, it is the lack of all three adrenal steroids (cortisol, aldosterone, and adrenal androgens) that contributes to the clinical features. Early in the disease process, patients present with gradually progressive symptoms that may be insidious in onset. These patients are often identified by recognition of a combination of symptoms, signs, and laboratory findings that involve multiple organ systems (Table 2). All patients with adrenocorticol deficiency have weakness and fatigue (100%), weight loss of 4–20 kg (100%), and anorexia (100%), probably caused by the role of cortisol in appetite regulation. The most distinctive physical finding is the hyperpigmentation (92%) found in non-sun-exposed areas such as the gingiva, axilla, or creases in the palms of the hands. The hyperpigmentation is caused by cosecretion of melanocyte-stimulating hormone (MSH) with the excess ACTH. Vitiligo (4%) may also occur in the presence of hyperpigmentation as part of the autoimmune disease and is due to autoimmune destruction of melanocytes.

Gastrointestinal symptoms occur in most patients and vary from anorexia to nausea, abdominal discomfort, vomiting, and diarrhea *(12)*. Fluid loss from these symptoms may exacerbate hypotension, which is present in 80–90% of patients. Hypotension may present with dizziness or orthostatic changes and occasionally syncope. The lack of cortisol effect on vascular tone and the lack of aldosterone effect on sodium resorption in the kidney may combine to produce severe hypotension *(13)*. Clinically, patients develop salt craving (20%) to compensate for this lack of aldosterone, with stories of patients chipping and eating 50-lb salt blocks in an attempt to maintain vascular volume.

Routine Laboratory Findings

Electrolyte disturbances are found in 92% of patients, with hyponatremia the most common (88%). Without aldosterone there is salt wasting, so urine sodium is inappropriately high; combined with the finding of hyponatremia, this may be misdiagnosed as the syndrome of inappropriate antidiuretic hormone (SIADH). The combination of hyponatremia and hyperkalemia owing to loss of mineralocorticoid effect on sodium/potassium exchange should strongly suggest adrenal

Table 2
Early Findings in Adrenal Insufficiency

Early symptoms	Early signs	Test of choice	Treatment
Primary adrenal insufficiency			
Fatigue, weakness, weight loss, anorexia	Electroylyte abnormalities (hyponatrenia, hyperkalemia) orthostatic hypotension, hyperpigmentation	Early AM cortisol, short ACTH stimulation test	Hydrocortisone (20 mg in AM and 10 mg in PM), Florinef (0.1 mg/d)
Secondary adrenal insufficiency			
Weight loss, fatigue, symptoms of hypothyroidism or hypogonadism, headache	Pituitary mass effect with visual field defects, hypothyroidism, hypogonadism	Low-dose (1 µg) ACTH stimulation test, free T4, gonadal hormones Insulin-induced hypoglycemia measuring cortisol response	Hydrocortisone (20 mg in AM and 10 mg in PM) Often other hormones such as thyroid and gender hormones, but not Florinef

ACTH, adrenocorticotropic hormone.

insufficiency. Hypoglycemia is an uncommon feature but may be provoked by fever, nausea, or vomiting in patients with Addison's disease.

Other laboratory features include normocytic normochromic anemia, relative lymphocytosis and eosinophilia (recall the case of John F. Kennedy), and mild hypercalcemia in 6% of patients. Chest x-ray reveals a small heart, and abdominal x-rays may show adrenal calcification owing to damage to the adrenals. Abdominal computed tomography (CT) may show enlargement of the adrenal glands in tuberculosis, malignant tumor, metastases, or adrenal hemorrhage, whereas small or absent adrenal glands are characteristic of autoimmune destruction.

Secondary Adrenocorticol Insufficiency

The presentation of secondary adrenal insufficiency is similar to that of primary adrenal insufficiency except that the adrenal glands remain intact and it is either hypothalamic CRH or pituitary ACTH secretion that is deficient. Clinically, this difference is seen as the lack of hyperpigmentation (owing to excess ACTH and MSH secretion in Addison's disease) and absent features of mineralocorticoid deficiency, since the adrenal glands can still directly respond to

Table 3
Tests for Adrenal Insufficiency

Initial testing to rule out adrenal insufficiency
  1. 24-h urinary free cortisol
  2. Early AM serum cortisol
  Either test will rule out adrenal insufficiency if normal (serum cortisol > 20 mg/dL),
    but if low, should be followed with a provocative test to confirm adrenal
    insufficiency.
Provocative testing
  Primary adrenal insufficiency: rapid ACTH stimulation giving 250 μg of synthetic
    ACTH im or iv and measuring cortisol before and 30 min after ACTH. Serum
    cortisol > 20 mg/dL at basal or post ACTH stimulation is normal.
  Secondary adrenal insufficiency: Low-dose (1 μg) ACTH stimulation test or insulin-
    induced hypoglycemia (see text). Serum cortisol > 18 mg/dL is normal either basal
    or post stimulation. An alternative is the overnight metyrapone (dose based on
    weight—see text) test with a plasma 11-deoxycortisol at 8 AM > 7 mg/dL normal.

ACTH, adrenocorticotropic hormone.

hyperkalemia and low plasma volume through the renin-angiotensin system. Thus hypotension, salt wasting, and hyperkalemia are uncommon. Symptoms of fatigue, weight loss, weakness, nausea, myalgias, and hypoglycemia remain, because of cortisol deficiency.

Depending on the etiology of secondary adrenocorticol deficiency, patients may present with symptoms suggestive of a pituitary mass (headache, visual field disturbances) or symptoms suggestive of loss of other pituitary hormones—most commonly hypogonadism and hypothyroidism. Because hypothyroidism is more common and easier to diagnose, signs and symptoms of either primary or secondary adrenal insufficiency may be clear only after thyroid hormone replacement. Patients who develop weight loss, anorexia, or hypotension after thyroid replacement should be tested for adrenal insufficiency.

DIAGNOSTIC EVALUATION

Initial diagnostic testing (Table 3) will depend on the severity of symptoms on presentation. In severe life-threatening cases, therapy with glucocorticoids such as dexamethasone as well as volume replacement with normal saline should be started, with diagnostic testing delayed.

In patients in whom adrenal insufficiency is to be ruled out, 24-h urinary free cortisol or plasma cortisol between 8 and 9 AM may be measured. If the 24-h urinary free cortisol is normal or the plasma cortisol is greater than 20 μg/dL (14), then adrenal insufficiency is excluded. In an acute emergency room or intensive care setting, plasma cortisol should be greater than 20 μg/dL at any time owing to the stress of the medical condition, but if time allows, a rapid ACTH stimulation test should be done.

Rapid ACTH Stimulation Test

In most patients dynamic testing is recommended, and the rapid ACTH stimulation test is the procedure of choice *(14,15)*. This test should be the initial diagnostic test in either primary or secondary adrenal insufficiency. Corticotropin (250 µg) is given intravenously or intramuscularly, and plasma cortisol is measured before and 30 (or preferably) 60 min after the injection. If the patient is hypotensive and possibly not perfusing peripheral tissue, the intravenous route is preferred. Because the test requires minimally only 30 min and bypasses the hypothalamic/pituitary axis, in life-threatening situations, dexamethasone can be administered and will not affect results if the ACTH stimulation test is done within 48 h of starting dexamethasone. A cortisol value of 20 µg/dL or more (either basal or stimulated) excludes primary adrenal insufficiency *(15)* but may not exclude secondary adrenal insufficiency with decreased (not absent) pituitary ACTH reserve (*see* discussion just below).

An abnormal cortisol response to ACTH stimulation establishes adrenal insufficiency. Measurement of ACTH at the same time as the baseline cortisol (before administration of synthetic ACTH) will distinguish primary adrenal insufficiency from secondary, which has inappropriately low ACTH levels with an absent response of cortisol.

Patients with severe secondary adrenal insufficiency do not respond to the rapid ACTH stimulation test because of adrenal atrophy owing to loss of the trophic effect of ACTH. However, patients with mild or recent onset secondary adrenal insufficiency may have a normal adrenal response to the usual high dose of exogenous ACTH. There are three tests to diagnose early or partial secondary adrenal insufficiency. The most established test is to induce hypoglycemia with insulin *(16)* and to measure cortisol response, but this is unpleasant at best and potentially dangerous. An overnight metyrapone (an agent that blocks the final step in cortisol production and results in elevated levels of 11-deoxycortisol) test is simpler and carries a lower risk *(17)*, but the drug is not always available. A single oral dose of metyrapone based on weight (2.0 g for ≤70 kg, 2.5 g for 70–90 kg, and 3.0 g for >90 kg) is given at midnight with a snack to reduce gastrointestinal upset. Blood for cortisol and 11-deoxycortisol is drawn at 8 AM. A level of 11-deoxycortisol of 7 µg/dL or more is normal, with less than 7 µg/dL in patients with either primary or secondary adrenal insufficiency (This test cannot distinguish primary from secondary.) Recently, a low-dose, intravenous ACTH (1 µg vs 250 µg in the rapid test) stimulation test *(18)* with cortisol levels checked at 0, 20, and 30 min has been proposed to replace the insulin and metyrapone tests for secondary adrenal insufficiency. The argument against using the 1-µg dose to diagnose all patients with adrenal insufficiency is that it may miss mild primary adrenal insufficiency.

Radiographic procedures are not diagnostic and should be done only after the diagnosis has been established by hormone tests. However, head magnetic resonance imaging should be done in patients with headache or visual field distur-

Table 4
Treatment of Adrenal Insufficiency

Acute Adrenal Crisis
  1. Fluids: 5% glucose in 0.9% saline (vigorous at first, e.g., 2 L in 3–4 h)
  2. Hydrocortisone iv: 100 mg as soon as possible then q6h for 24–48 h (this dose of
     hydrocortisone has enough salt-retaining ability so that mineralocorticoid
     therapy is not necessary)
Chronic adrenal insufficiency
  Primary adrenal insufficiency:
  1. Hydrocortisone 20 mg in AM and 10 mg in PM (alternatives include cortisone
     acetate 25 mg in AM and 12.5 mg in PM, or prednisone 5 mg in AM and 2.5 mg
     in PM)
  2. Florinef (9-α-fluorocorticoid) 0.1 mg
  Secondary adrenal insufficiency:
  Same glucocorticoid but patients do not need mineralocorticoid replacement

bances to rule out pituitary or hypothalamic tumor. X-rays are generally not useful
in patients with primary adrenal insufficiency caused by autoimmune disease. In
all other cases, a CT of the abdomen may reveal enlarged adrenal glands, which
may need to be biopsied by CT-guided fine needle for the diagnosis.

TREATMENT

Treatment guidelines are outlined in Table 4.

Acute Adrenal Crisis

Acute adrenal insufficiency is a medical emergency. It may occur in a patent
with known adrenal insufficiency in the setting of acute illness caused by infection, trauma, or surgery without appropriate stress dosing of glucocorticoid, or
(if the patient cannot retain injested glucocorticoids) because of nausea and
vomiting, or, finally, as a presentation of undiagnosed adrenal insufficiency.
Symptoms develop rapidly and include nausea, vomiting, and abdominal pain
that may mimic an acute abdomen. Fever is usually present and may be very high
owing to glucocorticoid deficiency itself or an underlying infection, which may
exacerbate the glucocorticoid deficiency. Eventually, dehydration with severe
hypotension leads to vascular collapse and death. As an initial presentation,
these symptoms of abdominal pain, fever, and hypotension may appear to be
an acute surgical abdomen and may lead to unnecessary and possibly fatal surgery. Evidence of chronic physical changes (weight loss, hyperpigmentation,
fatigue) or hyponatremia, hyperkalemia, hypoglycemia, or eosinophilia should
suggest primary adrenal disease. In the setting of anticoagulant therapy, adrenal
hemorrhage causing destruction of the glands may present with severe abdominal pain and rapidly developing signs of acute adrenal insufficiency *(19)*.

Therapy should not be delayed in the acute setting for laboratory confirmation. Since death results from shock and vascular collapse, intravenous rehydration with saline 0.9% and 5% glucose should be vigorous. Blood should be drawn for electrolytes, cortisol, and ACTH. A rapid ACTH stimulation test will provide additional information, and dexamethasone 4–8 mg may be given as initial glucocorticoid replacement since it will not interfere with the ACTH stimulation test or cortisol assay. If time permits, an ACTH level should be drawn before dexamethasone since ACTH will be suppressed after the dexamethasone is given.

After the ACTH stimulation test is completed, a preparation of glucocorticoid with mineralocorticoid activity is recommended. Hydrocortisone 100 mg intravenously every 6 h is the drug of choice *(20)* and, combined with saline fluid replacement, will provide adequate mineralocorticoid activity. Hydrocortisone can be tapered to 50 mg every 6 h on the second day if recovery is satisfactory and the precipitating illness has been identified. In the absence of complications, treatment can be tapered to replacement levels within 3–5 d.

Chronic Adrenal Insufficiency

The treatment for chronic primary adrenal insufficiency includes replacement of both glucocorticoid and mineralocorticoid. In secondary (pituitary/hypothalmic) adrenal insufficiency, only glucocorticoid replacement is necessary because the adrenal gland is still intact and can respond directly to hyperkalemia and hypovolemia through the renin/angiotension system to stimulate mineralocorticoid secretion.

The glucocorticoid of choice is cortisol (hydrocortisone) dosed at 20 mg in the AM and 10 mg in the PM, usually between 4 and 6 PM to mimic the normal circadian rhythm of glucocorticoids *(21)*. Cortisone acetate is equally acceptable at 25 mg in the AM and 12.5 mg in the PM. Adequacy of glucocorticoid replacement is based primarily on clinical judgment. Direct assay of ACTH is only rarely used since serum ACTH measurement is not as sensitive an index of glucocorticoid replacement as thyroid-stimulating hormone (TSH) is for thyroid hormone replacement. Excess replacement of glucocorticoid may lead to weight gain or cushinoid features; inadequate doses result in persistent weakness, fatigue, and excess pigmentation.

Mineralocorticoid activity is replaced by 9-α-fluorocorticoid (Florinef) 0.05–0.2 mg/d. Adequate mineralocorticoid therapy is obtained when blood pressure (including loss of orthostatic drop in blood pressure) potassium, and renin levels return to normal. Excessive therapy results in sodium retention (hypertension, edema) and hypokalemia, and underreplacement results in persistent hypotension, hyperkalemia, and hyperreninenia. Many patients have a variable seasonal need for mineralocorticoid, requiring none or 0.05 mg in the winter, 0.1 mg/d in the summer, and 0.2 mg when the weather is very hot (>90°F) and humid.

Glucocorticoid Coverage for Stress

In response to acute illness, trauma, or surgical intervention, there is increased secretion of CRH, ACTH, and finally cortisol. Patients with primary or secondary adrenal insufficiency will not be able to increase cortisol production and require both physiologic and supplemental stress therapy with glucocorticoid. Because of the large variation in cortisol production in healthy patients under stress, it is difficult to predict cortisol needs of patients exactly during stressful conditions.

A recent review (22) suggests that the conventional recommendations for stress doses of 200–300 mg of hydrocortisone for any procedure or medical illness should be discouraged. Excess amount and duration of the glucocorticoid may result in poor wound healing, immunosuppression, hyperglycemia, and excess sodium retention with volume overload.

Instead of the one-dose-fits-all protocol, these authors recommend corticosteroid supplementation based on the level of medical or surgical stress. Patients who should receive supplementation are all those with primary or secondary adrenal insufficiency, including patients currently receiving more than physiologic glucocorticoid treatment equivalent to more than 5 mg/d of prednisone. All these patients plus those receiving less than 5 mg/d of prednisone who undergo any procedure or have a medical illness require their usual daily glucocorticoid therapy either orally or intravenously. Patients who take less than physiologic replacement (prednisone ≤5 mg/d) do not require additional supplementation since their adrenal glands remain responsive to ACTH release and do respond to stress by increasing endogenous ACTH.

For minor illness (fever < 100°F, nausea but able to take in fluids and medications) or procedures that take less than 1 h under local anesthesia, only replacement therapy is required and is given prior to the procedure. For moderate illness including bacterial pneumonia, severe gastroenteritis, or prolonged fever as well as cholecystectomy or hemicolectomy, 50–75 mg of hydrocortisone is given on the day of the procedure or acute illness with tapering over 1–2 d to replacement doses. Prior studies have shown that severe illness or surgery increases daily production of cortisol, eliminating the diurnal pattern; however levels, return to normal within 24–48 h after surgery or illness.

With major illness such as pancreatitis or major surgery, patients should receive 100–150 mg on the day of the procedure and tapering over 1–2 d. For critically ill patients 50–100 mg of hydrocortisone every 6 h or 0.18 mg/kg/h as a continuous infusion to be continued as needed is sufficient. Cortisol in doses of 50 mg/d or more has enough intrinsic mineralocorticoid effect so that additional mineralocorticoid supplementation is not needed, especially when saline is being administered.

This dosing of supplemental corticosteroid based on level of surgical or medical stress is based on cortisol production rates studied during stress, not clinical outcome studies. Previous recommendations of 100 mg iv hydrocortisone for minor procedures or illness, and 100 mg iv every 6 h for major surgery or illness appear excessive. Too much and too long administration of supplemental therapy may cause adverse effects such as delayed wound healing, immunosuppression, and hyperglycemia.

Special Treatment Considerations

Although primary adrenal insufficiency is rare, secondary adrenal insufficiency after withdrawal of supraphysiologic corticosteroid therapy is common, and both are potentially fatal conditions if unrecognized and untreated. With the introduction of glucocorticoid replacement in the late 1940s, the survival of patients with adrenal insufficiency now approaches that of the normal population. However, owing to the lack of cortisol production in response to stress, certain everyday life-type experiences must be recognized and treated in patients with adrenal insufficiency to avoid life-threatening conditions. Education of the patient and their family members is crucial to avoid adrenal crisis. Table 5 outlines some special considerations, with recommendations for patients, family members, and caregivers.

During pregnancy, replacement of both glucocorticoid and mineralocorticoid usually does not change *(23)*. Occasionally increased sodium intake is required in the second and third trimester and, less commonly, an increase in glucocorticoid or mineralocorticoid requirement. During labor and delivery, special attention to hydration with a saline infusion and administration of 50–100 mg cortisol orally or iv in divided doses over 24 h should be given.

Each patient should carry an identification bracelet or card in case of an accident so that prompt administration of corticosteroid can be given in an emergency, especially if mental capacity has been diminished. Patients and close family members should be able to administer intramuscular dexamethasone 4 mg/mL, available as a Decadron emergency kit. When patients develop nausea and vomiting and are unable to keep the oral cortisol down after two or three attempts, the dexamethasone injection will allow 6–8 h of replaced glucocorticoid, hopefully to allow recovery from reversible gastroenteritis. If the patient develops signs of dehydration, fluid replacement with iv saline will be required in a clinic or hospital setting. Patients should be encouraged to recognize symptoms of dehydration early and to seek medical care.

CONCLUSIONS

Diagnosis of adrenal insufficiency is often delayed because of nonspecific and misleading symptoms. As the process progresses, symptoms worsen, and an acute crisis may be precipitated by surgery, trauma, or infection. Being aware of glucocorticoid use in the previous 12 mo is essential to recognize the most

Table 5
Special Considerations

Daily recommendations
  1. Education of patient and family about critical need for daily cortisol. If unable to take or retain (nausea, vomiting), patients should have access to a Decadron Emergency kit for im administration of 4 mg dexamethazone.
  2. Identification bracelet or card
  3. Extra salt or mineralocorticoid when weather is very hot (>90°F) or humid
Stress recommendations
  1. Minor illness (maintain fluid intake, fever <100°F, nonbacterial infections) or medical procedure lasting less than 1 h: replace only physiologic dose of gluocorticoid.
  2. Moderate illness (fever >100°F, bacterial infections) or procedures (cholecysectomy): 50–75 mg of hydrocortisone per day, tapering quickly
  3. Severe illness or surgery: 100–150 mg/d of hydrocortisone
  4. Critical illness: 50–100 mg q6h or continuous infusion of 0.18 mg/kg/h of hydrocortisone

common cause of secondary adrenal insufficiency. Recognizing clinical features in multiple systems such as metabolic (hypoglycemia, weight loss), gastrointestinal (nausea, anorexia), cardiovascular (postural hypotension), electrolyte (hyponatremia, hyperkalemia, salt craving), and hyperpigmentation is the key to early diagnosis of adrenal insufficiency.

Since the introduction of glucocorticoid therapy, survival in patients with primary or secondary adrenal insufficiency has depended on diagnosis and appropriate therapy, including patient education and coverage for stress. Deaths from adrenal insufficiency are rare in diagnosed and appropriately treated patients; thus finding, educating, and treating these patients can be very rewarding.

REFERENCES

  1. Laurenti S, Vecchi L, Santeusanio F, Falorni A. Is the prevalence of Addison's disease under-estimated? J Clin Endocrinol Metab 1999;84:1762–1763.
  2. Hench PS, Slocumb CH, Polley MF, Kendall EC. Effect of cortisone and pituitary adrenocorticotropic hormone (ACTH) on rheumatic diseases. JAMA 1950;144:1327–1335.
  3. Loughlin KR. John F. Kennedy and his adrenal disease. Urology 2002;59:165–169.
  4. Weir E, Fleming R. Case report: microcardia secondary to chronic adrenocortical insufficiency. Can Med Assoc J 2001;165:1585–1586.
  5. Irvine WJ, Barnes EW. Adrenocortial insufficiency. J Clin Endocrinol Metab 1972;1: 549–556.
  6. Falorni A, Nikoshkov A, Laurenti S, et al. High diagnostic accuracy for idiopathic Addison's disease with a sensitive radiolabeling assay for antibodies against recombinant human 21-hydroxylase. J Clin Endocrinol Metab 1995;80:2752–2755.
  7. Laurenti S, Arvat E, Candeloro P, et al. Low dose (1 μg) ACTH test in the evaluation of adrenal dysfunction in pre-clinical Addison's disease. Clin Endocrinol 2000;53:107–115.
  8. Trence DL, Morley JE. Polyglandular autoimmune syndromes. Am J Med 1984;77:107–116.

9. Augbourg P. Adrenoleukodystrophy and other peroxisomal diseases. Curr Opin Genet Dev 1994;4:407–411.
10. Spiegel RJ, Vigershy RA, Oliff AI, Echelberger CK, Brubon J, Poplack DG. Adrenal suppression after short term corticosteroid therapy. Lancet 1979;1:630–633.
11. Albert SG, Slavin RG. Adrenal insufficiency in an adult on inhaled corticosteroids; recovery of adrenal function with inhaled nedocromil sodium. Ann Allergy Asthma Immunol 1998;81:582–584.
12. Tobin MV, Aldridge SA, Morris AI, Belchetz PE, Gilmore IT. Gastrointestinal manifestations of Addison's disease. Am J Gastroenterol 1989;84:1302–1308.
13. Walker BR, Connacher AA, Webb DJ, Edwards CRW. Glucocorticoids and blood pressure: a role for the cortisol/cortisone shuttle in the control of vascular tone Clin Sci 1992;83:171–178.
14. Grinspoon SK, Buller BMK. Laboratory assessment of adrenal insufficiency. J Clin Endocrinol Metab 1994;79:923–931.
15. Oelkers W, Diedrich S, Bahr V. Diagnosis and therapy surveillance in Addison's disease: rapid adrenocorticotropin (ACTH) test and measurement of plasma ACTH, renin activity, and aldosterone. J Clin Endocrinol Metab 1992;75:259–264.
16. Parvord SR, Girach A, Price DE, Absalom SR, Falconer-Smith J, Howlett TA. A retrospective audit of combined pituitary function test using the insulin stress test, TRH and GnRH in a distinct laboratory. Clin Endocrinol (Oxf) 1992;36:135–139.
17. Steiner H, Bahr V, Exner P, Oelkers PW. Pituitary function tests: comparison of ACTH and 11-deoxycortisol response in the metyrapone test and with the insulin hypoglycemia test. Exp Clin Endocrinol 1994;102:33–38.
18. Thaler LM, Blevins LS. The low dose (1 μg) achenocorticotropin stimulation test in the evaluation of patients with suspected central adrenal insufficiency. J Clin Endocrinol Metab 1999;83:2726–2729.
19. Rao RH, Vagnucci AH, Amico JA. Bilateral massive adrenal hemorrhage: early recognition and treatment. Ann Intern Med 1989;110:227–235.
20. Miller WL, Chrousos GP. The adrenal cortex. In: Felig P, Frohman L, eds. Endocrinology and Metabolism, 4th ed. McGraw-Hill, New York, 2001, pp. 461–475.
21. Oelkers W. Adrenal insufficiency. N Engl J Med 1996;16:1206–1212.
22. Coursin DB, Wood KE. Corticosteroid supplementation for adrenal insufficiency. JAMA 2002;287:236–240.

14 Cushing's Syndrome

D. Lynn Loriaux, MD, PhD

CONTENTS

EARLY DIAGNOSIS AND TREATMENT

The period between the onset of the signs and symptoms of Cushing's syndrome and its definitive diagnosis averages 5 yr *(1)*. Thus, the idea of an early diagnosis is somewhat of an oxymoron. The diagnosis requires a convincing combination of clinical findings and biochemical abnormalities *(2–8)*. The obvious combination is an established clinical picture coupled with some reliable measure of an elevated cortisol production rate. The diagnosis can be made in the absence of evidence for an increased cortisol production rate if the clinical picture is unequivocal, and in the absence of a convincing clinical picture if the urine free cortisol excretion is greater than 300 µg/day *(9–11)*. The various combinations of clinical presentation and cortisol production rate can be lumped into four differential diagnostic categories. These relationships can be seen in Fig. 1.

This figure shows the basic categories into which Cushing's syndrome can be divided. Patients in square 1 have typical Cushing's syndrome *(9–11)*. Patients in square 2 have what may be called catabolic Cushing's syndrome *(11–14)*, and patients in square 3 could be thought of as having atypical Cushing's syndrome *(15–19)*. The subjects in square 4 are, of course, normal with regard to adrenal function. The differential diagnosis of each type of Cushing's syndrome is shown

From: *Contemporary Endocrinology: Early Diagnosis and Treatment of Endocrine Disorders*
Edited by: R. S. Bar © Humana Press Inc., Totowa, NJ

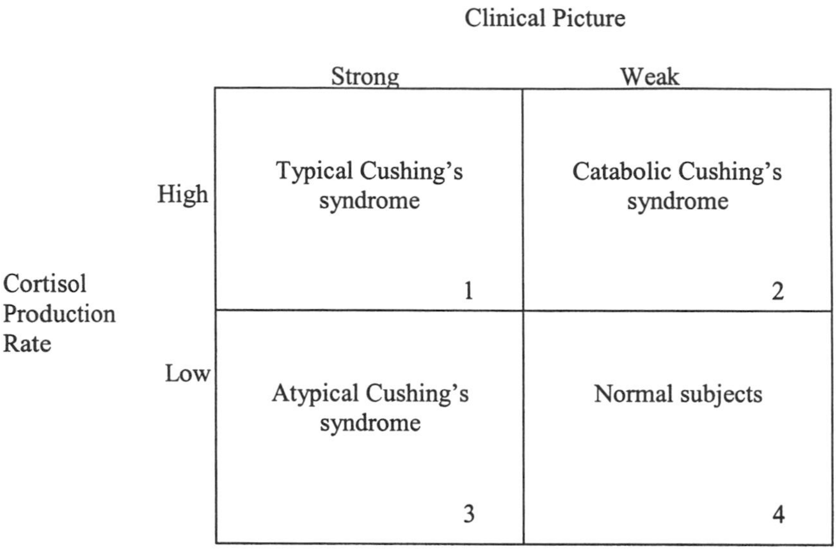

Clinical Picture

Fig. 1. Cortisol production rate and clinical picture in Cushing's syndrome.

in Table 1, and the rough sensitivity and specificity of the signs and symptoms of Cushing's syndrome are shown in Table 2 *(20)*.

Four tools are used to work through the differential diagnosis *(21–26)*. The first is a photographic record of the progress of the clinical picture. Driver's license, photo IDs, and family snapshots can all be helpful. Laboratory tools include the urinary free cortisol excretion, plasma adrenocorticotropic hormone (ACTH) level, plasma ACTH level following corticotrophin-releasing hormone (CRH) stimulation, and, most recently, salivary cortisol *(27–31)*. In addition, the inferior petrosal sinus sampling procedure (IPSS) measuring ACTH simultaneously in a peripheral vein and in the right and left inferior petrosol sinuses is the standard way of defining the anatomic site of ACTH hypersecretion *(32,33)*.

DIFFERENTIAL DIAGNOSIS OF ACTH-DEPENDENT VERSUS ACTH-INDEPENDENT CUSHING'S SYNDROME

If circulating ACTH can be measured in a patient with established Cushing's syndrome, the patient has ACTH-dependent disease *(34)*. The best test for this is the CRH-stimulated plasma ACTH (CRH at 1 µg/kg is administered by slow intravenous push, and plasma ACTH is measured at 5, 10, and 30 min. Any ACTH value > 10 pg/mL secures the diagnosis of ACTH-dependent disease.)

Pituitary versus ectopic ACTH secretion is defined by the ACTH gradient between peripheral blood and blood draining the pituitary gland (inferior petrosal sinus blood). In this test it is also wise to employ CRH stimulation of ACTH

Table 1
Differential Diagnosis of Cushing's Syndrome[a]

Typical Cushing's syndrome
    ACTH-dependent Cushing's syndrome
        ACTH-secreting pituitary microadenoma
        Ectopic ACTH secretion (bronchial carcinoid most common)
        Exogenous ACTH administration
    ACTH-independent Cushing's syndrome
        Adrenal adenoma
        Adrenal carcinoma
        Micronodular adrenal dysplasia
        Exogenous glucocorticoid administration—iaotrogenic Cushing's syndrome
    Catabolic Cushing's syndrome
    Ectopic ACTH secretion (usually small cell cancer of the lung but also other aggressive
        pluripotential cancers)
    Atypical Cushing's syndrome
        Exogenous glucocorticoid administration
        Periodic or intermittent Cushing's syndrome

[a]Common signs and symptoms of Cushing's syndrome associated with their approximate sensitivity and specificity are shown in Table 2.

Table 2
Signs and Symptoms of Cushing's Syndrome

	Sensitivity	*Specificity*
Signs		
Weight gain	+ + +	+
Plethora	+ +	+
Thin skin	+	+
Striae	+	+
Supraclavicular	+	+ +
Fat pad hypertrophy	+	+ + +
Proximal muscle weakness	+	+ + +
Symptoms		
Depression	+ + +	+
Fatigue	+ +	+
Weakness	+	+

+, low; ++, moderate; +++, high.

secretion, in which case, any gradient, central to peripheral, greater than 2.8 secures the diagnosis of pituitary Cushing's syndrome, or Cushing's disease.

ACTH-independent causes of Cushing's syndrome are distinguished one from the other by magnetic resonance imaging (MRI) *(35–37)*. Unilateral adrenal enlargement suggests adenoma or carcinoma *(38,39)*. Bilateral enlargement suggests primary pigmented micronodular dysplasia, and bilateral atrophy of the adrenal glands suggest factitious or iatrogenic disease.

TREATMENT

The appropriate treatment for Cushing's syndrome is dictated by the specific diagnosis *(38,39)*. Cushing disease is treated first by transsphenoidal micro-adenectomy *(40–42)*. This is successful 95% of the time in the hands of a skilled and experienced neurosurgeon. If that fails, a second transsphenoidal exploration is usually indicated. If that fails, pituitary irradiation *(40,42)* or, perhaps more commonly, laparoscopic bilateral adrenalectomy is the treatment of choice *(43–48)*. Catabolic Cushing's syndrome should be treated by attacking the underlying malignancy. This therapy can be augmented with competitive inhibitors of adrenal steroidgenesis. Ketoconazole is currently the agent of first choice *(49,50)*. Usually complete blockade is achieved at a dose of 800 mg/d or less. The most common reason for failure with this agent is drug-induced hepatitis. If this occurs, heralded by rising transaminase levels, the remaining option is laparoscopic bilateral adrenalectomy *(48)*. Atypical Cushing's syndrome should be treated by withdrawing the offending agent, usually a synthetic glucocorticoid.

There is one important general principle in the treatment of Cushing's syndrome. When treatment is successful, the patient will be left with adrenal insufficiency, which is a lethal condition. All patients with Cushing's syndrome in the postintervention period should be "covered" with a replacement dose of glucocorticoid until the effects of treatment can be assessed: 25 mg/d of hydrocortisone, 5 mg/d of prednisone, or 0.5 mg/d dexamethasone. If plasma cortisol can be measured on the morning after the intervention, the treatment has failed to cure the patient, and replacement glucocorticoids usually can be withdrawn.

What are the indications for early intervention? These are shown in Table 3. Patients with a urinary free cortisol (UFC) of greater than 2000μg/d are at risk for steroid psychosis. (Never perform a dexamethasone suppression test in such a patient). Serious life-threatening systemic infection can sometimes manifest only as hypotension leading to unexpected cardiovascular collapse. These patients should receive early intervention. Medically, this is ketoconazole. It should be tried first and used to "hold the line" until definitive surgical therapy can be provided.

Surgical wound dehiscence in this setting will require a reduction in glucocorticoid effect for healing to occur. The only effective treatment for steroid psychosis is to reduce circulating glucocorticoid concentrations *(50)*. The other diverse neuropsychic disturbances of glucocorticoid excess, from cognitive abnormalities to steroid psychosis, must also be considered in the evaluation of Cushing's syndrome *(51–56)*.

Table 3
Indications for Early Treatment
of Cushing's Syndrome

1. UFC excretions above 2000 µg/d
2. Sepsis
3. Psychosis
4. Wound dehiscence
5. Severe proximal muscle weakness

UFC, urinary free cortisol.

REFERENCES

1. Norton JA, Li M, Gillary J, Le HN. Cushing's syndrome. Curr Prob Surg 2001;38:488–545.
2. Wright-Pascoe R, Charles CF, Richards R, Fletcher P, Hanchard B, Kelly D. A clinicopathological study of Cushing's syndrome at the University Hospital of the West Indies and a review of the literature. West Ind Med J 2001;50:55–61.
3. Newell-Price J, Jorgensen JO, Grossman A. The diagnosis and differential diagnosis of Cushing's syndrome. Horm Res 1999;51(suppl 3):81–94.
4. Bollanti L, Riondino G, Strollo F. Endocrine paraneoplastic syndromes with special reference to the elderly. Endocr J UK 2001;14:151–157.
5. Ross RJ, Trainer PJ. Endocrine investigation: Cushing's syndrome. Clin Endocrinol 1998;49:153–155.
6. Cavagnini F, Pecori Giraldi F. Epidemiology and follow-up of Cushing's disease. Ann Endocrinol 2001;62:168–172.
7. Clayton LH, Dilley KB. Cushing's syndrome. Am J N 1998; 98:40–41.
8. Newell-Price J. Grossman AB. The differential diagnosis of Cushing's syndrome. Ann Endocrinol 2001;62:173–179.
9. Grigsby PW. Pituitary adenoma. Front Radiat Ther Oncol 2001;35:48–56.
10. Klee GG. Maximizing efficacy of endocrine tests: importance of decision-focused testing strategies and appropriate patient preparation. Clin Chem 1999;45:1323–1330.
11. Vierhapper H. Adrenocortical tumors: clinical symptoms and biochemical diagnosis. Eur J Radiol 2002;41:88–94.
12. Landman RE, Horwith M, Peterson RE, Khandji AG, Wardlaw SL. Long-term survival with ACTH-secreting carcinoma of the pituitary: a case report and review of the literature [Review]. J Clin Endocrinol Metab 2002;87:3084–3089.
13. dePerrot M, Spilopoulos A, Fischer S, Totsch M, Keshavjee S. Neuroendocrine carcinoma (carcinoid) of the thymus associated with Cushing's syndrome. Ann Thorac Surg 2002;73:675–681.
14. Boscaro M, Barzon L, Fallo F, Sonino N. Cushing's syndrome. Lancet 201;357:783–791.
15. Invitti C, Pecori Giraldi F, Cavagnini F, Sonzogni A. Usual association of adrenal angiosarcoma and Cushing's disease. Horm Res 2001.56:124–129.
16. Danese RD, Aron DC. Cushing's syndrome and hypertension. Endocrinol Metab Clin North Am 1994;23:299–324.
17. Hou L, Harshbarger T, Herrick MK, Tse V. Suprasellar adrenocorticotropic hormone-secreting ectopic pituitary adenoma: a case report and literature review. Neurosurgery 2002;50:618–625.
18. Holthouse DJ, Robbins PD, Kahler R, Knuckey N, Pullan P. Corticotroph pituitary carcinoma: case report and literature review. Endocr Pathol 2001;12:329–341.

19. Findling JW, Raff H. Diagnosis and differential diagnosis of Cushing's syndrome. Endocrinol Metab Clin North Am 2001;30:729–747.
20. Perry RR, Nieman LK, Cutler GB Jr, et al. Primary adrenal causes of Cushing's syndrome. Diagnosis and surgical management. Ann Surg 1989;210:59–68.
21. Castro M, Elias PC, Martinelli CE Jr, Antonini SR, Santiago L, Moreira AC. Salivary cortisol as a tool of physiological studies and diagnositic strategies. Braz J Med Biol Res 2000;33:1171–1175.
22. Katz J, Bouloux PM. Cushing's: how to make the diagnosis. Practitioner 1999;234:118–122, 124.
23. Goldfarb DA. Contemporary evaluation and management of Cushing's syndrome. World J Urol 1999;17:22–25.
24. Boscaro M, Barzon L, Sonino N. The diagnosis of Cushing's syndrome: atypical presentations and laboratory shortcomings. Arch Intern Med 2000;160:3045–3053.
25. Kirk LF Jr, Hash RB, Katner HP, Jones T. Cushing's disease: clinical manifestations and diagnostic evaluation. Am Fam Physician 2000;62:1119–1127, 1133–1134.
26. Miyachi Y. Pathophysiology and diagnosis of Cushing's syndrome. Biomed Pharmacother 2000;54(suppl 1):113s–117s.
27. Perry LA, Grossman AB. The role of the laboratory in the diagnosis of Cushing's syndrome. Ann Clin Biochem 1997;34:345–359.
28. Wood PJ, Barth JH, Freedman DB, Perry L, Sheridan B. Evidence for the low dose dexamethasone suppression test to screen for Cushing's syndrome: recommendations for a protocol for biochemistry laboratories. Ann Clin Biochem 1997;34:222–229.
29. Raff H, Raff JL, Findling JW. Late-night salivary cortisol as a screening test for Cushing's syndrome. J Clin Endocrinol Metab 1998;83:2681–2686.
30. Meier CA, Biller BM. Clinical and biochemical evaluation of Cushing's syndrome. Endocrinol Metab Clin North Am 1977;26:741–762.
31. Baker JT. Adrenal disorders. A primary care approach. Lippincotts Primary Care Pract 1997;1:527–536.
32. Pecori Giraldi F, Invitti C, Cavagnini F. Inferior petrosal sinus sampling ten years down the road. J Endocrinol Invest 2000;23:325–327.
33. Findling JW, Raff H. Newer diagnostic techniques and problems in Cushing's disease. Endocrinol Metab Clin North Am 1999;28:191–210.
34. Newell-Price J, Trainer P, Besser M, Grossman A. The diagnosis and differential diagnosis of Cushing's syndrome and pseudo-Cushing's states. Endocr Rev 1998;19:647–672.
35. Lockhart ME, Smith JK, Kenney PJ. Imaging of adrenal masses. Eur J Radiol 2002;41:95–112.
36. Takamura T, Nagai Y, Taniguchi M, et al. Adrenocorticoptropin-independent unilateral adrenocortical hyperplasia with Cushing's syndrome: immunohistochemical studies of steroidogenic enzymes, ultrastructural examination and a review of the literature. Pathol Int 2001;5:118–122.
37. Miyajima A, Nakashima J, Tachibana M, Baba S, Nakamura K, Murai M. ACTH-independent bilateral macronodular adrenocortical hyperplasia caused Cushing's syndrome. Urol Int 1997;58:259–261.
38. Veznedaroglu E, Armonda RA, Andrews DW. Diagnosis and therapy for pituitary tumors. Curr Opin Oncol 1999;11:27–31.
39. Zin-ul-Miraj M, Usmani GN, Yaqub MM, Ashraf S. Cushing's syndrome caused by an adrenal adenoma. J Pediatr Surg 1998;33:644–646.
40. Hardy J. Cushing's disease: Pituitary microsurgery. Curr Ther Endocrinol Metab 1997;6:63–65.
41. Ludecke DK, Flitsch J, Knappe UJ, Saeger W. Cushing's disease: a surgical view. J Neurooncology 2001;54:151–166.
42. Lissett CA, Shalet SM. Management of pituitary tumors: strategy for investigation and follow-up. Horm Res 2000;53(suppl 3):65–70.

43. Kazaryan AM, Mala T, Edwin B. Does tumor size influence the outcome of laparoscopic adrenalectomy? J. Laparoendoscop Adv Surg Techn 2001;11:1–4.
44. Sung GT, Gill IS. Laparoscopic adrenalectomy. Semin Laparoscop Surg 2000;7:211–222.
45. Godellas CV, Prinz RA. Surgical approach to adrenal neoplasms: laparoscopic versus open adrenalectomy. Surg Oncol Clin North Am 1998;7:807–817.
46. Lanzi R, Montorsi F, Losa M, et al. Laparoscopic bilateral adrenalectomy for persistent Cushing's disease after transsphenoidal surgery. Surgery 1998;123:144–150.
47. Schell SR, Talamini MA, Udelsman R. Laparoscopic adrenalectomy. Adv Surg 1997;31:333–350.
48. McCallum RW, Connell JM. Laparoscopic adrenalectomy. Clin Endocrinol (Oxf) 2001;55:435–36.
49. Berwaerts J, Verhelst J, Mahler C, Abs R. Cushing's syndrome in pregnancy treated by ketoconazole: case report and review of the literature. Gynecol Endocrinol 1999;13:175–182.
50. Pies R. Differential diagnosis and treatment of steroid-induced affective syndromes. Gen Hosp Psychiatry 1995;17:353–61.
51. Sonino N, Fava GA. Psychiatric disorders associated with Cushing's syndrome. Epidemiology, pathophysiology and treatment. Drugs 2001;15:361–373.
52. Belanoff JK, Gross K, Yager A, Schatzberg AF. Corticosteroids and cognition. J Psychiatr Res 2001;35:127–145.
53. Sapolsky RM. Glucocorticoids and hippocampal atrophy in neuropsychiatric disorders. Arch Gen Psychiatry 2000;57:925–935.
54. Brown ES, Rush AJ, McEwen BS. Hippocampal remodeling and damage by corticosteriods: implications for mood disorders. Neuropsychopharmacology 1999;21:474–484.
55. Sonino N, Fava GA. Psychosomatic aspects of Cushing's disease. Psychother Psychosom 1998;67:140–146.
56. Sonino N. From the lesson of Harvey Cushing to current knowledge: psychosocial aspects of endocrine disease. Psychother Psychosom 1997;66:113–116.

15 Hypercalcemia and Hypocalcemia

Arna Gudmundsdottir, MD, and Gregory Doelle, MD

Contents

CALCIUM HOMEOSTASIS

Ninety-nine percent of total body calcium is within bone; 1% of this is rapidly exchangeable with extracellular calcium. Extracellular calcium is a substrate for bone mineralization. In the circulation, calcium is bound to proteins, principally albumin; however, 50% circulates as ionized calcium. Ionized calcium is biologically active, and its concentration is tightly regulated. Interactions of parathyroid hormone (PTH) and 1,25-dihydroxyvitamin D [1,25(OH)$_2$D] precisely regulate ionized calcium concentration and mineral metabolism.

PTH is secreted primarily as an 84-amino acid peptide. Synthetic PTH 1–34 is fully active. PTH controls the concentration of ionized calcium in extracellular fluid by binding to the type 1 PTH receptor in target tissues *(1)*. The parathyroid cell in turn responds to both the absolute level of ionized calcium and the rate of change of ionized calcium *(2)* by binding calcium at its cell surface. The calcium sensor on the parathyroid cell surface *(3)* is a member of the G-protein-coupled family of receptors. Inactivating mutations of the calcium sensing receptor have been described *(4)*, and calcimimetic compounds that bind to this receptor and inhibit PTH secretion may ultimately be useful in the treatment of disorders of parathyroid gland activity *(5)*.

From: *Contemporary Endocrinology: Early Diagnosis and Treatment of Endocrine Disorders*
Edited by: R. S. Bar © Humana Press Inc., Totowa, NJ

At the level of the kidney, PTH stimulates calcium reabsorption in the thick ascending limb and distal tubular segments. PTH has little effect on calcium reabsorption in the proximal tubule. Phosphate reabsorption, however, is strongly inhibited by PTH. Quantitatively, inhibition of phosphate reabsorption at the proximal tubule is most important. PTH also stimulates synthesis of $1,25(OH)_2D$ in the proximal tubule by activating 25-hydroxyvitamin D [25(OH)D] 1-α-hydroxylase and by inhibiting 24-hydroxylase *(6)*. In bone, PTH increases the number and the activity of osteoclasts and thus stimulates bone resorption. The net effect of PTH on bone varies, however, with dose and method of PTH administration *(7,8)*. Bone resorption predominates in primary hyperparathyroidism and with continuous administration of PTH. Intermittent administration of PTH favors bone formation and may find application in the treatment of osteoporosis *(9)*.

Vitamin D is available to humans via adequate sunlight exposure and also through fortified nutritional sources. Vitamin D_2 (plant origin; ergocalciferol) and vitamin D_3 (animal origin; cholecalciferol) have equivalent biologic potencies. In the liver, vitamin D undergoes 25-hydroxylation to 25(OH)D. The half-life of 25(OH)D is 2–3 wk. The final step in the production of active hormone is 1-α-hydroxylation in the kidney to form $1,25(OH)_2D$. 1-α-Hydroxylation, unlike 25-hydroxylation, is tightly controlled. PTH and hypophosphatemia are the major inducers of renal 1-α-hydroxylase, whereas calcium decreases its activity.

The biologic activity of $1,25(OH)_2D$ occurs through binding to a nuclear receptor. The vitamin D receptor forms a heterodimer with the retinoid X receptor and binds to specific DNA sequences to control transcription *(10)*. Although less potent on a molar basis, 25(OH)D can also bind to the receptor and can thus mediate the hypercalcemic effects of vitamin D intoxication. Although the vitamin D receptor is expressed in most tissues, the major physiologic effect of vitamin D binding to its receptor involves regulation of intestinal calcium transport. $1,25(OH)_2D$ also regulates transcription of the bone matrix proteins, stimulates differentiation of osteoclasts, and increases osteoclastic bone resorption.

Serum concentrations of calcium and phosphate are maintained within precise limits. Both PTH and $1,25(OH)_2D$ regulate mineral ion levels. These, in turn, regulate PTH and $1,25(OH)_2D$ secretion. Furthermore, PTH and $1,25(OH)_2D$ regulate the production of each other. As a result of these homeostatic mechanisms, states of calcium deficiency or excess are associated with maintenance of nearly normal serum calcium concentrations as changes in levels of both PTH and $1,25(OH)_2D$, lead to homeostatic changes in intestinal calcium absorption, renal calcium reabsorption, and bone resorption.

Table 1
Serum Calcium Levels

Condition	Calcium (mg/dL)
Normal serum calcium	8.5–10.5
Mild hypercalcemia	<12
Moderate hypercalcemia	12–14
Severe hypercalcemia	>14

HYPERCALCEMIA

Clinical Features

The symptoms of hypercalcemia correlate well with the degree of elevation of the serum calcium and rapidity of its increase (Table 1). Patients with mild hypercalcemia are frequently asymptomatic or not aware of the subtle symptoms they may have until the hypercalcemia has been corrected (11,16). Chronic hypercalcemia, even if severe, may also result in minimal symptoms.

The signs and symptoms are similar regardless of the etiology of the hypercalcemia. The most common symptoms of hypercalcemia are neurologic, renal, and gastrointestinal. The neurologic symptoms include weakness, lethargy, depression, and even coma in severe cases. Renal effects include polyuria from hypercalciuria-induced nephrogenic diabetes insipidus, decreased glomerular filtration rate (GFR), hyperchloremic acidosis, nephrocalcinosis, and stones. The gastrointestinal symptoms may include nausea, vomiting, constipation, and anorexia.

Differential Diagnosis

The two most common causes of hypercalcemia, malignancy and primary hyperparathyroidism, account for more than 90% of the cases (12). In hypercalcemia of malignancy the underlying malignancy is generally already evident and the patient is ill with classical symptoms of hypercalcemia. Unless the cause of the hypercalcemia is obvious, the next step is measurement of serum PTH. It is useful to classify hypercalcemia as PTH-dependent or non-PTH-dependent. A high or even inappropriately normal value in the presence of hypercalcemia confirms the diagnosis of primary hyperparathyroidism. Exceptions to this rule are patients with hypercalcemic disorders related to lithium or thiazide diuretic use, patients who have hyperparathyroidism along with other hypercalcemic disorders, or the few patients who have benign familial hypercalcemia. These conditions are distinguished by careful history taking and measurements of uri-

Table 2
Causes of Hypercalcemia

Primary hyperparathyroidism
  Sporadic
  Familial
Familial hyperparathyroid syndromes
  Associated with MEN-1 or MEN-2A
  Familial (benign) hypocalciuric hypercalcemia
Hypercalcemia of malignancy
  Humoral hypercalcemia of malignancy
    PTHrP secretion (solid tumors)
    $1,25(OH)_2D_3$ production (lymphomas)
Ectopic secretion of PTH
  Osteolytic bone lesions (multiple myeloma, leukemia, lymphoma)
Secondary and tertiary hyperparathyroidism
Sarcoidosis and other granulomatous diseases
Endocrinopathies
  Thyrotoxicosis
  Adrenal insufficiency
  Pheochromocytoma
  VIPoma
Drug induced
  Vitamin A intoxication
  Vitamin D intoxication
  Thiazide diuretics
  Lithium
  Milk-alkali syndrome
  Estrogens, androgens, tamoxifen
Miscellaneous causes
  Immobilization
  Acute renal failure
  Idiopathic hypercalcemia of infancy
  ICU hypercalcemia
  Serum protein disorders

ICU, intensive care unit; MEN, multipe endocrine neoplasia; PTH, parathyroid hormone; PTHrP, PTH related peptide; VIPoma, vasoactive intestinal protein-secreting tumor.

nary calcium. Hypercalcemia of malignancy is usually a result of secretion of PTH-related peptide (PTHrP) by the tumor, and patients virtually always have suppressed or undetectable levels of intact PTH. Negative PTHrP does not rule out hypercalcemia of malignancy, since certain tumors cause hypercalcemia by other means. Table 2 lists the causes of hypercalcemia.

Primary Hyperparathyroidism

INCIDENCE AND ETIOLOGY

Primary hyperparathyroidism is caused by excess secretion of PTH from one or more of the parathyroid glands. It is caused by a benign, solitary adenoma 80% of the time and less commonly by hyperplasia of all four parathyroid glands. Four-gland disease is seen in association with multiple endocrine neoplasia type 1 or 2 but may also occur sporadically. Parathyroid carcinoma is extremely rare, occurring in less than 0.5% of cases of hypercalcemia *(13)*. In adenomas, the parathyroid cell loses its sensitivity to calcium for unclear reasons. In hyperplasia, the sensitivity appears intact, but the number of cells is much increased. The peak incidence of primary hyperparathyroidism is the fifth to sixth decade of life, with a female to male ratio of 3:1 *(14)*. It remains distinctly unusual in children. The incidence of primary hyperparathyroidism increased dramatically in the 1970s with the introduction of the automated screening tests, but a continued decline has recently been reported *(15)*. Currently the prevalence rates are about 1–4 per 1000 *(14)*.

SIGNS AND SYMPTOMS

Most people are presumably asymptomatic at the time of diagnosis. However, many have physical or neuropsychological disabilities that improve after surgical cure of their hyperparathyroidism *(11,16)*. The classical symptoms related to skeletal and renal complications are rarely seen today. *Osteitis fibrosa cystica*, with bone cysts and brown tumors of the long bones, is seen in well under 5% of patients *(17)*. Primary hyperparathyroidism is associated with bone loss largely at cortical sites *(14)*. A large study that followed 121 patients prospectively for more than 10 yr showed that bone mineral density (BMD) was stable in most of the patients and in fact improved in patients who underwent parathyroid surgery. However, in a subgroup of patients who did not undergo surgery, BMD decreased by more than 10% in 20% of the patients *(18)*. The data on fracture incidence among patients with primary hyperparathyroidism is conflicting; some studies have not shown an increase in fracture incidence, whereas others have *(14,19)*. The incidence of kidney stones has declined from 33% to less than 20% in the last 4 decades *(20)*. Hypercalciuria, defined as daily calcium excretion of more than 250 mg in women and more than 300 mg daily in men, is seen in up to 30% of patients *(17)*. Peptic ulcer disease and pancreatitis are virtually never seen any more.

DIAGNOSIS

The diagnosis is established by laboratory tests, circulating PTH being the most definitive test to make the diagnosis. The PTH will be inappropriately elevated in most cases. Most patients also have high serum calcium and even more have high serum ionized calcium concentrations *(21)*. The serum phosphorus tends to be in the lower range of normal, and alkaline phosphatase activity may be elevated.

TREATMENT

Surgical excision of the abnormal parathyroid tissue is the only definitive way to cure primary hyperparathyroidism. The rate of progression of hyperparathyroidism is slow, however, and we lack predictive indices that indicate who among the asymptomatic are at risk for complications of this disease *(18)*. Thus, there has been some controversy regarding the indications for surgery. To address this issue, in 1990 the National Institutes of Health held a consensus conference on asymptomatic primary hyperparathyroidism *(22)*. It was agreed that people with mild disease who were asymptomatic could be followed safely with medical monitoring. Table 3 lists the indications for surgery in asymptomatic patients with primary hyperparathyroidism. Some physicians recommend surgery for almost all patients with hyperparathyroidism for the following reasons: surgical risks are low, monitoring costs are substantial, and quality of life improves after surgical cure even in mild cases *(23)*. Surgical treatment also improves both subjective symptoms and complications, such as nephrolithiasis and osteopenia *(18)*. Surgical methodology has improved remarkably in recent years *(24)*. The location of an adenoma or the presence of parathyroid hyperplasia can be confirmed by technetium-99m sestamibi imaging. Then serum PTH can be measured 10 min after removal of an abnormal parathyroid gland to indicate whether the patient has been cured or whether additional exploration is needed. Parathyroid surgery can therefore often be done in about an hour as an outpatient procedure.

No calcimimetic drugs are currently commercially available and, therefore many patients must choose between an operation or no treatment. Drugs that inhibit bone resorption, such as bisphosphonates, can decrease hypercalcemia, but unfortunately PTH secretion may increase. Estrogens are an exception; they increase bone density and may decrease serum calcium concentration slightly in postmenopausal women *(25)*. In patients who do not undergo surgery, surveillance is necessary. Adequate hydration and ambulation are always encouraged. All diuretics should be avoided, and dietary intake of calcium should be moderate. Routine medical follow-up usually includes visits twice yearly with serum calcium measurements, yearly measurements of 24-h urinary calcium excretion, yearly bone densitometry, and yearly creatinine *(17)*. Long-term survival in these patients is not adversely affected *(26)*.

Familial Hyperparathyroid Syndromes

MEN-1

In the rare instance in which hyperparathyroidism is not from sporadic tumor, it may be hereditary, the most common variety being multiple endocrine neoplasia type 1 (MEN-1). MEN-1 is inherited in an autosomal dominant fashion owing to an inactivating mutation of a tumor suppressor gene recently mapped to chro-

Table 3
Indications for Surgery in Asymptomatic Primary Hyperparathyroidism

Raised serum calcium (>2.85 mmol/L or >11.4 mg/dL)
History of episode of life-threatening hypercalcemia
Reduced creatinine clearance (<70% of that for age-matched healthy people)
Kidney stone(s)
Raised 24-h urinary calcium excretion (400 mg)
Substantial reduction of bone mass (>2 SD below mean for age, sex, and ethnic group)
Patient requests surgery
Patient unable to be followed up for monitoring
Age <50 yr

mosome 11q13 *(27)*. The gene product is called Menin. MEN-1 occurs in both sexes equally; in general, affected patients are younger then those with sporadic hyperparathyroidism. By the age of 40, hyperparathyroidism is seen in 85% of cases, Zollinger-Ellison syndrome in 35%, and prolactinoma in 25%. Other tumors are seen less often *(28)*. Hyperparathyroidism in MEN-1 is usually a multiglandular disorder involving all four glands. Because of four-gland involvement, a common approach is to resect three and a half glands or to remove all four glands and autotransplant tissue into the forearm muscles.

MEN-2A

MEN-2 is caused by an activating mutation in the *RET* proto-oncogene on chromosome 10q11.2. It is an autosomal dominant disorder that can be diagnosed by commercially available molecular genetic tests using polymerase chain reaction (PCR) *(29)*. Hyperparathyroidism is caused by diffuse parathyroid hyperplasia and is less common in MEN-2 than in MEN-1. The major clinical findings in this syndrome are medullary thyroid carcinoma (MTC), seen in almost all cases, and bilateral pheochromocytoma, seen in approximately half of affected individuals. It is important that patients do not undergo parathyroidectomy with undiagnosed pheochromocytoma, which can prove to be lethal.

HYPERPARATHYROIDISM-JAW TUMOR SYNDROME

Hyperparathyroidism-jaw tumor syndrome (HPT-JT) is an autosomal dominant disorder characterized by early-onset, recurrent parathyroid tumors and fibroosseous jaw tumors. Parathyroid carcinoma and renal tumors occur less frequently. Bony lesions in the maxilla and mandible look like punched-out or cystic lesions on radiographs. These differ from the classic brown tumors seen with primary hyperparathyroidism by their lack of osteoclasts *(30)*.

Familial Hypocalciuric Hypercalcemia

Familial hypocalciuric (or benign) hypercalcemia (FHH) is an autosomal dominant disorder characterized by lifelong asymptomatic hypercalcemia with below-normal urinary calcium excretion. It is caused by an inactivating mutation of the calcium-sensing receptor gene *(31)*. This results in insensitivity of the parathyroid cells to inhibition by serum calcium. Hypercalcemia is usually mild, and the PTH level is normal or slightly elevated. The urinary calcium level is usually less than 50 mg/24 h, and the calcium/creatinine clearance ratio is less than 0.01. Clinically it is important to distinguish FHH from primary hyperparathyroidism to avoid unnecessary surgery *(32)*. This may be difficult based on biochemical tests alone, since these can overlap. In that setting family studies become necessary to make the diagnosis *(33)*. Children of one or two parents with this disorder may develop neonatal severe hypercalcemia, a life-threatening condition that requires total parathyroidectomy.

Hypercalcemia of Malignancy

Hypercalcemia is the most common paraneoplastic endocrine syndrome. It is caused by an increase in osteoclast-mediated resorption, most often induced by circulating factors secreted by the tumor. The vast majority of cases are caused by the overexpression of PTHrP. PTHrP was first described in the late 1980s. Compared with the 84-amino acid peptide PTH, it is considerably longer, with three isoforms and 139–173 amino acids. However, the amino acid sequence at the amino terminus bears a strong homology to PTH and binds with equal affinity to the PTH/PTHrP-1 receptor in bone and kidney. Normal physiologic functions of PTHrP are still being investigated. The hormone is found in a wide variety of cell types and exhibits diverse functions, most of which are unrelated to calcium homeostasis.

The most common malignancies associated with PTHrP-induced hypercalcemia are squamous cell carcinomas of the lung, esophagus, head, neck, cervix, vulva, and skin. It is also seen in renal, bladder, and ovarian carcinomas. Breast cancer can cause hypercalcemia by humoral mechanisms or through skeletal metastatic involvement. In addition, patients are usually volume-depleted as a result of their hypercalcemia and have poor oral intake owing to their underlying disease. They are unable to concentrate their urine, which leads to a decrease in the filtered load of calcium as well as a reduction in fractional excretion of calcium. Other calcitropic hormones can also cause this syndrome. Ectopic PTH production has been described but is extremely rare. Increased levels of 1,25-$(OH)_2D$, thought to be caused by increased 1-α-hydroxylase activity in lymphoproliferative cells, can occur in hematologic malignancies. Prostaglandins can also contribute to the hypercalcemia of malignancy.

Only 30% of patients with multiple myeloma develop hypercalcemia even though most of them have extensive bone destruction, possibly because of locally produced osteolytic factors rather than humoral mediators. It has been suggested that myeloma cells in the marrow express cytokine-like factors such as tumor necrosis factor (TNF)-α, TNF-β, interleukin (IL)-1α, IL-1β, IL-6, and PTHrP, which act locally to stimulate the osteoclasts *(34)*. Most patients with adult T-cell leukemia/lymphoma (ATL) resulting from human T-cell lymphotropic virus type-1 (HTLV-1) infection develop humoral hypercalcemia of malignancy *(35)*. Animal studies have suggested that this is owing to tumor-derived PTHrP.

Treatment goals are to reduce the osteoclastic bone resorption, reduce tumor burden, and facilitate renal clearance of calcium. Bisphosphonates have become the standard therapy to reduce bone resorption and decrease hypercalcemia in malignancy. Bisphosphonates may also prevent the progression of bone metastases, particularly in multiple myeloma *(36)*. Glucocorticoids are useful in reducing hypercalcemia of malignancy as well, particularly when it is caused by multiple myeloma or excess $1,25(OH)_2D$, as in sarcoidosis. Severe hypercalcemia, as often seen in malignancy, needs to be aggressively treated with intravenous normal saline and a loop diuretic while the patient's cardiovascular status is closely monitored.

Tertiary Hyperparathyroidism and Refractory Secondary Hyperparathyroidism

In patients with chronic renal failure, secondary hyperparathyroidism tends to last longer and to be more severe than in patients with other hypocalcemic disorders, such as dietary vitamin D deficiency. Eventually, refractory secondary hyperparathyroidism can develop into a tertiary hyperparathyroidism characterized by oversecretion of PTH and hypercalcemia. Factors that lead to stimulation of the parathyroid glands in uremia are hypocalcemia, hyperphosphatemia, $1,25(OH)_2D_3$ deficiency, and vitamin D receptor (VDR) downregulation *(37)*. Mild secondary hyperparathyroidism is reversible when these are corrected. These patients generally have PTH levels above 150–200 pg/mL, whereas patients with tertiary hyperparathyroidism have PTH levels above 1500 pg/mL. That is rarely seen today, but the risk is related to duration of end-stage renal disease (ESRD) requiring hemodialysis. PTH-induced hypercalcemia is commonly seen postoperatively after successful renal transplantation, particularly in patients with long-standing secondary hyperparathyroidism. This can be dangerous to the renal graft but usually subsides within months to a few years *(21)*.

Patients with chronic renal disease can develop hyperparathyroid uremic bone disease, characterized by excess bone resorption. The treatment for this is calcium or $1,25(OH)_2D$ to decrease the PTH secretion. Other patients have an adynamic bone disease with low bone activity or osteomalacia that has minimal parathyroid hypersecretion (38).

Resistant secondary hyperparathyroidism in ESRD is difficult to treat. Active vitamin D (calcitriol) is indicated for prevention and treatment of secondary hyperparathyroidism but must be monitored to avoid hypercalcemia and hyperphosphatemia (39). Calcimimetic compounds are promising, and a recent report of one such agent was found to be beneficial in primary hyperparathyroidism (5). Surgical therapy is indicated in symptomatic patients with non-suppressible PTH levels (40).

Miscellaneous Causes of Hypercalcemia

SARCOIDOSIS AND OTHER GRANULOMATOUS DISEASES

Hypercalcemia occurs in about 10% of patients with sarcoidosis, and hypercalciuria is about three times more frequent (41). Kidney stones develop in about 10% of patients and are usually pure calcium oxalate stones (42). Pulmonary macrophages from affected individuals contain 25(OH)D 1-α-hydroxylase activity that is not readily inhibited by calcium or 1,25(OH)2D. Glucocorticoids suppress the 1-α-hydroxylase activity and provide effective treatment for both the disease and this complication of it.

Other granulomatous diseases associated with abnormal vitamin D metabolism include tuberculosis, coccidioidomycosis, histoplasmosis, leprosy, pulmonary eosinophilic granulomatosis, and lymphomas.

ENDOCRINOPATHIES

Because of the hypermetabolic state in hyperthyroidism, the bone is in a high-turnover state. This may result in mild hypercalcemia, elevated alkaline phosphatase, or, more commonly, hypercalciuria. The phosphorus is in the upper range of normal, and PTH is usually suppressed.

Hypercalcemia can be seen in acute adrenal crisis and responds well to glucocorticoids. Pheochromocytoma is occasionally complicated by hypercalcemia owing to PTHrP secretion.

DRUG-INDUCED HYPERCALCEMIA

Thiazide diuretics can cause a mild increase in serum calcium. If the hypercalcemia persists, primary hyperparathyroidism needs to be ruled out.

Individuals who ingest large doses of vitamin D may develop hypercalcemia. This is easily diagnosed by elevated levels of 25(OH)D. The $1,25(OH)_2D$ levels are often normal because of reduced PTH levels from the hypercalcemia. Hypercalciuria is invariably seen. Treatment (including rehydration, reduced calcium intake, and glucocorticoids in addition to withdrawing the vitamin D) may be prolonged, especially if the condition is caused by the lipophilic nonhydroxiphilic vitamin D.

Excessive ingestion of vitamin A is usually owing to self-medication and can lead to osteoporosis and fractures. How vitamin A stimulates bone resorption is not clear.

The milk-alkali syndrome is characterized by alkalosis, renal impairment, and nephrocalcinosis. It is usually caused by large quantities of calcium along with an absorbable alkali, such as the absorbable antacids used for peptic ulcer disease.

IMMOBILIZATION

Bed rest for any reason will lead to accelerated bone resorption and hypercalcemia in individuals with a high rate of bone turnover. This includes children, young adults, patients with Paget's disease of bone, and patients with hyperthyroidism. The hypercalcemia reverses with the resumption of normal weightbearing.

Treatment of Hypercalcemia

When deciding on time of therapy initiation for hypercalcemia one needs to consider the underlying cause and the patient's symptoms *(43)*. When the serum calcium is greater than 14 mg/dL, therapy should be initiated regardless of symptoms. Moderate hypercalcemia (12–14 mg/dL) is treated aggressively if the patient is having clinical signs or symptoms consistent with hypercalcemia. Initially general measures should be instituted, consisting of rehydration with normal saline. Hypercalcemia impairs the urinary concentrating ability, leading to polyuria and dehydration. For correction, this may require 3–4 L of saline over a 24–48-h period. After the extracellular fluid volume has been replaced, small doses of furosemide (10–20 mg) may be given to avoid hypernatremia and volume overload. Potassium and magnesium must be monitored and replaced as necessary. Dialysis is reserved for more severe cases.

Specific approaches are based on the underlying disorder. The drug of first choice is usually pamidronate. It is the most potent bisphosphonate available and acts by inhibiting osteoclastic bone resorption. The initial dose is 60–90 mg by intravenous infusion over 4–24 h. The hypocalcemic effects of pamidronate may persist for 1–6 wk, and then it can be redosed. Administration in large volume (500 mL or more) is recommended because precipitated calcium bisphosphonate carries the risk of nephrotoxicity. It should be used cautiously if baseline creatinine exceeds 2.5 mg/dL. In the case of impaired renal function or severe hypercalcemia, salmon calcitonin may be administered subcutaneously, 4–8 IU/kg every 6–8 h, but it only lowers serum calcium by 1–3 mg/dL and usually loses its effect after 3 d. This has the most rapid onset of action of the calcium-lowering drugs but is not suitable for chronic use since the patients will become insensitive to it. Plicamycin is another agent that lowers calcium effectively in most patients, even after a single dose. Plicamycin has significant complications (renal, hepatic, bone marrow), particularly after repeated dosing. Glucocorticoids are an

Table 4
Causes of Hypocalcemia

Hypoparathyroidism
  Postsurgical
  Congenital
    DiGeorge syndrome
    Autoimmune polyglandular syndrome type 1
  Infiltrative
    Hemochromatosis
    Wilson's disease
  Impaired PTH secretion
    Hypomagnesemia
    Activating mutations of calcium sensor
  PTH resistance
    Hypomagnesemia
    Pseudohypoparathyroidism type Ia and Ib
Vitamin D deficiency
Anticonvulsant therapy
Vitamin D-dependent rickets type I
Vitamin D-dependent rickets type II
Miscellaneous causes
  Hungry bone syndrome
  Osteoblastic metastases
  Administration of citrated blood products
  Pancreatitis
  Critical illness

PTH, parathyroid hormone.

effective treatment for hypercalcemia, particularly if caused by multiple myeloma, lymphoma, sarcoidosis, or intoxication with vitamin D or vitamin A. Other available antiresorptive agents are the bisphosphonate etidronate and gallium nitrate. They are less effective than pamidronate and are therefore in little use at present.

HYPOCALCEMIA

Clinical Features

Neuromuscular irritability accounts for the predominant symptoms of hypocalcemia. Circumoral paresthesias, paresthesias in the digits, latent tetany (Chvostek's sign and Trousseau's sign), or spontaneous tetany can be seen. Generalized seizures and laryngeal spasm may occur and can be life-threatening. Electrocardiographic changes (QT prolongation) are common, whereas cardiac arrhythmias are less common. Chronic hypocalcemia generally develops gradually and often without symptoms. When associated with hyperphosphatemia, chronic hypocalcemia can lead to basal ganglia calcification and, less frequently, extrapyramidal signs and symptoms (44). Cataracts may form. Osteomalacia may result from chronic hypocalcemia in association with hypophosphatemia. Chronic hypocalcemia is most often attributable to deficiencies of either PTH or $1,25(OH)_2D$, or resistance to these hormones. Table 4 lists the causes of hypocalcemia.

Hypoparathyroidism

Hypocalcemia caused by PTH deficiency is characterized by low serum calcium concentration and hyperphosphatemia, reflecting loss of PTH effects at the level of bone and kidney. With modern PTH assays, PTH concentrations are usually low or undetectable, but may be inappropriately normal. $1,25(OH)_2D$ concentration is low because of lack of PTH and lack of hypophosphatemia, both of which stimulate renal 1-α-hydroxylase activity.

The most common cause of PTH deficiency is surgical hypoparathyroidism, the result of removal of parathyroid tissue or disruption of blood supply to the parathyroid glands. Infiltrative diseases [iron overload (45), copper deposition (46)] are uncommon causes of hypoparathyroidism. DiGeorge syndrome is a sporadic disorder associated with incomplete development of branchial pouches and varying degrees of parathyroid hypoplasia. DiGeorge syndrome results from mutations of an unknown gene at chromosome 22q11 (47). The autosomal recessive type 1 polyglandular syndrome includes hypoparathyroidism in association with mucocutaneous candidiasis and adrenocortical insufficiency. The syndrome is caused by a mutation in AIRE, autoimmune regulator gene of unknown function (48). Profound hypomagnesemia can lead to impaired secretion of PTH as well as target organ resistance to PTH. Finally, activating mutations of the calcium-sensing receptor can cause autosomal dominant hypocalcemia with normal PTH concentrations and hypercalciuria (49).

Pseudohypoparathyroidism

Pseudohypoparathyroidism (PHP) was first described by Albright in 1942. Variants of PHP have since been identified. Molecular defects in the gene encoding the α-subunit of the stimulatory G-protein (Gs_α) contribute to three different forms of this disease, PHP-Ia, pseudo-PHP, and PHP-Ib.

PTH signaling is mediated by the type 1 PTH receptor, which acts on a stimulatory guanine-nucleotide-binding protein (Gs). Gs is composed of three subunits (α, β, and γ). The Gs_α subunit is encoded by the GNAS1 gene and mediates cyclic AMP stimulation by PTH.

PHP-Ia is characterized by resistance to PTH and skeletal and developmental abnormalities termed Albright's hereditary osteodystrophy. These abnormalities include short stature, round face, obesity, brachydactyly, and mental retardation. PTH resistance is caused by inactivating mutations of Gs_α (50) inherited

Table 5
Pseudohypoparathyroidism (PHP)

Type	PTH resistance	AHO	Pathophysiology
PHP Ia	+	+	*GNAS1* mutation
PseudoPHP	–	+	*GNAS1* mutation/imprinting
PHP Ib	+	–	*GNAS1* mutation?

AHO, Albright's hereditary osteodystrophy; PTH, parathyroid hormone.

as an autosomal dominant trait. Resistance to thyroid-stimulating hormone (TSH) is also common in this disorder. Pseudo-PHP typically occurs in families with PHP-Ia and is characterized by phenotypic abnormalities similar to those of patients with PHP-Ia, but these individuals demonstrate normal regulation of calcium and phosphate homeostasis. This disorder also involves inactivating mutations of *GNAS1*, but hormone resistance is thought to be suppressed by "paternal imprinting" (i.e., the *GNAS1* gene is inherited from the father and the mutant copy is suppressed in selected tissues) *(51)*. PHP-Ib is characterized by resistance to PTH, no resistance to thyrotropin, and absence of features of AHO. This disorder is thought to occur by mutation in or near *GNAS1 (52)*. Gs$_\alpha$ activity is normal in individuals with PHP-Ib (Table 5).

Vitamin D-Related Disorders

The primary cause of hypocalcemia in vitamin D deficiency or resistance is impaired intestinal absorption of calcium. In addition to hypocalcemia, vitamin D deficiency is characterized by hypophosphatemia and secondary hyperparathyroidism, and thus differentiation from hypoparathyroidism is usually straightforward from a laboratory standpoint.

Vitamin D deficiency results from lack of solar exposure and decreased intake or impaired absorption of vitamin D. Early vitamin D deficiency is detected when levels of 25(OH)D are low, generally below 15 ng/mL. In addition to nutritional deficiency, phenytoin and other anticonvulsant medications *(53)* can accelerate hepatic inactivation of vitamin D.

Renal parenchymal damage can result in deficiency of 1,25(OH)$_2$D. This leads to impaired intestinal absorption of calcium. Hyperphosphatemia further lowers 1,25(OH)$_2$D and serum calcium. Calcium-containing antacids serve as phosphate binders and also attenuate the hypocalcemic stimulus to PTH secretion. In the setting of renal parenchymal disease, use of calcitriol [1,25(OH)$_2$D] is frequently necessary to maintain absorption of calcium and to prevent the development of secondary hyperparathyroidism.

Vitamin D-dependent rickets is an autosomal recessive disorder of vitamin D activation characterized by normal or elevated levels of 25(OH)D and low levels of 1,25(OH)$_2$D in the setting of hypocalcemia, rickets, and secondary hyperparathyroidism. This disorder typically responds to physiologic replacement doses of calcitriol *(54,55)*. Vitamin D-dependent rickets type II (vitamin D-resistant rickets) is a rare autosomal recessive disorder characterized by hypocalcemia, hypophosphatemia, elevated PTH concentration, and elevated levels of $1,25(OH)_2D$. This disorder results from mutation of the vitamin D receptor gene *(56)*. Presentation is similar to that of vitamin D-dependent rickets; alopecia has been described in some kindreds *(57)*. Treatment of vitamin D-dependent rickets type II is challenging, with variable response to pharmacologic doses of vitamin D or calcitriol *(58)*.

Treatment of Hypocalcemia

The treatments available for patients with hypocalcemia and hypoparathyroidism include calcium salts, vitamin D and vitamin D analogs, and thiazide diuretics. Acute hypocalcemia requires prompt attention and is best treated with intravenous calcium and calcitriol. Calcium products available for acute therapy include calcium gluconate and calcium chloride. Calcium gluconate is preferred, as calcium chloride can cause severe tissue necrosis with extravasation. Initial treatment of acute hypocalcemia should consist of 100–300 mg of elemental calcium infused over 15–20 min. An alternative is to provide a continuous infusion of 3 mg/kg/h of elemental calcium, with close monitoring of serum calcium levels. If hypomagnesemia is present, magnesium replacement is required.

Treatment of chronic hypocalcemia is determined by the underlying disorder. Oral calcium (providing 1–3 g of elemental calcium daily) is essential in all circumstances. Vitamin D therapy is dictated by the disorder causing hypocalcemia. Calcitriol is preferred in disorders with impaired 1-α-hydroxylation (renal failure, hypoparathyroidism, vitamin D-dependent rickets), and is given in doses of 0.25–1.0 μg daily. Nutritional vitamin D deficiency can be treated with vitamin D 50,000 U daily for 1–2 wk followed by weekly treatment until stores are replaced. Vitamin D at 800 IU should be provided chronically. The normal daily requirement of vitamin D is 400 IU.

Calcitriol will increase serum calcium levels within 1–2 d and is preferred for initial inpatient treatment to minimize duration of hospitalization. Calcitriol has an equally short half-life and is preferred in situations when vitamin D intoxication is a concern.

Patients with hypocalcemia need to be monitored closely to assess response to treatment. Correction of hypocalcemia should lead to correction of secondary hyperparathyroidism, if present, and serum PTH should be measured several weeks after initiation of therapy. In the setting of secondary hyperparathyroidism, serum alkaline phosphatase and PTH may remain elevated for 6–12 mo. During treatment with calcium and vitamin D or vitamin D analog, 24-h urine calcium excretion should be measured to assess risk of nephrolithiasis. With

Table 6
Calcium-Containing Compounds

Compound	Elemental calcium content
Oral	
Calcium carbonate	500 mg/1250 mg
Calcium acetate[a]	169 mg/667 mg
Calcium citrate	200 mg/950 mg
Calcium lactate	90 mg/650 mg
Calcium glubionate	115 mg/5 mL syrup
Parenteral	
Calcium gluconate	93 mg/10 mL (10% solution)
Calcium chloride	27 mg/10 mL (10% solution)

[a]Approved for treatment of hyperphosphatemia only.

treatment of hypoparathyroidism, avoidance of hypercalciuria is difficult owing to loss of PTH-mediated calcium reabsorption. Addition of a thiazide diuretic may minimize renal calcium loss.

Table 6 lists the available therapeutic calcium-containing preparations.

SCREENING

Although most individuals with disorders of blood calcium concentration are asymptomatic, sometimes serum calcium measurement is indicated. Individuals should be screened for hypercalcemia in the setting of nephrocalcinosis and nephrolithiasis, with evidence of osteopenia at sites of predominantly cortical bone, as well as for signs and symptoms suggesting hypercalcemia. Although these are uncommon or nonspecific, they include band keratopathy, anorexia, constipation and abdominal pain, possibly peptic ulcer disease, and pancreatitis, as well as a variety of nonspecific neuropsychiatric symptoms. It seems reasonable to monitor serum calcium periodically in patients taking calcium or vitamin D supplements and in persons taking medications that can potentially alter blood calcium concentrations.

Screening for hypocalcemia should be performed routinely following thyroidectomy and neck dissection, in the setting of osteopenia in excess of that expected for age, and in the setting of malabsorption or hypomagnesemia. Individuals with the phenotypic appearance of Albright's hereditary osteodystrophy should have serum calcium (and probably PTH) measured. Persons with chronic mucocutaneous candidiasis should be screened for hypocalcemia since polyglandular autoimmune syndrome type 1 may present with cutaneous manifestations prior to development of hypoparathyroidism.

REFERENCES

1. Juppner H. Receptors for parathyroid hormone and parathyroid hormone-related peptide: exploration of their biological importance. Bone 1999;25:87–90.
2. Grant FD, Conlin PR, Brown EM. Rate and concentration dependence of parathyroid hormone dynamics during stepwise changes in serum ionized calcium in normal humans. J Clin Endocrinol Metab 1990;71:370–378.
3. Brown EM, Gamba G, Riccardi D et al. Cloning and characterization of an extracellular Ca(2+)-sensing receptor from bovine parathyroid. Nature 1993;366:575–580.
4. Pollak MR, Brown EM, Chou YH, et al. Mutations in the human Ca(2+)-sensing receptor gene cause familial hypocalciuric hypercalcemia and neonatal severe hyperparathyroidism. Cell 1993;75:1297–1303.
5. Silverberg SJ, Bone HG, Marriott TB, et al. Short-term inhibition of parathyroid hormone secretion by a calcium-receptor agonist in patients with primary hyperparathyroidism. N Engl J Med 1997;337:1506–1510.
6. Fraser Dr, Kodicek E. Unique biosynthesis by kidney of a biological active vitamin D metabolite. Nature 1970;228:764–766.
7. Ishizuya T, Yokose S, Hori M, et al. Parathyroid hormone exerts disparate effects on osteoblast differentiation depending on exposure time in rat osteoblastic cells. J Clin Invest 1997;99:2961–2970.
8. Schiller PC, D'Ippolito G, Roos BA, Howard GA. Anabolic or catabolic responses of MC3T3-E1 osteoblastic cells to parathyroid hormone depend on time and duration of treatment. J Bone Miner Res 1999;14:1504–1512.
9. Neer RM, Arnaud CD, Zanchetta JR, et al. Effects of parathyroid hormone (1-34) on fractures and bone mineral density in postmenopausal women with osteoporosis. N Engl J Med 2001;344:1434–1441.
10. Kliewer SA, Umesono K, Mangelsdorf DJ, Evans RM. Retinoid X receptor interacts with nuclear receptors in retinoic acid, thyroid hormone and vitamin D3 signalling. Nature 1992;355:446–449.
11. Burney RE, Jones KR, Christy B, Thompson NW. Health status improvement after surgical correction of primary hyperparathyroidism in patients with high and low preoperative calcium levels. Surgery 1999;125:608–614.
12. Shane E. Hypercalcemia: pathogenesis, clinical manifestations, differential diagnosis, and management. In: Favus MJ, ed. Primer on the Metabolic Bone Diseases and Disorders of Mineral Metabolism. Lippincott Williams & Wilkins, Philadelphia, 1999, pp.183–187.
13. Shane E. Parathyroid carcinoma. J Clin Endocrinol Metab 2001;86:485–493
14. Khan A, Bilezikian J. Primary hyperparathyroidism: pathophysiology and impact on bone. Can Med Assoc J 2000;163:184–7
15. Wermers RA, Khosla S, Atkinson EJ, Hodgson SF, O'Fallon WM, Melton LJ 3rd. The rise and fall of primary hyperparathyroidism: a population-based study in Rochester, Minnesota, 1965–1992. Ann Intern Med 1997;126:433–440.
16. Chan AK, Duh Q-Y, Katz MH, Siperstein AE, Clark OH. Clinical manifestations of primary hyperparathyroidism before and after parathyroidectomy: a case-control study. Ann Surg 1995;222:402–414.
17. Bilezikian, JP. Primary hyperparathyroidism. In: Favus MJ, ed. Primer on the Metabolic Bone Diseases and Disorders of Mineral Metabolism. Lippincott Williams & Wilkins, Philadelphia, 1999, pp.187–192.
18. Silverberg SJ, Shane E, Jacobs TP, Siris E, Bilezikian JP. A 10-year prospective study of primary hyperparathyroidism with or without parathyroid surgery. N Engl J Med 1999;341:1249–1255.

19. Khosla S, Melton LJ 3rd, Wermers RA, Crowson CS, O'Fallon Wm, Riggs Bl. Primary hyperparathyroidism and the risk of fracture: a population-based study. J Bone Miner Res 1999;14:1700–1707.
20. Silverberg SJ, Shane E, Jacobs TP, et al. Nephrolithiasis and bone involvement in primary hyperparathyroidism. Am J Med 1990;89:327–334.
21. Marx SJ. Hyperparathyroid and hypoparathyroid disorders. N Engl J Med 2000;343:1863–1875.
22. National Institutes of Health. Consensus development conference statement. J Bone Miner Res 1991;6(suppl 2):S9–13.
23. Siminoski K. Asymptomatic hyperparathyroidism: is the pendulum swinging back? Can Med Assoc J 2000;163:173–175.
24. Irvin GL, Prudhomme DL, Deriso GT, Sfakianakis G, Chandarlapaty SK. A new approach to parathyroidectomy. Ann Surg 1994;219:574–579; discussion 579–581.
25. Grey AB, Stapleton JP, Evans MC, Tatnell MA, Reid IR. Effect of hormone replacement therapy on bone mineral density in postmenopausal women with mild primary hyperparathyroidism: a randomized, controlled trial. Ann Intern Med 1996;125:360–368.
26. Wermers RA, Khosla S, Atkinson EJ, et al. Survival after the diagnosis of hyperparathyroidism: a population-based study. Am J Med 1998;104:115–122.
27. Chandrasekharappa SC, Guru SC, Manickam P, et al. Positional cloning of the gene for multiple endocrine neoplasia-type 1. Science 1997;276:404–407.
28. Marx SJ, Spiegel AM, Skarulis MC, Doppman JL, Collins FS, Liotta LA. Multiple endocrine neoplasia type 1: clinical and genetic topics. Ann Intern Med 1998;129:484–494.
29. Ledger GA, Khosla S, Lindor NM, Thibodeau SN, Gharib H. Genetic testing in the diagnosis and management of multiple endocrine neoplasia type II. Ann Intern Med 1995;122:118–124
30. Jackson CE, Norum RA, Boyd SB, et al. Hereditary hyperparathyroidism and multiple ossifying jaw fibromas: a clinically and genetically distinct syndrome. Surgery 1990;108:1006–1013
31. Pollak MR, Brown EM, Chou YH, et al. Mutations in the human Ca(2+)-sensing receptor gene cause familial hypocalciuric hypercalcemia and neonatal severe hyperparathyroidism. Cell 1993;75:1297–1303
32. Marx SJ, Stock JL, Attie MF, et al. Familial hypocalciuric hypercalcemia: recognition among patients referred after unsuccessful parathyroid exploration. Ann Intern Med 1980;92:351–356
33. Law WM Jr, Heath H III. Familial benign hypercalcemia (hypocalciuric hypercalcemia): clinical and pathogenetic studies in 21 families. Ann Intern Med 1985;102:511–519
34. Lust JA, Donovan KA. The role of interleukin-1 beta in the pathogenesis of multiple myeloma. Hematol Oncol Clin North Am 1999;13:1117–1125
35. Richard V, Lairmore MD, Green PL, et al. Humoral hypercalcemia: severe combined immunodeficient/beige mouse model of adult T-cell lymphoma independent of human T-cell lymphotropic virus type-1 tax expression. Am J Pathol 2001;158:2219–2228
36. Berenson JR. New advances in the biology and treatment of myeloma bone disease. Semin Hematol 2001;38(2 suppl 3):15–20
37. Indridason OS, Quarles LD. Tertiary hyperparathyroidism and refractory secondary hyperparathyroidism. In: Favus MJ, ed. Primer on the Metabolic Bone Diseases and Disorders of Mineral Metabolism. Lippincott Williams & Wilkins, Philadelphia, 1999, pp. 198–202.
38. Sherrard DJ, Hercz G, Pei Y, et al. The spectrum of bone disease in end-stage renal failure— an evolving disorder. Kidney Int 1993;43:436–442
39. Schomig M, Ritz E. Management of disturbed calcium metabolism in uraemic patients: 1. use of vitamin D metabolites. Nephrol Dial Transplant 2000;15(suppl 5):18–24
40. Schomig M, Ritz E. Management of disturbed calcium metabolism in uraemic patients: 2. indications for parathyroidectomy. Nephrol Dial Transplant 2000;15(Suppl 5):25–29
41. Sharma OP. Vitamin D, calcium, and sarcoidosis. Chest 1996;109:535–539
42. Rodman JS, Mahler RJ. Kidney stones as manifestation of hypercalcemic disorders. Hyperparathyroidism and sarcoidosis. Urol Clin North Am 2000;27:275–285.

43. Bushinsky DA, Monk RD. Calcium. Lancet 1998;352:306–311.
44. Tambyah PA, Ong BK, Lee KO. Reversible parkinsonism and asymptomatic hypocalcemia with basal ganglia calcification from hypoparathyroidism 26 years after thyroid surgery. Am J Med 1994;94:444–445.
45. Gertner JM, Broadus AE, Anast CS, et al. Impaired parathyroid response to induced hypocalcemia in thalassemia major. J Pediatr 1979;95:210–213.
46. Carpenter TO, Carnes DL, Anast CS. Hypoparathyroidism in Wilson's disease. N Engl J Med 1983;309:873–877.
47. Novelli A, Sabani M, Caiola A, et al. Diagnosis of DiGeorge and Williams syndromes using FISH analysis of peripheral blood smears. Mol Cell Probes 1999;13:303–307.
48. Bjorses P, Halonen M, Palvimo JJ, et al. Mutations in the AIRE gene. Effects on subcellular location and transactivation function of the autoimmune polyendocrinopathy-candidiasis-ectodermal dystrophy protein. Am J Hum Genet 2000;66:378–392.
49. Pearce SHS, Williamson C, Kifor O, et al. A familial syndrome of hypocalcemia with hypercalciuria due to mutations in the calcium-sensing receptor. N Engl J Med 1996;335:1115–1122.
50. Spiegel AM. Mutations in G proteins and G protein-coupled receptors in endocrine disease. J Clin Endocrinol Metab 1996;81:2434–2442.
51. Yu S, Yu D, Lee E, et al. Variable and tissue specific hormone resistance in heterotrimeric Gs protein alpha-subunit (Gs_α) knockout mice is due to tissue-specific imprinting of the Gs_α gene. Proc Natl Acad Sci 1998;95:8715–8720.
52. Liu J, Litman D, Rosenberg MJ, et al. A GNAS1 imprinting defect in pseudohypoparathyroidism type IB. J Clin Invest 2000;106:1167–1174.
53. Hahn TJ, Hendin BA, Scharp CR, Haddad JG Jr. Effects of chronic anticonvulsant therapy on serum 25-hydroxycalciferol levels in adults. N Engl J Med 1972;287:900–904.
54. Fraser D, Kooh SW, Kind HP, et al. Pathogenesis of hereditary vitamin-D-dependent rickets. An inborn error of vitamin D metabolism involving defective conversion of 25-hydroxyvitamin D to 1 alpha, 25-dihydroxyvitamin D. N Engl J Med 1973;289:817–822.
55. Reade TM, Scriver CR, Glorieux FH, et al. Response to crystalline 1 alpha-hydroxyvitamin D3 in vitamin D dependency. Pediatr Res 1975;9:593–599.
56. Hughes MR, Malloy PJ, O'Malley BW, et al. Genetic defects of the 1,25-dihydroxyvitamin D3 receptor. J Recept Res 1991;11:699–716.
57. Chen TL, Hirst MA, Cone CM, et al. 1,25-Dihydroxyvitamin D resistance, rickets, and alopecia: analysis of receptors and bioresponse in cultured fibroblasts from patients and parents. J Clin Endocrinol Metab 1984;59:383–388.
58. Bell NH. Vitamin D-dependent rickets type II. Calcif Tissue Int 1980;31:89–91.

16 Pheochromocytoma

Karel Pacak, MD, PhD, DSc,
Graeme Eisenhofer, PhD,
Jacques W. M. Lenders, MD, PhD,
and Christian A. Koch, MD, FACE, FACP

INTRODUCTION

Pheochromocytomas are catecholamine-producing tumors that occur in about 0.05–0.1% of patients with hypertension. There are about 500–1600 pheochromocytoma cases per year in the United States *(1)*. Pheochromocytomas arise from chromaffin cells, usually within the adrenal medulla. In about 10% of cases, these tumors develop from extraadrenal sites, most commonly from chromaffin tissue adjacent to sympathetic ganglia of the neck, mediastinum, abdomen, and pelvis. These extraadrenal chromaffin tissue tumors are often referred to as paragangliomas *(2)*. Approximately 10% of pheochromocytomas are familial and in most cases are secondary to multiple endocrine neoplasia type 2, von Hippel-Lindau syndrome, or neurofibromatosis type 1 (for review, *see* refs. *3–5*). Familial tumors are often multicentric and bilateral and less prone to become malignant *(6–10, 101, 102)*. Between 10 and 25% of patients develop metastases, with a life expectancy of 3–5 yr *(11,12)*. Distinguishing benign from malignant pheochromocytoma is not possible based on histopathologic features. Malignant

From: *Contemporary Endocrinology: Early Diagnosis and Treatment of Endocrine Disorders*
Edited by: R. S. Bar © Humana Press Inc., Totowa, NJ

pheochromocytoma is diagnosed based on the presence of metastatic lesions at sites where chromaffin cells are not present (e.g., liver, lungs, lymphatic nodes, and bones).

CLINICAL PRESENTATION

Most of the clinical features of pheochromocytoma result from metabolic and hemodynamic actions of norepinephrine and epinephrine secreted by the tumor *(1,5,13)*. Hypertension is the most common clinical sign. Headache, excessive truncal sweating, and palpitations are the most common symptoms. Although pallor is found only in a small number of patients, the presence of this sign is highly suspicious for pheochromocytoma and, together with hypertension and excessive sweating, provides a high probability of the diagnosis. Some patients may also suffer from anxiety, unusual nervousness, constipation, low energy level, and exhaustion after attacks (Table 1). Differential diagnoses include panic and anxiety syndromes, hypernoradrenergic hypertension, supraventricular tachycardia, baroreflex failure, postural tachycardia syndrome, cluster or migraine headache, hypertensive encephalopathy, hypoglycemia, carcinoid tumor, adrenomedullary hyperplasia, and hyperthyroidism. Pheochromocytomas must also be considered in any patient with an adrenal incidentaloma, regardless of signs and symptoms. Unusual symptoms related to paroxysmal blood pressure elevation or sudden arrhythmia during diagnostic procedures (e.g., endoscopy, catheterization), anesthesia, food, or dietary supplements should promptly arouse a suspicion of pheochromocytoma. In children, the differential diagnosis of hypertension should also include renal diseases, renal artery stenosis, and coarctation of the aorta *(14–16)*.

Pheochromocytomas in pregnancy may be confused with toxemia and preeclampsia. The diagnosis should be particularly considered when the hypertension is episodic or associated with suggestive symptoms *(17,18)* and especially when proteinuria and leg edema are not present. In pregnant patients with unrecognized pheochromocytoma, fatal hypertensive crises and arrhythmia can be caused by anesthesia, vaginal delivery, abdominal palpation, uterine contractions, trauma, and hemorrhage into the tumor or vigorous fetal movement *(17–19)*.

BIOCHEMICAL DIAGNOSIS

Diagnosis of a pheochromocytoma depends on biochemical evidence of excessive catecholamine (norepinephrine and epinephrine) production by the tumor. This is usually achieved by measurements of catecholamines and catecholamine metabolites in plasma or urine. However, catecholamines are normally produced by the sympathetic nervous system and the adrenal medulla and are not specific to pheochromocytoma. Thus, a variety of physiologic conditions involving sympathoadrenomedullary activation cause increased levels of catecholamines and their metabolites.

Table 1
Diagnosis of Pheochromocytoma

Reasons for early screening for pheochromocytoma
    Severe uncontrolled hypertension
    Severe headache
    Excessive truncal sweating
    Frequent palpitations (especially under rest conditions)
    Pallor, especially with high blood pressure and palpitations
    Severe anxiety, unusual nervousness, or panic attacks
Outcomes of early diagnosis and treatment
    Prevents hypertensive crises
    Prevents lethal arrhythmias
    Prevents myocardial infarction
    Prevents stroke
    May decrease likelihood of developing metastatic disease

Pheochromocytomas may also be "silent," that is, they may not secrete catecholamines in amounts sufficient to produce a positive test result for measurement of urine or plasma catecholamines or the associated typical clinical signs and symptoms (20–22). Furthermore, many pheochromocytomas secrete catecholamines episodically; between episodes, plasma levels or urinary excretion of catecholamines may be normal. Thus, plasma levels and urinary outputs of catecholamines are normal in about 5–15% of patients with pheochromocytoma and do not reliably exclude or confirm the presence of a tumor. Finally, reliable 24-h urine collections may be difficult to obtain, especially in children. Correction of urinary results for creatinine excretion adds another confounder owing to creatinine's dependence on diet, muscle mass, physical activity, and diurnal variation (23–26).

A new biochemical test was recently introduced involving measurements of plasma free metanephrines (normetanephrine and metanephrine) which offers advantages over other tests for diagnosis of pheochromocytoma (3,20,22,27–31). Plasma free (unconjugated) metanephrines are produced in tumor tissue by the actions of catechol-O-methyltransferase on catecholamines (Fig. 1) that leak from storage vesicles within tumor cells. Free metanephrines are produced constantly and *independently* of catecholamine release; they therefore show larger and more consistent increases above normal than plasma catecholamines and appear to exclude reliably the presence of all but the smallest of pheochromocytomas (approx 99% sensitivity, approx 89% specificity). Thus, if plasma concentrations of free normetanephrine and metanephrine are negative, no other tests are necessary (1,3). Measurements of plasma free metanephrines reduce a risk of missed diagnosis of pheochromocytoma, minimize the need to run multiple

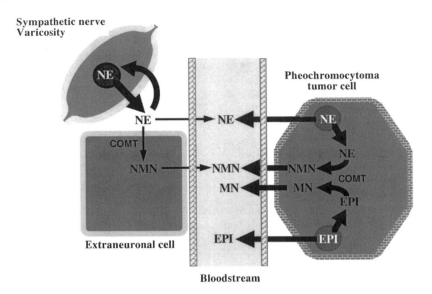

Fig. 1. The catechol-O-methyltransferase (COMT) that is present in a pheochromocytoma cell converts norepinephrine (NE) and epinephrine (EPI) to normetanephrine (NMN) and metanephrine (MN), respectively. A small portion of NMN can be also derived from the action of COMT in extraneuronal cells.

diagnostic tests to exclude a tumor, and provide a very cost-effective approach for diagnosis *(22)*. Plasma free metanephrines also provide a sensitive tool for detection of pheochromocytomas in children. However, age-appropriate reference ranges should be used, and gender differences should be considered *(32)*.

To measure plasma levels of metanephrines and catecholamines correctly, patients should abstain from caffeinated beverages and alcohol for 24 h and avoid acetaminophen, which interferes with the normetanephrine assay, for at least 5 d prior to the blood draw. Patients should also avoid smoking for a few hours before testing. After an overnight fast (water permitted), the blood sample should be drawn through an indwelling intravenous cannula with the subjects rested in supine position for at least 20 min after insertion of the cannula.

Measurements of urinary excretion of fractionated metanephrines performed by modern high-performance liquid chromatography (HPLC) methods also provide a reasonably sensitive biochemical test for the diagnosis of pheochromocytoma. However, this test is less specific than measurements of plasma free metanephrines (Table 2). Our observations show that if plasma concentrations of either free normetanephrine or metanephrine are about five and two times above the upper reference limit, respectively; the diagnosis of pheochromocytoma is confirmed biochemically, and no other biochemical tests are necessary.

Table 2
Sensitivities and Specificities of Individual Biochemical Plasma
and Urine Tests for Diagnosis of Sporadic and Familial Pheochromocytoma

Test	Sensitivity (%)		Specificity (%)	
	Hereditary	Sporadic	Hereditary	Sporadic
Plasma tests				
Free metanephrines	97	99	96	82
Catecholamines	69	92	89	72
Urine tests				
Fract. Metanephrines	96	97	82	45
Total metanephrines	60	88	97	89
Catecholamines	79	91	96	75
VMA	46	77	99	86

VA, vanillylmandelic acid; *see* ref. 22.

In patients with an elevation of plasma free normetanephrine or metanephrine between the value of five or two times above the upper reference limit, respectively, and the upper reference limit, further tests such as clonidine or glucagon tests may be necessary to confirm the diagnosis *(1,33–37)*.

A threefold increase in plasma norepinephrine levels 2 min after glucagon administration indicates a norepinephrine-producing pheochromocytoma with a high degree of specificity. Unfortunately, this test has not been validated for epinephrine responses in patients with epinephrine-secreting tumors, but our unpublished observations show that patients with such tumors have high epinephrine responses (usually at least five times above the upper reference limit).

The clonidine suppression test is particularly useful in patients with increased plasma norepinephrine, in whom it is unclear whether the increase is attributable to sympathetic activation or catecholamine release from a tumor. Clonidine is administered orally in a dose of 0.3 mg/70 kg of body weight. Lack of a decrease in norepinephrine (below the upper reference limit and <50% compared with baseline value) 3 h after clonidine administration is highly suggestive of a pheochromocytoma. Our preliminary results suggest that the clonidine test coupled with measurements of plasma free normetanephrine is very useful in patients with elevated plasma free normetanephrine levels and normal or only marginally increased plasma norepinephrine levels. In those patients, norepinephrine may decrease after clonidine, whereas normetanephrine rarely decreases with a pheochromocytoma.

Both clonidine and glucagon tests should be carried out by experienced clinicians because of several adverse effects associated with the administration of these drugs to patients who can harbor pheochromocytoma. For example, clinicians should be aware of rapid increase in heart rate and blood pressure after glucagon administration and marked hypotension in some patients after clonidine administration. Severe hypertension usually requires treatment with phentolamine, and hypotension is treated with fluid administration and Trendelenburg positioning. To avoid more severe hypotension, we suggest that a patient stop taking antihypertensive medications the evening before the test, and in obese patients we do not increase the clonidine dose above 0.4 mg.

We do not recommend glucagon or clonidine tests in pregnant patients. If values from biochemical tests are clearly elevated, the tumor is confirmed; if there is only moderate or small elevation of plasma free metanephrines, we recommend either repeating the test or proceeding directly to localization of pheochromocytoma.

Finally, in patients with renal failure, pheochromocytoma can probably be reliably diagnosed based on measurements of plasma free metanephrines, in contrast to conjugated metanephrines, which are usually elevated because of dependence of their clearance on renal excretion.

We currently recommend HPLC measurements of plasma free normetanephrine and metanephrine levels as the initial biochemical test (Fig. 2). In medical centers where measurements of plasma free metanephrines are not available, we recommend that initial biochemical tests for exclusion of a pheochromocytoma should include HPLC measurements of 24-h urinary normetanephrine and metanephrine.

At the present time, there are no other reliable plasma markers to diagnose the presence of pheochromocytoma. Chromogranin A, once a promising marker for the presence of pheochromocytoma (38), is often falsely negative and if elevated (e.g., in patients with renal failure) can be falsely positive.

LOCALIZATION

Conventional imaging studies such as computed tomography (CT) or magnetic resonance imaging (MRI) are the most appropriate imaging modalities for initial localization of pheochromocytoma, since both offer high sensitivity for the detection of this tumor (39–43). Both CT and MRI, however, have inadequate specificity to identify a mass positively as a pheochromocytoma. In contrast to these methods, [123]I- or ^{131}I-labeled metaiodobenzylguanidine (MIBG) scintigraphy offers high specificity (>99%) for detection of pheochromocytoma. However, the sensitivity of MIBG scintigraphy is low (<85%). Although ^{123}I-MIBG is superior to ^{131}I-MIBG for the detection of this tumor, this isotope is currently used in only few medical institutions in the United Sates (44,45).

6-[^{18}F]Fluorodopamine positron emission tomography (PET), represents a new diagnostic tool for the early localization of pheochromocytoma (1,3,46,47). 6-[^{18}F]Fluorodopamine is a positron-emitting analog of dopamine. After intravenous injection (currently 1 mCi is used) 6-[^{18}F]fluorodopamine is transported

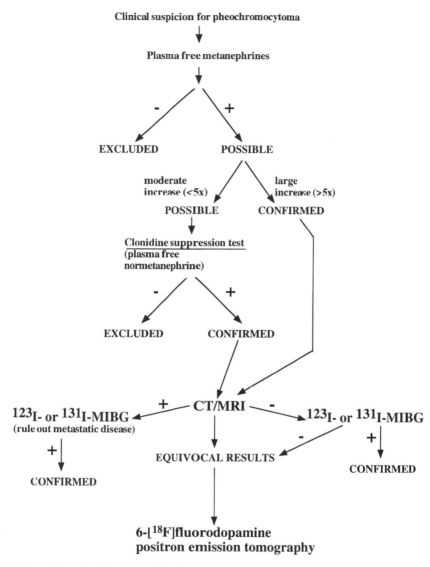

Fig. 2. Algorithm showing use of biochemical tests and imaging studies for diagnosis and localization of pheochromocytoma.

rapidly, actively, and avidly into catecholamine-synthesizing cells by the cellular membrane norepinephrine transporter system *(48–51)*. From the cytoplasm, 6-[^{18}F]fluorodopamine is translocated via an intracellular vesicular transporter system into sympathetic vesicles, and accumulation of 6-[^{18}F]fluorodopamine in these vesicles enables visualization of chromaffin cells. Since pheochromocytoma cells also express these transporter systems, 6-[^{18}F]fluorodopamine can be used for the detection of the tumor.

Based on recent studies *(3,46)*, 6-[^{18}F]fluorodopamine PET scanning can detect and localize pheochromocytomas with high sensitivity. Our preliminary results also suggest that 6-[^{18}F]fluorodopamine PET scanning is superior in the localization of pheochromocytoma to other nuclear imaging modalities including ^{131}I-MIBG scintigraphy and [^{111}In-DTPA-D-Phe]-pentetreotide (octreotide) (unpublished observations). Because of the limited availability of PET scanners and costs related to PET imaging, at the present time we recommend using 6-[^{18}F]fluorodopamine PET scanning in difficult cases in which biochemical tests are positive but conventional imaging studies cannot localize the tumor. Other positron-emitting imaging agents have also been used with some success to visualize pheochromocytoma, including ^{18}F-fluorodeoxyglucose, ^{11}C-hydroxy-ephedrine, and ^{11}C-hydroxyephedrine *(52–54)*. None of these agents is ideal since false-positive or-negative results may occur.

Somatostatin receptor scintigraphy using octreotide, an analog of somatostatin, is also used to localize pheochromocytomas *(55–57)*. However, the conventional 6–12-mCi dose of octreotide localizes pheochromocytoma in less than 30% of cases *(55)*. In contrast, in patients with a malignant pheochromocytoma, Octreoscan can be very useful in the detection of metastases, especially in patients with negative MIBG scans *(55)*. Based on experience at the National Institutes of Health (NIH), we do not recommend Octreoscan as the first-line imaging test for the localization of pheochromocytoma. An Octreoscan should be reserved for patients in whom conventional imaging studies cannot locate the tumor, MIBG scintigraphy is negative, and 6-[^{18}F]fluorodopamine PET scanning is not available. Thus, in patients with metastatic pheochromocytoma, octreotide scintigraphy should be used in those patients in whom further treatment is planned using this compound and in whom the MIBG scan is negative.

In pregnancy, MRI or ultrasound represent the best approach for localizing pheochromocytoma since both methods entail little or no radiation exposure to the fetus. MRI is preferable since this imaging modality has very good sensitivity and specificity. Moreover, the gravid uterus after 24 wk of gestation presents a problem for accurate sonographic examination *(17–19)*.

TREATMENT

Surgery provides the only effective curative treatment for solitary pheochromocytoma. Laparoscopy is the surgical method of choice in most patients *(58–70)*. Because of the potentially severe and even fatal consequences of surgical anesthesia-induced release of catecholamines by a tumor, it is imperative that patients with pheochromocytoma be appropriately prepared for the surgical procedure. Adequate blood pressure control should be achieved preferably by using α- and β-adrenergic and/or calcium channel blockers *(3,5,13,71–79)*.

For α-adrenergic blockers, we recommend using phenoxybenzamine with the starting dose of 10 mg twice a day. The dose is adjusted based on blood pressure monitoring, and in some patients a dose over 150 mg per day is required. Clinicians should be aware of phenoxybenzamine-induced postural hypotension; 50–70% of patients have orthostatic hypotension even without α-blockers. Follow the orthostatic blood pressure and treat with intravascular volume expansion until orthostatic blood pressure is gone. β-adrenergic blockers should be used after adequate α-blockade is achieved. We recommend using atenolol at a starting dose of 12.5 mg once or twice a day. The dose is adjusted based on heart rate, which should not exceed 80 beats per minute if treated appropriately.

For calcium channel blockers, we recommend using amlodipine (Norvasc®) with a starting dose of 10 mg once a day *(5,80)*. Administration of α-methyl-para-tyrosine (metyrosine, Demser™) to block synthesis of catecholamines may also be appropriate in patients with active tumors, especially when α- and β-blockers cannot adequately control symptoms and signs of catecholamine excess *(3,81–87)*. The starting dose for metyrosine is usually 250 mg twice to four times a day; in patients undergoing surgery, the drug is given about 2 wk prior to the procedure. The maximum dose is 4 g/d. Such high doses, however, should be used cautiously since metyrosine can deplete catecholamine synthesis in the brain, which is associated with sedation and depression. At our institution, at midnight before surgery, 1 mg/kg of phenoxybenzamine and 1 g metyrosine are given. Hypertensive crisis should be treated with an intravenous bolus of 5 mg phentolamine (Regitine®) with repeated doses every 2 min until hypertension is adequately controlled. Phentolamine can also be given as a continuous infusion. Sodium nitroprusside and labetelol are other drugs that can be given intravenously in patients presenting with hypertensive crisis.

To minimize adverse effects of paroxysmal hypertension and arrhythmias in pregnant patients with pheochromocytoma, it is important to use combined α- and β-adrenoceptor blockade. Phenoxybenzamine can be used for α-adreno-ceptor blockade (starting dose usually 10 mg two times a day followed by 10-mg increments) until there is a desired blood pressure response. Phenoxybenzamine should be followed by atenolol 25 mg once a day or propranolol 20 mg three times a day to maintain a heart rate about 80–100 beats per minute. Using appropriate blockade, the fetal and maternal morbidity and mortality are markedly decreased.

In patients with pheochromocytoma presenting late in pregnancy, surgery should be delayed until fetal maturity is reached. The tumor should then be removed after cesarean delivery. Vaginal delivery is not recommended since it may cause marked catecholamine release from tumor manipulation. At least 1–2 wk should be allowed for effects of adequate blockade before surgery. If patients present in early pregnancy, two options are available. First, the patient can be treated with appropriate medication. Second, if medication cannot control symptoms and signs of catecholamine excess, the pheochromocytoma should be removed. Both options have their risks, and these need to be weighed against the clinical condition of patient and fetus. Surgery is best done early in the second trimester (before 23 wk gestation) when spontaneous abortion is less likely to occur as a result of the procedure; additionally, the size of the uterus will not preclude surgical procedures. Spinal and epidural anesthesia are contraindicated since they may cause prolonged hypotension and have also been associated with marked catecholamine release by the tumor.

Currently, there is no effective treatment for malignant pheochromocytoma. In some patients surgical mass reduction to achieve lower catecholamine levels or alleviation of symptoms from local tumor growth is important as palliative treatment *(88)*. As per several reports, combination chemotherapy, most commonly with cyclophosphamide, vincristine, and dacarbazine, produces remission *(89–91)*. Recent unpublished data suggest, however, that remission is achieved in less than 50% of patients (T. Fojo, personal communications). Recently, paclitaxel as a single agent has been used for treatment of metastatic pheochromocytoma *(92)*. Radiotherapies using ^{131}I-labeled MIBG have practically the same effect as chemotherapy *(93–99)*. Recent experiments showing that cisplatin and doxorubicin increase uptake of MIBG into pheochromocytoma cells are a promising avenue as the future therapeutic option for some patients with metastatic pheochromocytoma *(88)*. Currently, a few clinical trials with indium- or ytrium-labeled octreotide are in progress *(56,88)*. External radiation is used in patients with skeletal metastatic disease, and chemoembolization is limited to patients with, e.g., liver metastatic disease *(100)*. However, none of these treatment modalities have proved curative. Clinicians using chemotherapy should be aware of potentially fatal complications arising from excessive catecholamine release as tumor cells are destroyed (usually within the first 24 h). With the use of MIBG, a major complication is bone marrow suppression, usually 4 wk after initiation of therapy.

REFERENCES

1. Pacak K, Chrousos GP, Koch CA, Lenders JW, Eisenhofer G. Pheochromocytoma: progress in diagnosis, therapy, and genetics. In: Margioris A, Chrousos GP, eds. Adrenal disorders, 1st ed., vol 1. Humana Press, Totowa, NJ, 2001, pp. 479–523.
2. Erickson D, Kudva YC, Ebersold MJ, et al. Benign paragangliomas: clinical presentation and treatment outcomes in 236 patients. J Clin Endocrinol Metab 2001;86:5210–5216.
3. Pacak K, Linehan WM, Eisenhofer G, Walther MM, Goldstein DS. Recent advances in genetics, diagnosis, localization, and treatment of pheochromocytoma. Ann Intern Med 2001;134:315–329.
4. Young WF Jr. Pheochromocytoma: issues in diagnosis & treatment. Compr Ther 1997; 23:319–326.
5. Bravo E. Evolving concepts in the pathophysiology, diagnosis, and treatment of pheochromocytoma. Endocr Rev 1994;15:356–368.

6. Koch CA, Vortmeyer AO, Huang SC, Alesci S, Zhuang Z, Pacak K. Genetic aspects of pheochromocytoma [Review]. Endocr Regul 2001;35:43–52.
7. Neumann HP. Genetics of hypertension: the pheochromocytoma model. Clin Invest 1994; 72:729–730.
8. Neumann HP, Bender BU, Januszewicz A, Janetschek G, Eng C. Inherited pheochromocytoma. Adv Nephrol Necker Hosp 1997;27:361–376.
9. Neumann HP, Berger DP, Sigmund G, et al. Pheochromocytomas, multiple endocrine neoplasia type 2, and von Hippel-Lindau disease. N Engl J Med 1993;329:1531–1538.
10. Scopsi L, Castellani MR, Gullo M, et al. Malignant pheochromocytoma in multiple endocrine neoplasia type 2B syndrome. Case report and review of the literature. Tumori 1996;82:480–484.
11. Proye C, Vix M, Goropoulos A, Kerlo P, Lecomte-Houcke M. High incidence of malignant pheochromocytoma in a surgical unit. 26 cases out of 100 patients operated from 1971 to 1991. J Endocrinol Invest 1992;15:651–663.
12. John H, Ziegler WH, Hauri D, Jaeger P. Pheochromocytomas: can malignant potential be predicted? Urology 1999;53:679–683
13. Manger W, Gifford R. Clinical and Experimental Pheochromocytoma. Blackwell Science, Cambridge, MA, 1996.
14. Londe S. Causes of hypertension in the young. Pediatr Clin North Am 1978;25:55–65.
15. Londe S, Goldring D. High blood pressure in children: problems and guidelines for evaluation and treatment. Am J Cardiol 1976;37:650–657.
16. Londe S, Goldring D. Childhood blood pressure and hypertension in office practice. Compr Ther 1977;3:66–74.
17. Ahlawat SK, Jain S, Kumari S, Varma S, Sharma BK. Pheochromocytoma associated with pregnancy: case report and review of the literature. Obstet Gynecol Surv 1999;54:728–737.
18. Harper MA, Murnaghan GA, Kennedy L, Hadden DR, Atkinson AB. Phaeochromocytoma in pregnancy. Five cases and a review of the literature. Br J Obstet Gynaecol 1989;96:594–606.
19. Keely E. Endocrine causes of hypertension in pregnancy—when to start looking for zebras. Semin Perinatol 1998;22:471–484.
20. Lenders JW, Keiser HR, Goldstein DS, et al. Plasma metanephrines in the diagnosis of pheochromocytoma. Ann Intern Med 1995;123:101–109.
21. Shawar L, Svec F. Pheochromocytoma with elevated metanephrines as the only biochemical finding. J La State Med Soc 1996;148:535–538.
22. Lenders JW, Pacak K, Walther MM, et al. Biochemical diagnosis of pheochromocytoma: which test is best? JAMA 2000;287:1427–1434.
23. Calles-Escandon J, Cunningham JJ, Snyder P, et al. Influence of exercise on urea, creatinine, and 3-methylhistidine excretion in normal human subjects. Am J Physiol 1984;246:E334–338.
24. Curtis G, Fogel M. Creatinine excretion: diurnal variation and variability of whole and part-day measures. A methodologic issue in psychoendocrine research. Psychosom Med 1970;32:337–350.
25. Neubert A, Remer T. The impact of dietary protein intake on urinary creatinine excretion in a healthy pediatric population. J Pediatr 1998;133:655–659.
26. Wang ZM, Gallagher D, Nelson ME, Matthews DE, Heymsfield SB. Total-body skeletal muscle mass: evaluation of 24-h urinary creatinine excretion by computerized axial tomography. Am J Clin Nutr 1996;63:863–869.
27. Eisenhofer G, Friberg P, Pacak K, et al. Plasma metadrenalines: do they provide useful information about sympatho-adrenal function and catecholamine metabolism? Clin Sci 1995;88:533–542
28. Eisenhofer G, Keiser H, Friberg P, et al. Plasma metanephrines are markers of pheochromocytoma produced by catechol-O-methyltransferase within tumors. J Clin Endocrinol Metab 1998;83:2175–2185

29. Eisenhofer G, Pecorella W, Pacak K, Hooper D, Kopin I, Goldstein D. The neuronal and extraneuronal origins of plasma 3-methoxy-4-hydroxyphenylglycol in rats. J Auton Nerv Syst 1994;50:93–107

30. Eisenhofer G. Free or total metanephrines for diagnosis of pheochromocytoma: what is the difference? Clin Chem 2001;47:988–989.

31. Eisenhofer G, Walther M, Keiser HR, Lenders JW, Friberg P, Pacak K. Plasma metanephrines: a novel and cost-effective test for pheochromocytoma. Braz J Med Biol Res 2000;33:1157–1169.

32. Weise M, Merke D, Pacak K, Walther MM, Eisenhofer G. Utility of plasma free metanephrines for detecting childhood pheochromocytoma. J Clin Endocrinol Metab 2002;87:1955–1960.

33. Siqueira-Filho AG, Sheps SG, Maher FT, Jiang NS, Elveback LR. Glucagon-blood catecholamine test: use in isolated and familial pheochromocytoma. Arch Intern Med 1975;135:1227–1231

34. Bravo EL. Pheochromocytoma. Current concepts in diagnosis, localization, and management. Prim Care 1983;10:75–86.

35. Bravo EL. Effects of clonidine on sympathetic function. Chest 1983;83:369–371.

36. Bravo EL, Tarazi RC, Fouad FM, Vidt DG, Gifford RW Jr. Clonidine-suppression test: a useful aid in the diagnosis of pheochromocytoma. N Engl J Med 1981;305:623–626.

37. Grossman E, Goldstein D, Hoffman A, Keiser H. Glucagon and clonidine testing in the diagnosis of pheochromocytoma. Hypertension 1991;17:733–741.

38. Hsiao R, Neumann H, Parmer R, Barbosa J, O'Connor D. Chromogranin A in familial pheochromocytoma: diagnostic screening value, prediction of tumor mass, and post-resection kinetics indicating two-compartment distribution. Am J Med 1990;88:607–613.

39. Fink IJ, Reinig JW, Dwyer AJ, Doppman JL, Linehan WM, Keiser HR. MR imaging of pheochromocytomas. J Comput Assist Tomogr 1985;9:454–458

40. Schmedtje JF Jr, Sax S, Pool JL, Goldfarb RA, Nelson EB. Localization of ectopic pheochromocytomas by magnetic resonance imaging. Am J Med 1987;83:770–772

41. Sisson JC, Frager MS, Valk TW, et al. Scintigraphic localization of pheochromocytoma. N Engl J Med 1981;305:12–17

42. Kloos RT, Gross MD, Francis IR, Korobkin M, Shapiro B. Incidentally discovered adrenal masses. Endocr Rev 1995;16:460–484.

43. Kloos RT, Korobkin M, Thompson NW, Francis IR, Shapiro B, Gross MD. Incidentally discovered adrenal masses. Cancer Treat Res 1997;89:263–292.

44. Furuta N, Kiyota H, Yoshigoe F, Hasegawa N, Ohishi Y. Diagnosis of pheochromocytoma using [^{123}I]-compared with [^{131}I]-metaiodobenzylguanidine scintigraphy. Int J Urol 1999;6:119–124.

45. Eisenhofer G, Pacak K, Goldstein DS, Chen C, Shulkin B. ^{123}-MIBG scintigraphy of catecholamine systems: impediments to applications in clinical medicine [Letter]. Eur J Nucl Med 2000;27:611–612

46. Pacak K, Eisenhofer G, Carrasquillo JA, Chen CC, Li ST, Goldstein DS. 6-[^{18}F]fluorodopamine positron emission tomographic (PET) scanning for diagnostic localization of pheochromocytoma. Hypertension 2001;38:6–8.

47. Pacak K, Fojo T, Goldstein DS, et al. Radiofrequency ablation: a novel approach for treatment of metastatic pheochromocytoma. J Natl Cancer Inst 2001;93:648–649.

48. Goldstein DS, Coronado L, Kopin IJ. 6-[Fluorine-18]fluorodopamine pharmacokinetics and dosimetry in humans. J Nucl Med 1994;35:964–973.

49. Goldstein DS, Eisenhofer G, Dunn BB, et al. Positron emission tomographic imaging of cardiac sympathetic innervation using 6-[^{18}F]fluorodopamine: initial findings in humans. J Am Coll Cardiol 1993;22:1961–1971.

50. Goldstein DS, Holmes C. Metabolic fate of the sympathoneural imaging agent 6-[^{18}F]fluorodopamine in humans. Clin Exp Hypertens 1997;19:155–161.

51. Goldstein DS, Holmes C, Stuhlmuller JE, Lenders JW, Kopin IJ. 6-[^{18}F]fluorodopamine positron emission tomographic scanning in the assessment of cardiac sympathoneural function—studies in normal humans. Clin Auton Res 1997;7:17–29.

52. Shulkin B, Wieland D, Schwaiger M, et al. PET scanning with hydroxyephedrine: a new approach to the localization of pheochromocytoma. J Nucl Med 1992;33:1125–1131.

53. Shulkin B, Wieland D, Shapiro B, Sisson J. PET epinephrine studies of pheochromocytoma. J Nucl Med 1995;36:22P–23P.

54. Shulkin BL, Thompson NW, Shapiro B, Francis IR, Sisson JC. Pheochromocytomas: Imaging with 2-[fluorine-18]fluoro-2-deoxy-D-glucose PET. Nucl Med 1999;212:35–41.

55. van der Harst E, de Herder WW, Bruining HA, et al. [(123)I]metaiodobenzylguanidine and [(111)In]octreotide uptake in benign and malignant pheochromocytomas. J Clin Endocrinol Metab 2001;86:685–693.

56. Kopf D, Bockisch A, Steinert H, et al. Octreotide scintigraphy and catecholamine response to an octreotide challenge in malignant phaeochromocytoma. Clin Endocrinol (Oxf) 1997;46:39–44.

57. Koriyama N, Kakei M, Yaekura K, et al. Control of catecholamine release and blood pressure with octreotide in a patient with pheochromocytoma: a case report with in vitro studies. Horm Res 2000;53:46–50.

58. Gagner M, Breton G, Pharand D, Pomp A. Is laparoscopic adrenalectomy indicated for pheochromocytomas? Surgery 1996;120:1076–1079; discussion 1079–1080.

59. Gagner M, Pomp A, Heniford B, Pharand D, Lacroix A. Laparoscopic adrenalectomy. lessons learned from 100 consecutive procedures. Ann Surg 1997;226:238–247.

60. Guazzoni G, Montorsi F, Bocciardi A, et al. Transperitoneal laparoscopic versus open adrenalectomy for benign hyperfunctioning adrenal tumors: a comparative study. J Urol 1995;153:1597–1600.

61. Linos D, Stylopoulos N, Boukis M, Souvatzoglou A, Raptis S, Papadimitriou J. Anterior, posterior, or laparoscopic approach for the management of adrenal diseases? Am J Surg 1997;173:120–125.

62. Reinig J, Doppman J, Dwyer A, Johnson A, Knop R. Adrenal masses differentiated by MR. Radiology 1986;158:81–84.

63. Vargas H, Kavoussi L, Bartlett D, et al. Laparoscopic adrenalectomy: a new standard of care. Urology 1997;49:673–678.

64. Walther M, Herring J, Choyke P, Linehan W. Laparoscopic partial adrenalectomy in patients with hereditary forms of pheochromocytoma. J Urol 2000;164:14–17.

65. Thompson G, Grant C, van Heerden J, et al. Laparoscopic versus open posterior adrenalectomy: a case-control study of 100 patients. Surgery 1997;122:1132–1136.

66. Janetschek G, Neumann HP. Laparoscopic surgery for pheochromocytoma. Urol Clin North Am 2001;28:97–105.

67. Radmayr C, Neumann H, Bartsch G, Elsner R, Janetschek G. Laparoscopic partial adrenalectomy for bilateral pheochromocytomas in a boy with von Hippel-Lindau disease. Eur Urol 2000;38:344–348.

68. Neumann HP, Reincke M, Bender BU, Elsner R, Janetschek G. Preserved adrenocortical function after laparoscopic bilateral adrenal sparing surgery for hereditary pheochromocytoma. J Clin Endocrinol Metab 1999;84:2608–2610.

69. Neumann HP, Bender BU, Reincke M, Eggstein S, Laubenberger J, Kirste G. Adrenal-sparing surgery for phaeochromocytoma. Br J Surg 1999;86:94–97.

70. Janetschek G, Finkenstedt G, Gasser R, et al. Laparoscopic surgery for pheochromocytoma: adrenalectomy, partial resection, excision of paragangliomas. J Urol 1998;160:330–334.

71. Gifford RW Jr, Manger WM, Bravo EL. Pheochromocytoma. Endocrinol Metab Clin North Am 1994;23:387–404.

72. Ross JH. Pheochromocytoma. Special considerations in children. Urol Clin North Am 2000;27:393–402.

73. Walther M, Keiser H, Linehan W. Pheochromocytoma: evaluation, diagnosis, and management. World J Urology 1999;17:35–39.
74. Bravo EL, Gifford RW Jr. Current concepts. Pheochromocytoma: diagnosis, localization and management. N Engl J Med 1984; 311:1298–1303.
75. Bravo EL, Gifford RW Jr. Pheochromocytoma. Endocrinol Metab Clin North Am 1993;22:329–341.
76. Reddy VS, O'Neill JA Jr, Holcomb GW, 3rd, et al. Twenty-five-year surgical experience with pheochromocytoma in children. Am Surg 2000; 66:1085–1091; discussion 1092.
77. Young WF Jr. Management approaches to adrenal incidentalomas. A view from Rochester, Minnesota. Endocrinol Metab Clin North Am 2000;29:159–185.
78. Poopalalingam R, Chin EY. Rapid preparation of a patient with pheochromocytoma with labetolol and magnesium sulfate. Can J Anaesth 2001;48:876–880.
79. Kinney MA, Warner ME, vanHeerden JA, et al. Perianesthetic risks and outcomes of pheochromocytoma and paraganglioma resection. Anesth Analg 2000;91:1118–1123.
80. Bravo EL. Pheochromocytoma. Curr Ther Endocrinol Metab 1997;6:195–197
81. Atuk NO. Pheochromocytoma: diagnosis, localization, and treatment. Hosp Pract (Off Ed) 1983;18:187–202.
82. Decoulx M, Wemeau JL, Racadot-Leroy N, Grimbert I, Proye C, Plane C. [Alpha-methyl-paratyrosine in the treatment of malignant pheochromocytoma]. Rev Med Interne 1987;8:383–388.
83. Hauptman JB, Modlinger RS, Ertel NH. Pheochromocytoma resistant to alpha-adrenergic blockade. Arch Intern Med 1983;143:2321–2323.
84. Miller D, Robblee JA. Perioperative management of a patient with a malignant pheochromocytoma. Can Anaesth Soc J 1985;32:278–282.
85. Rivero Sanchez M, Selgas Gutierrez R, Lorenzo Aguiar MD, et al. [Effect of alpha-methyl-paratyrosine on the urinary excretion of catecholamines in patients with pheochromocytoma]. Rev Clin Esp 1981;161:235–239.
86. Sand J, Salmi J, Saaristo J, Auvinen O. Preoperative treatment and survival of patients with pheochromocytomas. Ann Chir Gynaecol 1997;86:230–232
87. Steinsapir J, Carr AA, Prisant LM, Bransome ED Jr. Metyrosine and pheochromocytoma. Arch Intern Med 1997;157:901–906.
88. Kopf D, Goretzki PE, Lehnert H. Clinical management of malignant adrenal tumors. J Cancer Res Clin Oncol 2001;127:143–155.
89. Averbuch SD, Steakley CS, Young RC, et al. Malignant pheochromocytoma: effective treatment with a combination of cyclophosphamide, vincristine, and dacarbazine. Ann Intern Med 1988;109:267–273.
90. Keiser HR, Goldstein DS, Wade JL, Douglas FL, Averbuch SD. Treatment of malignant pheochromocytoma with combination chemotherapy. Hypertension 1985;7:I18–24.
91. Mundschenk J, Kopf D, Lehnert H. [Therapy of malignant pheochromocytoma. Invitation to participate in a randomized multicenter study (letter)]. Dtsch Med Wochenschr 1998;123:32–33.
92. Kruijtzer CM, Beijnen JH, Swart M, Schellens JH. Successful treatment with paclitaxel of a patient with metastatic extra-adrenal pheochromocytoma (paraganglioma). A case report and review of the literature. Cancer Chemother Pharmacol 2000;45:428–431
93. Loh KC, Fitzgerald PA, Matthay KK, Yeo PP, Price DC. The treatment of malignant pheochromocytoma with iodine-131 metaiodobenzylguanidine (^{131}I-MIBG): a comprehensive review of 116 reported patients. J Endocrinol Invest 1997;20:648–658
94. Lumbroso J, Schlumberger M, Tenenbaum F, Aubert B, Travagli JP, Parmentier C. [^{131}I]metaiodobenzylguanidine therapy in 20 patients with malignant pheochromocytoma. J Nucl Biol Med 1991;35:288–291
95. Schlumberger M, Gicquel C, Lumbroso J, et al. Malignant pheochromocytoma: clinical, biological, histologic and therapeutic data in a series of 20 patients with distant metastases. J Endocrinol Invest 1992;15:631–642

96. Shapiro B, Sisson JC, Eyre P, Copp JE, Dmuchowski C, Beierwaltes WH. ^{131}I-MIBG—a new agent in diagnosis and treatment of pheochromocytoma. Cardiology 1985;72:137–142

97. Shapiro B, Sisson JC, Shulkin BL, Gross MD, Zempel S. The current status of radioiodinated metaiodobenzylguanidine therapy of neuro-endocrine tumors. Q J Nucl Med 1995;39:55–57.

98. Shapiro B, Sisson JC, Wieland DM, et al. Radiopharmaceutical therapy of malignant pheochromocytoma with ^{131}I]metaiodobenzylguanidine: results from ten years of experience. J Nucl Biol Med 1991;35:269–276

99. Shapiro B, Gross MD, Shulkin B. Radioisotope diagnosis and therapy of malignant pheochromocytoma. Trends Endocrinol Metab 2001;12:469–475.

100. Takahashi K, Ashizawa N, Minami T, et al. Malignant pheochromocytoma with multiple hepatic metastases treated by chemotherapy and transcatheter arterial embolization. Intern Med 1999;38:349–354.

101. Koch CA, Pacak K,, Chrousos GP. The molecular pathogenesis of hereditary and sporadic adrenocortical and adrenomedullary tumors. J Clin Endocrinol Metab 2002;87:5367–5384.

102. Koch CA, Vortmeyer AO, Zhuang Z, Brouwers FM, Pacak K. New insights into the genetics of familial chromaffin cell tumors. Ann NY Acad Sci 2992;970:11–28.

17 Hypogonadism in Men and Women

John H. MacIndoe, MD

INTRODUCTION

Basic Gonadal Physiology and Terminology

The gonads in both sexes serve the same dual functions, namely, the production of gametes and sex steroids. These functions are clinically quiescent in children but subsequently are induced at puberty and then maintained through much of adulthood by the glycoprotein pituitary gonadotropins leutinizing hormone (LH) and follicle-stimulating hormone (FSH). By historical convention these names refer to events and structures within the ovary, but their structures are identical in both men and women and their functions in each gender are largely similar. The secretions of these gonadotropins are largely regulated by classic feedback inhibition from circulating gonadal products, with LH being excreted by the sex steroid levels in blood and FSH by proteins (inhibins) produced by developing gametes (Fig. 1). When inadequate gonadal function results from a defect within the gonad itself, the condition is referred to as *primary* gonadal failure. Hypogonadism resulting from pituitary or hypothalamic defects is referred to as *secondary* and *tertiary* gonadal failure, respectively. Despite the later distinction, many authors continue to refer to either pituitary or hypothalamic failure as secondary or "central" hypogonadism.

From: *Contemporary Endocrinology: Early Diagnosis and Treatment of Endocrine Disorders*
Edited by: R. S. Bar © Humana Press Inc., Totowa, NJ

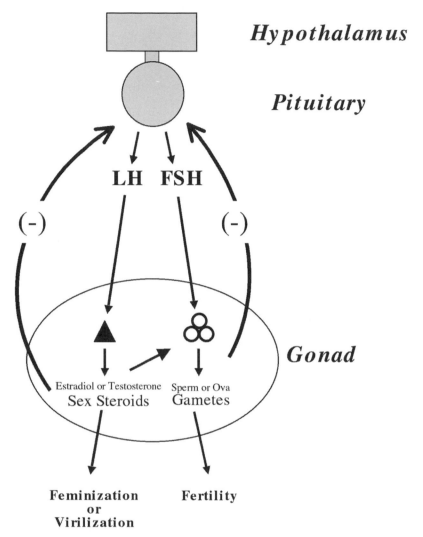

Fig. 1. Schematic depiction of the hypothalamic-pituitary-gonadal axis. Pituitary secretion of luteinizing hormone (LH) and follicle-stimulating hormone (FSH) subject to negative feedback, largely from the products resulting from their specific actions on the gonad.

Scope

Although there are several congenital causes of hypogonadism, which result in incomplete or absent pubertal development and subsequent hypogonadism, in this chapter we limit the discussion of hypogonadal disorders to those that develop in postpubertal individuals. In addition, we do not discuss issues regarding the infertility that accompanies most types of hypogonadism in the adult, but rather focus on the recognition and management of sex steroid deficiencies.

GONADAL FAILURE IN WOMEN

Premenopausal Women

The production of estrogen rises during the first half of the menstrual cycle in concert with the maturation of ovarian follicles to ovulation and then, during the second half, reaches a plateau as progesterone secretion rises with the formation of the corpus luteum. If the ovulated egg fails to be fertilized and achieve uterine implantation, the corpus luteum ceases to function, the levels of both steroids fall, and menses ensues. Persistent amenorrhea is the earliest and most obvious clinical sign of estrogen deficiency, but it also may be seen in other conditions of pituitary-ovarian dysfunction in which estrogen secretion may be normal. Two approaches can be used to distinguish between these general etiologies. They can be used alone or in concert, the latter being my preference. The laboratory evaluation of amenorrhea should include a pregnancy test and assays of serum LH, FSH, estradiol, and prolactin. At the same time, one can institute a "progesterone challenge" test by instructing the patient to take 10 mg of oral progestin, usually medroxyprogesterone acetate (MPA; Provera™), daily for 10 d.

The development of menses during or following withdrawal of the progestin provides evidence of adequate underlying estrogen production since uterine bleeding usually can occur only if the endometrium has been previously stimulated by estrogen. A menstrual response therefore excludes the presence of gonadal failure. However, the absence of uterine bleeding *per se* does not prove the presence of hypogonadism. Repeated plasma estradiol values below 20 pg/mL should be considered evidence of estrogen deficiency. Elevated gonadotropins in that setting would suggest a primary ovarian failure, whereas normal or frankly low values would indicate a defect in the hypothalamic-pituitary axis. The presence of hyperprolactinemia, a relatively common cause of amenorrhea, should lead to the consideration of underlying primary hypothyroidism, a hypothalamic lesion, or a pituitary adenoma. A variety of medications may also elevate prolactin levels sufficiently to disturb menses *(1)*.

Estrogen replacement is considered of prime importance in hypogonadal premenopausal women because of its role in maintaining bone mass and the normal structure and function of other estrogen target tissues, such as the breast and urogenital system. Such replacement can be instituted using standard postmenopausal hormone replacement therapy regimens, whereas some practitioners prefer using birth control medications for the sake of convenience. With either approach, monthly uterine bleeding should be maintained with a progesterone supplement to avoid the development of uterine hyperplasia and the risk of subsequent endometrial carcinoma resulting from unopposed chronic estrogen stimulation.

Menopausal Ovarian Failure

ESTROGEN DEFICIENCY

Menopause results from what might be considered a preprogrammed failure of ovarian function and is due to the gradual depletion of ovarian follicles. Although this process actually begins *in utero*, physiologic estrogen secretory patterns are maintained in most women until somewhere between 40 and 60 yr of age.

The first symptom of menopause is often vasomotor instability (hot flashes, warm flushes). These may begin after an interval of amenorrhea but usually surface earlier in the presence of irregular or even seemingly normal menstrual function. In most cases these episodes pass within 1–2 yr, but in a significant number of patients they may last for decades or disappear only to reappear years later. Although hot flashes are frequently considered a minor nuisance that will eventually pass, they may interfere significantly with normal REM sleep, thereby creating a state of relative sleep deprivation. Estrogen replacement therapy (ERT) represents the most effective approach to eliminating hot flashes. Relief is usually observed within 7–10 d after beginning such treatment. Other medications such as megestrol acetate (Megace™) *(2)*, clonidine *(3)*, selective serotonin reuptake inhibitors *(4)*, and veralipride *(5)*, have been reported to be effective in some but not all patients who are not able to take estrogen. The long-term consequences of estrogen deficiency include an accelerated rate of bone loss and, eventually, atrophy of vaginal tissues and the transitional epithelium lining the urethra. Estrogen deficiency has also been linked epidemiologically to a host of other disorders including colon cancer *(6)*, cognitive difficulties *(7)*, depression and anxiety *(8)*, and sexual dysfunction *(9)*.

The impact of ERT on cardiovascular function is currently increasingly controversial. Observational studies over the past several decades have suggested that estrogen replacement is associated with a significant decrease in coronary events *(10–14)*. However, prospective studies in patients who have had previous cardiac disease suggest that ERT may be linked to a slight increase in cardiovascular risk during the first year of use, with little subsequent coronary risk reduction *(15,16)*. Current ERT recommendations for women without known coronary disease or a coronary equivalent (diabetes, peripheral or symptomatic cerebrovascular disease) suggest that such replacement is safe but cannot be relied on to reduce coronary risk alone. Furthermore, women with coronary disease or a coronary equivalent who have been on estrogen for over 1 yr also do not appear to be at increased risk for coronary disease and thus should not be instructed to discontinue ERT solely for cardiovascular risk reduction *(17,18)*. Finally, a large prospective trial of PremPro™ being carried out by the Women's Health Initiative was recently halted by the safety monitoring board because of excessive morbidity in the drug treated group *(19)*. Despite an overall improvement in hip fractures and colorectal cancer, the use of Prempro™ (equine estrogen plus medroxyprogesterone acetate) was associated with an increased incidence of breast cancer, stroke, coronary heart disease and pulmonary embolism. The composite global index showed a small but significantly increased overall hazards ratio for treatment of 1.15 (1.03–1.28). Interestingly, a parallel study being carried out with Premarin™ (equine estrogen) alone in hysterectomized women has not been stopped, leaving in question whether the adverse effects seen in the Prempro study might be attributed to the presence of the synthetic progestin.

A variety of hormone replacement regimens are currently available. ERT can be performed with oral conjugated equine estrogen, esterified estrogens, micronized estradiol, or transdermal estradiol. There has been some growing support for the use of lower doses of these regimens that were traditionally used in the past because of data supporting similar efficacy with improved safety (20). The use of progesterone continues to be recommended for women with an intact uterus to prevent the long-term negative endometrial effects of unopposed estrogen. Several progesterones are approved for use, including MPA, which can be given for the first 10–15 d of each month at a dose of 10 mg/d or daily at 2.5 mg. Daily combined estrogen plus progesterone therapy has the potential advantage of providing the benefits of estrogens, the protection of progesterone, and little or no menstruation. The institution of such combination therapy in recently menopausal women has been associated with an increased frequency of unpredictable uterine bleeding, which generally resolves within 9 mo of treatment. Studies using norethindorine acetate (NA) as the progesterone suggest that unwanted uterine bleeding may be of shorter duration and that bone density is improved to a greater extent with NA vs MPA (21). Several fixed estrogen-progestin combinations are currently available including Prempro™ (conjugated equine estrogen plus MPA), Femhrt™ (ethinyl estradiol plus NA), and the transdermal combination, CombiPatch™ (micronized estradiol plus NA). Women with preexisting hypertriglyceridemia should be monitored closely for further increases in triglyceride values following the institution of estrogen replacement. Patients who demonstrate significant triglyceride increases with oral estrogens often experience lesser increases with transdermal preparations.

The recently reported safety results from Women's Health Initiative Prempro™ trial mentioned above has understandably created significant physician and patient concerns about the relative risk and benefits of HRT. My current practice is to advise continuing the use of ERT alone in women without a uterus, but to advise against the initiation or continued use of estrogen plus progestin combinations unless necessary to control hot flashes.

Androgen Replacement in Hypogonadal Women

Premenopausal circulating testosterone levels in women are approximately 10-fold lower than those seen in healthy men (22). They are maintained by the

Table 1
Who to Screen for Testosterone Deficiency

Adult women (receiving estrogen therapy or not)
  With a history of premenopausal pituitary, adrenal, or ovarian failure
  With postmenopausal complaints of reduced libido
Adult men (presenting with)
  Incomplete/absent secondary sexual development (for example, scanty beard
      development or reduced testicular size)
  Complaints of fatigue, reduced libido, and/or sexual dysfunction, especially those
      With chronic illness and complaints of fatigue, sexual dysfunction and/or reduced
        libido
      Receiving chronic supraphysiologic glucocorticoid treatment
      Over age 60
  A positive ADAM questionnaire response score

indirect production of testosterone from adrenal dehydroepiandrosterone (DHEA) and androstenedione and by the direct secretion of testosterone from the ovary. Adrenal DHEA secretion begins to decline in most women after the age of 30. This has been referred to as "adrenopause" and occurs at differing rates between individuals. Ovarian testosterone secretion declines by approximately 30% at menopause and then disappears almost entirely within the next decade. Although few studies have investigated the biologic effects of testosterone in women, several reports indicate that testosterone supplementation in ovariectomized women and some late menopausal patients results in a significant improvement in libido and sexual fantasy. More recent reports suggest, in addition, that testosterone supplementation may improve energy and depression (23) (Table 1).

Suspected testosterone deficiency is confirmed by a serum bioavailable or free testosterone value below the normal range for a premenopausal adult woman. As discussed later, these tests are more sensitive than the more commonly available total testosterone assay. Low-dose testosterone supplementation can be carried out using oral preparations containing methyl testosterone, sublingual testosterone, intramuscular long-acting testosterone esters, or compounded transdermal preparations. The most commonly used oral preparation is Estratest™, a combination of conjugated estrogens and methyl testosterone.

When administered alone, oral androgens have been shown to impact significantly on hepatic lipid metabolism by decreasing high-density lipoprotein (HDL) and increasing low-density (LDL). In contrast, estrogens alone both raise HDL and lower LDL. Lipid studies before and after the daily oral administration of 1.25 mg esterified estrogens and 2.5 mg of methyl testosterone (doses similar to those found in Estratest) showed significant decreases in total and HDL cholesterol and a decline in triglycerides *(24)*. This finding suggests that the conjugated estrogens in this preparation were not able to offset the deleterious HDL effects of the oral androgen.

Sublingual testosterone is rapidly absorbed into the systemic circulation but has a very short half-life. Thus repeated doses throughout the day would be required to maintain circulating levels of testosterone in a consistent physiologic range. A recent publication utilizing transdermal testosterone in hypoandrogenic women demonstrated effective restoration of high-normal serum free and bioavailable testosterone levels and midnormal premenopausal circulating testosterone levels, with improvements in libido, sexual function, and depression symptomatology. At this writing, however, neither the preparation used in that study nor other low-dose transdermal preparations have been approved for use by the Food and Drug Administration. Some clinicians have utilized compounding pharmacies to prepare reduced-strength topical testosterone creams or gels. However, there are no published studies regarding the efficacies or safety of these preparations.

I currently prefer to use intramuscular testosterone esters for female testosterone replacement. Intramuscular testosterone enanthate (Deletestryl™) or cypionate (Depotestosterone™) in doses of 20–50 mg intramuscularly every 10–14 d appears to reverse most sexual complaints, with only an approximate 10% incidence of mild hirsutism, which is usually reversed by lowering or discontinuing the medication. The much higher doses of testosterone supplementation used in men have occasionally been associated with increased fluid retention as well as increases in blood pressure and/or hemoglobin concentration. To date, however, these adverse long-term side effects have not been reported with low-dose testosterone supplementation in women.

RECOGNITION AND TREATMENT
OF HYPOGONADISM IN ADULT MEN

Somewhere between 4 and 5 million adult men in this country are believed to suffer from testosterone (T) deficiency. However, since these estimates are largely based on data using measurements of total testosterone (tT) values in blood, this incidence may be a significant underestimate (see the following discussion). Furthermore, only approximately 5% of recognized hypogonadal patients are currently receiving treatment, suggesting that T deficiency in adult men is both significantly underrecognized and undertreated.

The lack of T in men, like estrogen deficiency in women, has not been clearly linked to long-term increased mortality, but a number of metabolic derangements resulting from this condition are likely to have significant impact on quality of life (Table 1). These include loss of lean body and bone mass, increased fat mass, infertility, fatigue, depression, and loss of libido.

The appearance of primary gonadal failure in healthy mature men prior to their eighth decade is relatively uncommon and is usually linked to direct testicular damage resulting from gonadal radiation exposure, systemic chemotherapy, adult mumps orchitis, or castration. In contrast, secondary gonadal failure is relatively common. Hypothalamic or pituitary lesions (i.e., tumors or infiltrative diseases such as sarcoidosis or hemochromatosis) are relatively infrequent, whereas selective hypogonadotrophic hypogonadism appears to be a relatively common result of head trauma *(25)*. Physical stress owing to injury or illness has been linked to transient hypotestosteronemia. Emotional stress can also be a presumably reversible cause of secondary hypogonadism. Unquestionably, however, the most common cause of T deficiency in otherwise healthy men appears to be a physiologic process that accompanies aging. Gradual declines in T production have been shown to begin at about 40 yr of age in most healthy men. This stems from an apparent decrease in hypothalamic/pituitary feedback sensitivity to circulating T, which results in a gradual decline in T production in the face of normal serum LH and FSH concentrations. This secondary hypogonadism is often subtle, and it progresses until about age 70. Thereafter T levels continue to decline but are associated with increasing levels of LH, suggesting the appearance of an additional primary gonadal failure component in this age group. This phenomenon has been given several names, the most prevalent of which is andropause.

The gradual declines in T secretion observed in men aged 40–70 is often obscured clinically because it usually is not associated with major declines in circulating tT values. This occurs for two reasons. First, the normal range of tT is rather large, often spanning 250–1000 ng/mL. Small to moderate changes within this range, which, as noted above, occur without increases in gonadotropins, are easily missed or, if detected, considered to be clinically insignificant. A second reason is that the fractional conversion of T to estradiol increases with age in men. The resulting increases in circulating estrogen stimulate increased hepatic sex hormone binding globulin (SHBG) production. This results in an increase in tightly bound circulating T with reciprocal declines in free and loosely bound T. The blunted pituitary gonadotropins response to this gives rise to stable or slightly lower T production rates. This sequence of events results in fairly constant tT values despite continually declining circulating fractions of biologically active T.

Using longitudinal cross-sectional data from the Massachusetts Male Aging Study, a recent publication by Feldman et al. *(25)* has reported that tT drops by 0.8%/yr in men 40–70 yr old and that free testosterone (fT) and bioavailable testosterone (bvT; the sum of free and loosely bound hormone) decline by about 2% annually during the same period. However, data following the same subjects over time revealed a more pronounced drop in tT and fT or bvT of 1.6 and 2–3%/yr, respectively *(26)*. The extent to which these decreases in biologi-

Table 2
Androgen Deficiency in Aging Males (ADAM) Questionnaire[a]

1. **Do you have a decrease in sex drive?**
2. Do you have a lack of energy?
3. Do you have a decrease in strength and/or endurance?
4. Have you lost height?
5. Have you noticed a decreased enjoyment of life?
6. Are you sad and/or grumpy?
7. **Are your erections less strong?**
8. Has it been more difficult to maintain your erection throughout sexual intercourse?
9. Are you falling asleep after dinner?
10. Has your work performance deteriorated recently?

[a]Screening questionnaire for male hypogonadism. A positive response to questions 1 or 7, alone, or any three other questions, is considered preliminary evidence of hypogonadism.
Data from ref. 26.

cally active T result in reduced physiologic function remains ill defined and probably varies between individuals. Nevertheless, most authors agree that serum fT or bvT values in symptomatic patients, which fall below those seen in normal young men, are consistent with a diagnosis of hypogonadism.

Diagnosis

Given the relatively vague symptoms of hypogonadism, the search for T deficiency often begins only after the patient complains of erectile dysfunction or, less commonly, fatigue. Less frequently, it may be discovered during the evaluation of suspected hypopituitarism. The symptoms of hypogonadism include loss of libido, erectile dysfunction, fatigue, loss of stamina, and depression. These complaints are often minimized or completely withheld by patients during visits to health care providers for other reasons. They are uncovered much more frequently when health care providers incorporate specific questions about such symptoms or adopt a specifically designed screening questionnaire into their practice routines. Dr. John E. Morley at the St. Louis University School of Medicine *(9)* has developed one such instrument, the Androgen Deficiency in Aging Males (ADAM) questionnaire (Table 2). The presence of hypogonadism is strongly suggested by a positive answer to question number 1 or 7, or, alternatively, a positive answer to any three of the other questions. This test has recently been validated in a group of Canadian physicians *(27)*.

Circulating T in younger men exhibits a small but reproducible diurnal variation, with higher levels occurring in the morning. Biochemical evidence of hypotestosteronemia can be obtained by drawing a morning serum tT, fT, or bvT.

Given the impact of high SHBG on tT, tT values that return within the lower half of the normal range should be pursued with a measurement of either fT or bvT. I prefer to use bvT as the initial test, particularly in patients with obesity or either acute or chronic medical illnesses, since these conditions are often associated with additional influences on both SHBG and T production.

Serum tT values that clearly fall below the normal range for all ages usually represent unequivocal evidence of hypogonadism. However, this is not always true since conditions such as congenital SHBG deficiency (and even the presence of hyperinsulinemia) can on occasion lower SHBG adequately to produce sub-normal tT values. Several authorities consider that fT or bvT values below the normal range for a 30–40-yr-old man are compatible with hypogonadism as well, although this notion is somewhat more controversial (28). The presence of hypotestosteronemia should be pursued with measurement of LH, FSH, and prolactin. Since andropause alone is seldom associated with tT values below 150 ng/dL, patients demonstrating such values should be evaluated further for hypo-thalamic or pituitary lesions with magnetic resonance imaging of the head using thin cuts through the sella turcica.

Testosterone Treatment

Safe and effective androgen replacement therapy (ART) can be provided through the use of intramuscular long-acting testosterone esters, transdermal patches, or transdermal testosterone-containing gel (Table 3). Oral androgen replacement should be avoided because of the consistently deleterious effects of these preparations on LDL and HDL cholesterol levels and (less commonly) hepatic function.

Intramuscular T esters (cypionate, or enanthate) are initiated at doses of 200 mg im every 14 d or 100 mg every wk. Thereafter the dose and/or frequency of injections can be adjusted so that the total T value immediately preceding the next injection falls within the low- to midnormal range. This is the most inexpensive form of effective T replacement therapy. One potential disadvantage of this regimen, however, is that blood T frequently rises to values above 1000 ng/dL during the first few days following injection and then falls over time until the next dose. The resulting cyclic fluctuations in serum T that occur following repeated doses have been associated with concurrent mood swings in some individuals. Furthermore, the supraphysiologic T values attained early after each injection have been linked to a greater frequency of polycythemia than observed with other ART regimens (see Side Effects section below).

Nonscrotal transdermal T patches are currently available through two manu-facturers under the trade names Androderm™ and Testoderm TTS™. ART with these preparations is achieved by applying a 5-mg patch to nonscrotal skin daily. Blood levels rise to peak values within 4–6 h and thereafter remain in the mid to low physiologic range over the next 24 h. At present, a third alternative is the

Table 3
Testing and Treating Testosterone Deficiency in Symptomatic Men and Women

Screening (both genders)
  Serum bioavailable or free testosterone preferred over total testosterone (*see* text for discussion)
Starting treatment doses
  Women
    Testosterone ester (testosterone cypionate or -enanthate)
    20–50 mg im q 10–14 d
  Men
    Transdermal testosterone (preferred)
      Nonscrotal patch (5–7.5 mg/d)
      Alcohol-based testosterone gel (5–10 g/d)
        OR
    Testosterone ester 200 mg im q 10–14 d

daily application of T dissolved in an alcohol-based gel (Androgel™) to nonscrotal skin. It is available in packets containing either 2.5 or 5 g of 1% testosterone gel.

Although sexual dysfunction resulting from T deficiency appears to resolve at relatively low-dose T replacement, some authors suggest that the positive effects of T on bone and muscle may require consistent T values in the upper half of the normal range *(28)*. Therefore, serum total T should be monitored monthly during the initiation of transdermal ART, with dose titration upward until T levels above 500 ng/dL are achieved *(28)*.

Side Effects

The lipid effects reported for the ART therapies outlined above have been relatively minor and inconsistent between studies *(29)*. In contrast, both forms of treatment have been observed to stimulate red blood cell production and, in some patients, to produce frank polycythemia *(30,31)*. Current studies suggest that these responses may parallel the peak serum T concentrations achieved, since they are most commonly seen with the use of intramuscular T esters *(32,33)*. Patients most likely to develop significant hemoglobin changes appear to be elderly men and cigarette smokers of any age. Hemoglobin levels should be accessed at baseline, after 3 and 6 mo of treatment, and annually thereafter.

ART has also been infrequently linked to fluid retention and hypertension. When encountered, these effects generally occur within the first 1–3 mo of T replacement. Again, these effects appear to be more frequent with intramuscular T. It has been my anecdotal experience that patients who demonstrate these side effects, even with transdermal T therapy, may be managed successfully with twice-weekly 1000 U intramuscular injections of human chorionic gonadotropin, which stimulates testicular Leydig cell T secretion.

The prostate gland is a classical androgen target tissue, and concerns have been raised about the possible impact of ART on the subsequent development of benign prostatic hypertrophy and/or prostate cancer. Certainly a past history of prostate cancer is an absolute contraindication for T therapy. Prospective trials published to date have not demonstrated deleterious effects of ART on either potential complication in otherwise healthy men *(33)*. Prostate pathologies, however, are thought to evolve over the course of two or more decades, and currently published investigations cover observation periods far shorter. Thus, the long-term safety of ART has not been fully established. For this reason, a baseline prostate-specific antigen (PSA) and digital rectal examination should be performed in all patients who are ART candidates. A urologist should evaluate patients with elevated PSA before T replacement is begun. PSA values in men over 40 then should be monitored at 3 and 6 mo following the beginning of ART and annually thereafter. Digital rectal examination, blood pressure testing, and hemoglobin concentration assay should be performed annually in all ART patients as well.

Responses to ART

Symptoms of reduced libido and sexual dysfunction that result in hypogonadism should improve within a few weeks of instituting adequate T replacement. Strength and energy complaints may take somewhat longer to improve. Although there are several excellent studies showing beneficial affects of ART upon muscle mass, strength, sexual function, libido, and skeletal mass in men with severe hypogonadism *(34,35)*, fewer data are available regarding patients with more subtle T deficiency. Since ART is designed primarily to improve quality of life, it is my practice to discontinue such therapy after 3 mo in patients who find no symptomatic benefit.

REFERENCES

1. Tansey MJ, Schlechte JA. Pituitary production of prolactin and prolactin-suppressing drugs. Lupus 2001;10:660–664.
2. Loprinzi CL, Michalak JC, Quella SK. Megestrol acetate for the prevention of hot flashes. N Engl J Med 1994;331:347–352.
3. Pandya KJ, Raubertas RF, Flynn PJ, et al. Oral clonidine in postmenopausal patients with breast cancer experiencing tamoxifen-induced hot flashes: a University of Rochester Cancer Center Community Clinical Oncology Program study. Ann Intern Med 2000;132:788–793.
4. Stearns V, Isaacs C, Rowland J, et al. A pilot trial assessing the efficacy of paroxetine hydrochloride (Paxil) in controlling hot flashes in breast cancer survivors. Ann Oncol 2000;11:17–22.
5. David A, Don R, Tajchner G, Weissglas L. Veralipride: alternative antidopaminergic treatment for menopausal symptoms. Am J Obstet Gynecol 1988;158:1107–1115.

6. Moghissi KS. Hormone replacement therapy for menopausal women. Compr Ther 2000;26:197–202.
7. Yaffe K. Estrogens, selective estrogen receptor modulators, and dementia: what is the evidence? Ann NY Acad Sci 2001;949:215–222
8. Halbreich U, Kahn LS. Role of estrogen in the aetiology and treatment of mood disorders. CNS Drugs 2001;15:797–817
9. Bachmann G. Physiologic aspects of natural and surgical menopause. J Reprod Med 2001;46(3 suppl):307–315.
10. Grodstein F, Manson JE, Colditz GA, Willett WC, Speizer FE, Stampfer MJ. A prospective, observational study of postmenopausal hormone therapy and primary prevention of cardiovascular disease. Ann Intern Med 2000;133:933–941.
11. Bush TL, Barrett-Connor E, Cowan LD, et al. Cardiovascular mortality and noncontraceptive use of estrogen in women: results from the Lipid Research Clinics Program Follow-up Study. Circulation 1987;75:1102–1109.
12. Petitti DB, Perlman JA, Sidney S. Noncontraceptive estrogens and mortality: long-term follow-up of women in the Walnut Creek Study. Obstet Gynecol 1987;70:289–293.
13. Henderson BE, Paganini-Hill A, Ross RK. Decreased mortality in users of estrogen replacement therapy. Arch Intern Med 1991;151:75–78.
14. Psaty BM, Hackbert SR, Atkins D, et al. The risk of myocardial infarction associated with the combined use of estrogen and progestin in postmenopausal women. Arch Intern Med 1994;154:1333–1339.
15. Hulley S, Grady, D Bush T, et al., for the Heart and Estrogen/Progestin Replacement Study (HERS) Research Group. Randomized trial of estrogen plus progestin for secondary prevention of coronary heart disease in postmenopausal women. JAMA 1998;280:605–613.
16. Cherry N. Oestrogen therapy for prevention of reinfarction in postmenopausal women: a randomized placebo controlled trial. Lancet 2002;360:2001–2008.
17. Manson JE, Martin KA. Clinical practice. Postmenopausal hormone-replacement therapy. N Engl J Med 2001;345:34.
18. Mosca L, Collins P, Herrington DM, et al. Hormone replacement therapy and cardiovascular disease: a statement for healthcare professionals from the American Heart Association. Circulation 2001;104:499.
19. Writing group for the Women's Health Initiative investigators, Risks and benefits of estrogen plus progestin in healthy women; Principal results from the Women's Health Initiative Randomized Controlled Trial. JAMA 2002;288:321–333.
20. Utian WH, Shoupe D, Bachmann G, Pinkerton JV, Pickar JH. Relief of vasomotor symptoms and vaginal atrophy with lower doses of conjugated equine estrogens and medroxyprogesterone acetate. Fertil Steril 2001;75:1065–1079.
21. Ravn P, Bidstrup M, Wasnich RD, et al. Alendronate and estrogen-progestin in the long-term prevention of bone loss: four-year results from the early postmenopausal intervention cohort study. A randomized, controlled trial. Ann Intern Med 1999;131:935–942.
22. Bardin CW, Lipsett MB. Testosterone and androstenedione blood production rates in normal women and women with idiopathic hirsutism or polycystic ovaries. J Clin Invest 1967;46:891.
23. Shifren JL, Braunstein GD, Simon JA, et al. Transdermal testosterone treatment in women with impaired sexual function after oophorectomy. N Engl J Med 2000;343:682–688.
24. Watts, NB, Notelovitz, M, Timmons, MC, et al. Comparison of oral estrogens and estrogen plus androgen on bone mineral density, menopausal symptoms and lipid-lipoprotein profiles in surgical menopause. Obstet Gynecol 1995;85:529.
25. Benvenga S, Campenni A, Ruggeri RM, Trimarchi F. Hypopituitarism secondary to head trauma. J Clin Endocrinol Metab 2000;85:1353–1361.

26. Feldman HA, Longcope C, Derby CA, et al. Age trends in the level of serum testosterone and other hormones in middle-aged men: longitudinal results from the Massachusetts male aging study. J Clin Endocrinol Metab 2002;87:589–598.

27. Morley JE, Charlton E, Patrick P, et al. Validation of a screening questionnaire for androgen deficiency in aging males. Metabolism 2000;49:1239–242.

28. Summary of the Consensus Session from the 1st Annual Andropause Consensus 2000 Meeting, the Endocrine Society.

29. Singh AB, Hsia S, Alaupovic P, et al. The effects of varying doses of T on insulin sensitivity, plasma lipids, apolipoproteins, and C-reactive protein in healthy young men. J Clin Endocrinol Metab 2002;87:136–143.

30. Hajjar RR, Kaiser FE, Morley JE. Outcomes of long-term testosterone replacement in older hypogonadal males: a retrospective analysis. J Clin Endocrinol Metab 1997;82:3793–3796.

31. Viallard JF, Marit G, Mercie P, Leng B, Reiffers J, Pellegrin JL. Polycythaemia as a complication of transdermal testosterone therapy. Br J Haematol 2000;110:237–238.

32. Dobs AS, Meikle AW, Arver S, Sanders SW, Caramelli KE, Mazer NA. Pharmacokinetics, efficacy, and safety of a permeation-enhanced testosterone transdermal system in comparison with bi-weekly injections of testosterone enanthate for the treatment of hypogonadal men. J Clin Endocrinol Metab 1999;84:3469–3478

33. Bhasin S, ed. The Endocrine Society Clinical Bulletins in Andropause: Benefits and Risks of Treating Hypogonadism in the Aging Male, no. 2, 2002.

34. Gambineri A, Pasquali R. Testosterone therapy in men: clinical and pharmacological perspectives. J Endocrinol Invest 2000;23:196–214

35. Zitzmann M, Nieschlag E. Hormone substitution in male hypogonadism. Mol Cell Endocrinol 2000;161:73–88.

18 Osteoporosis and Osteomalacia

Whitney S. Goldner, MD,
and Joseph S. Dillon, MD

CONTENTS

OSTEOPOROSIS: *EARLY DIAGNOSIS AND MANAGEMENT*

Introduction

Osteoporosis is a metabolic bone disorder characterized by low bone mass and microarchitectural deterioration of bone tissue, leading to enhanced fragility and a consequent increase in fracture risk *(1).* Clinically, it is defined by evidence of osteopenia associated with a fracture, or history of fractures with minimal trauma. It is defined quantitatively as a bone mineral density (BMD) of less than 2.5 SD below the mean gender-matched maximal bone density *(1).*

Osteoporosis results from an imbalance between the rates of bone resorption and formation. Bone remodeling is a continuous process that occurs in an orderly fashion of bone resorption followed by bone formation (synthesis of bone matrix and its subsequent mineralization). The resorption and formation processes are tightly coupled in healthy bone. This entire cycle of bone formation takes approximately 8 mo *(2).* If the process of resorption and formation is not matched, there is remodeling imbalance, which results in continuous slow bone loss.

The causes of osteoporosis are considered either primary or secondary. The etiology of primary osteoporosis is mainly age-related estrogen deficiency secondary to menopause *(3).* After attaining peak bone mass in young adulthood (usually the second or third decade), bone mineral density remains fairly constant for men and women until middle life *(3).* Postmenopausal women have two

From: *Contemporary Endocrinology: Early Diagnosis and Treatment of Endocrine Disorders*
Edited by: R. S. Bar © Humana Press Inc., Totowa, NJ

phases of bone loss, whereas men have only one. The first phase in women is rapid and is secondary to a 90% decrease in estradiol at the time of menopause. It lasts for approximately 5–10 yr and results primarily in cancellous bone loss. It is estimated that over a decade there is a 20–30% loss in cancellous bone and a 5–10% loss in cortical bone. This phase merges with a slower phase of bone loss that is more generalized, continues indefinitely, and affects both men and women. The slow phase usually results in a 20–30% lifetime decline in both cancellous and cortical bone. Age-related increases in parathyroid hormone (PTH), as a result of decreased available calcium and vitamin D, are also thought to contribute to primary osteoporosis (2). Secondary osteoporosis occurs when a predisposing medical disorder directly, or indirectly, results in abnormal bone metabolism and eventual osteoporosis.

Osteoporosis, which affects approximately 10 million persons in the United States alone, is a major cause of morbidity and mortality in the aging population (4). Fractures are the most common cause of morbidity and mortality. These fractures are typically at the hip, spine, and distal forearm. The lifetime risk of a hip fracture in Caucasian women is 15–17.5%, with a comparable risk in Caucasian men of 5.5–6% (5–7). This compares with a 5% risk in African-American women and a 3% risk in African-American men (7). Hip fractures lead to an overall reduction in survival of about 15%, and most excess deaths are within the first 6 mo following a fracture (5,6). In addition to the increased mortality secondary to fractures, patients with fractures often have chronic back or hip pain, gait instability, kyphosis, and difficulties with activities of daily living. Preventive strategies, early intervention, and treatment have proved to be beneficial in reducing the number of long-term effects from osteoporosis.

Given the extent of the problem in the population, the severity of the complications for both the individual and society, and the demonstrated benefit of early intervention, it is important that clinicians recognize the risk factors, screen appropriately, and initiate therapy early in the course of the disorder. This chapter reviews issues related to screening, early diagnosis, and management of individuals with osteoporosis.

Risk Factors

Risk factors predisposing individuals to osteoporosis have been well characterized. Identifying these risk factors in patients facilitates early screening and advice about prophylaxis and treatment. The major risk factors are noted in Table 1 and are discussed further in the following paragraphs.

AGE

Age over 65 yr is directly associated with the occurrence of osteoporosis (8). Using a risk factor questionnaire and subsequent dual x-ray absorptiometry (DXA) scan, Weinstein and Ullery (8) showed that the mean age of individuals

Table 1
Risk Factors for Osteoporosis

Age
Environmental/lifestyle factors
Drugs
Malignancy
Connective tissue diseases
Organ transplant
Genetics
Menstrual status
Endocrine diseases
Gastrointestinal diseases
Chronic obstructive pulmonary disease
Anorexia nervosa

presenting with osteoporosis of the hip was 68.9 yr; for those presenting with osteoporosis of the vertebral spine, it was 66.6 yr. The American Academy of Clinical Endocrinologists (AACE) and the National Osteoporosis Foundation (NOF) currently recommend that all women over 65 yr be screened for osteoporosis (4,9). The National Institutes of Health (NIH) recommends screening based on clinical indications and personal risk factors rather than an absolute age (10).

GENETICS

Ethnic background is important when considering risk factors for osteoporosis. Some authors estimate that 30% of the postmenopausal Caucasian population is affected by osteoporosis (11). Caucasian and Asian women are at greater risk for osteoporosis than African-American, African-Caribbean, or Polynesian populations (11,12). African-Caribbean young adults have higher BMD than Caucasian adults at the lumbar spine, femoral neck, and total body (12). The same studies showed that men have higher baseline BMD than women at all sites, except for the femoral neck. African-American women and men also have lower fracture rates than Caucasian populations (7). African Americans have increased BMD, greater cross-sectional geometric properties in the femoral neck, and smaller endocortical diameter of the femoral neck. These properties allow the femoral neck to resist greater loading in African-American persons compared with Caucasians (13).

Family studies have demonstrated that mothers with osteoporotic fractures more commonly have daughters with lower bone density (14). The bone density deficit seems to be relatively specific to skeletal sites. This may imply that predisposition to osteoporotic fractures is partly owing to inherited factors in bone mass, density, and/or material quality of bone *(14)*. Bone geometry and hip axis length (the distance from the lateral surface of the trochanter to the inner surface of the pelvis) is also very important in the risk for hip fractures. Notably, Asian populations have shorter hip axis length, which results in stronger structure and fewer fractures in the hip compared with other sites *(2)*. The AACE currently recommends that women be screened for osteoporosis if any first-degree female relatives have been diagnosed with osteoporosis or have sustained low-trauma fracture *(9)*.

ENVIRONMENTAL AND LIFESTYLE FACTORS

Body Mass Index. Osteoporosis and body mass index (BMI) are inversely related. Women in the lowest tertile of BMI have approximately 10% lower BMD, in addition to increased bone resorption markers, compared with women in the highest tertile of BMI *(15)*. Overall, there is a difference of 20% in BMD between the extreme tertiles of BMI. Other investigators also find that low body weight and BMI are risk factors for osteoporosis and recommend that if a woman weighs less than 140 pounds at the time of menopause, she should be screened for osteoporosis *(8)*. The AACE recommends screening women who are postmenopausal and weigh less than 127 pounds *(9)*. Fortunately, the negative effect on BMD can be fully counteracted by hormone replacement therapy (HRT) or estrogen replacement therapy (ERT) if started at the onset of menopause *(15)*.

Tobacco Smoking. On average, smokers have 4% lower BMD that nonsmokers *(15)*. When a smoker also has a thin body habitus, the two have an additive effect on BMD *(15)*. Thin women who smoke cigarettes have 14% lower BMD than controls. The mechanism for this bone loss is controversial. Some studies suggest that smoking does not increase the risk for hip fracture in itself, but negates the protective skeletal effects of ERT or HRT *(16)*. Other studies show that smoking reduces the response to low-dose ERT (1 mg of estradiol) but not to high-dose treatment (2 mg of estradiol) *(15)*. This could indicate that high-dose estrogen is potent enough to overcome smoking as a risk factor. However, further studies are needed before recommending this therapy, since the combination of smoking and high-dose estrogen increases the risk of venous thromboembolism from estrogen.

Immobilization. Complete immobilization enhances bone resorption without adequate bone formation. Standing upright with postural shifting can usually prevent this process. Complete spinal cord injury patients have significantly lower BMD compared with incomplete spinal cord injury patients (who retain limited mobility) *(17)* and ambulatory controls *(18)*. By 12 mo after a complete spinal cord injury, there is a 28% decrease in radius BMD and a 15% decrease in tibia BMD *(19)*. Disuse osteoporosis is a phenomenon described in astronauts. It is bone loss that occurs with skeletal unloading, mainly affecting the bones most stressed by gravity. This phenomenon can also be seen in immobilized extremities and is termed regional osteoporosis *(20)*. Regional osteoporosis is clearly demonstrated when evaluating BMD in tetraplegics and paraplegics. Both groups have significantly reduced BMD (reduced 15% in the tibia) in the lower extremities, but only the tetraplegic group has reduced BMD in the upper extremities (reduced 28% in the radius). The paraplegics retain normal BMD in the spine and upper extremities *(19)*. Other studies have shown that BMD in the spine actually increases over time in paraplegics and quadraplegics *(21)*. This phenomenon of regional osteoporosis helps explain why spinal cord injury patients have an increased incidence of lower extremity fractures compared with other sites. Small studies have shown that early intervention with loading and weight-bearing exercises improves lower extremity BMD *(22)*.

MENSTRUAL STATUS

Estrogen inhibits bone resorption, and decreased exposure to estrogen can be a significant risk factor for osteoporosis in women. Anovulatory states are also a risk factor for osteoporosis. In anovulatory states, the unifying etiology for osteoporosis appears to be estrogen deficiency *(23)*. Gonadal failure can also cause accelerated bone loss. Amenorrheic girls with Turner's syndrome have significantly reduced BMD compared with eumenorrheic peers without Turner's syndrome *(24)*. The same study showed some improvement in BMD with the administration of estrogen. There is an association between wrist, hip, and vertebral fractures and later age of menarche *(25)*. Hence, it seems reasonable to believe that women with late initiation of menses or premature menopause are at increased risk for osteoporosis.

DRUGS

Glucocorticoids. Glucocorticoids impair bone remodeling by a combination of factors. Decreased osteoblast recruitment and differentiation, as well as increased bone resorption through enhancement of osteoclast activity, leads to decreased bone synthesis and increased resorption *(26)*. Other mechanisms include decreased intestinal calcium absorption, alterations in vitamin D metabolism, and increased renal calcium excretion. These changes result in increased intact PTH levels and secondary hyperparathyroidism *(27–29)*. Glucocorticoids have complex effects on vitamin D metabolism and activity, with increased 1,25-dihydroxy vitamin D but decreased vitamin D receptor expression or function *(26)*. Glucocorticoids indirectly inhibit the production of gonadotropic hormones. This results in a decrease in estrogen and androgen levels, which are important for bone preservation *(26)*.

Anticoagulants. Unfractionated heparin accelerates bone resorption and decreases the rate of cancellous bone formation, even when used for short periods *(30)*. Although osteoporosis was initially described with prolonged heparin therapy *(31)*, even low-dose unfractionated heparin for short periods may result in osteopenia *(32)*. Fortunately, low-molecular-weight (LMW) heparin may have less effect on bone density. A comparison of LMW and unfractionated heparin showed that the LMW heparin produced less osteopenia *(30)*. In contrast to unfractionated heparin, LMW heparin appears to decrease the rate of bone formation but does not affect bone resorption in cancellous bone.

Antiepileptics. Antiepileptic therapy can result in osteoporosis, osteomalacia, or both. Phenytoin and phenobarbital induce hepatic microsomal enzymes, causing enzymatic degradation of vitamin D *(33)*, resulting in demineralization of bone and osteomalacia. A study of institutionalized epileptics on phenytoin and phenobarbital showed a marked increase in fracture incidence compared with controls *(34)*. Reduced sunlight exposure and vitamin D intake may be additional risk factors in these patients, given their already impaired vitamin D metabolism *(33)*. Valproate monotherapy reduces axial and appendicular BMD in children on long-term antiepileptics. Since valproate does not induce hepatic enzymes, its mechanism for bone loss is unclear *(34)*. The effect of carbamazepine on bone metabolism is controversial, with some authors finding that it results in disordered bone metabolism and others finding no effect *(33,34)*.

Ethanol. Ethanol can cause osteoporosis directly or indirectly. Alcoholics have a reduced number of osteoblasts and a reduced rate of osteoid formation and subsequent mineralization *(35)*. Alcohol does not appear to have an effect on bone resorption *(35,36)*. Nutritional status may also play a role in alcoholic osteoporosis, since chronic alcohol intake is often associated with poor calcium and vitamin D intake *(37)*.

Chemotherapy. Chemotherapy may result in disrupted bone metabolism through many mechanisms. The most common etiology is chemotherapy-induced primary gonadal failure, resulting in hypogonadism and disordered bone metabolism. This commonly occurs when treating Hodgkin's or non-Hodgkin's lymphoma with alkylating agents and radiation *(38)*. There are also effects on the skeleton that are independent of gonadal function. Methotrexate causes uncoupling of bone turnover by inhibiting osteoblast proliferation *(38)*. Ifosfamide, an alkylating agent, often causes hypogonadism. However, it has also been shown to damage the renal proximal tubule, resulting in hypercalciuria, increased renal phosphate loss, and (rarely) hypophosphatemic rickets *(38)*. Cyclophosphamide increases the risk of osteoporosis by decreasing the total number of osteoblasts and osteoclasts. Glucocorticoids are often part of chemotherapy regimens, which compound the risk for osteoporosis.

Immunosuppressants. *See* Organ Transplant section below for a discussion of cyclosporine and tacrolimus, and *see* Glucocorticoid section above for a discussion of glucocorticoids.

Gonadotropin-Releasing Hormone Agonists. When gonadotropin-releasing hormone (GnRH) agonists are given in a pulsatile fashion, they stimulate the normal pituitary gonadotropin secretion. However, when given continuously, they suppress pituitary luteinizing hormone (LH) and follicle-stimulating hormone (FSH) secretion, inhibiting testosterone and estrogen production. Men with prostate cancer who are on continuous GnRH agonists have significantly lower BMD at the lateral lumbar spine and forearm, as well as increased markers of bone resorption compared with controls *(39)*.

ENDOCRINE DISEASES

Hypogonadism. Primary ovarian failure is the most common cause of postmenopausal or primary osteoporosis. However, all forms of hypogonadism are risk factors for osteoporosis. Hypogonadism can result from primary ovarian and testicular failure or hypothalamus-pituitary axis (HPA) dysfunction (as in anorexia nervosa or athletically-induced amenorrhea) *(37)*. Estrogen deficiency has been established as the etiology of osteoporosis in women with hypogonadism *(23)*. The etiology of osteoporosis in men is believed to be testosterone deficiency. Studies have shown severe osteopenia in men with idiopathic hypogonadotropic hypogonadism *(40)* and an improvement in bone mass with the reversal of hypogonadism and increased serum testosterone in hyperprolactinemic hypogonadal men (independent of prolactin levels) *(41)*. However, a recent study found that low serum testosterone had no relationship to BMD at any bone site, whereas estradiol levels were directly correlated with BMD *(42)*. This may imply that estrogen rather than testosterone plays a significant etiologic role in osteoporosis in hypogonadal men. This theory is supported in studies of males with aromatase deficiency and osteopenia who developed increased BMD and normal serum levels of estrogen and gonadotropins while receiving transdermal estrogen therapy *(43)*. Further studies are needed to evaluate the role of androgens and estrogens in BMD in males.

Hemochromatosis can cause hypogonadism and hence is a risk factor for osteoporosis. Both hypergonadotropic and hypogonadotropic hypogonadism may be seen in hemochromatosis, caused by either testicular or pituitary iron deposition *(44)*. Early detection and treatment of hemochromatosis should prevent these late complications.

Hyperparathyroidism. All forms of hyperparathyroidism can cause osteoporosis. PTH increases cancellous bone density by stimulating bone formation. However, it also increases bone resorption markers when used as treatment for osteoporosis *(45)*. Patients with hyperparathyroidism have cortical bone loss with either mild loss, or preservation of cancellous bone *(46,47)*. Hence, it is common for these patients to have a predominance of forearm compared with vertebral fractures *(37)*.

Hypercortisolemia. The mechanism for bone loss in Cushing's syndrome is the same as that seen with chronic exogenous glucocorticoid treatment (*see* Glucocorticoid section above). Usually the signs of Cushing's syndrome are apparent, but rarely patients may present with osteoporosis and compression fractures *(48)*. Thus it is important to consider the diagnosis of Cushing's syndrome in individuals presenting with osteoporosis.

Thyroid Disorders. Hyperthyroidism, either as a primary disease or as a result of treatment with thyroid hormone, is well established as an etiology of disordered bone metabolism *(49–51)*. Thyroid hormones stimulate bone resorption by increasing the number of osteoclasts, the number of resorption sites, and the ratio of resorptive to formative surfaces in cortical and cancellous bone *(50,51)*. There are usually more detrimental effects on cortical bone than on cancellous bone *(50,51)*. BMD is even further impacted if patients have additional risk factors (e.g., estrogen deficiency) for osteoporosis. Once euthyroid status is attained in an individual with hyperthyroidism, BMD improves slightly but does not go back to baseline, even after 2 yr of euthyroidism *(51)*.

Patients with thyroid cancer present a dilemma since they are treated with higher doses of thyroxine to suppress their thyroid-stimulating hormone (TSH). This presumably increases their risk for osteoporosis. However, studies have been conflicting and show either a rapid decline or no significant change in bone mass while patients are on therapy *(52)*. Bisphosphonate therapy increases BMD at the spine and hip in thyroid cancer patients on suppressive doses of thyroxine *(52)*. At present, we feel it is important to monitor free thyroxine and TSH levels frequently when a patient is on thyroid replacement or suppressive therapy and to determine therapy on an individual basis.

MALIGNANCY

Lymphoma, leukemia, multiple myeloma, systemic mastocytosis, and malignancy with bone metastases are the most common etiologies of malignancy-induced osteoporosis *(37)*. In general, any disease that infiltrates the bone marrow (lymphoma, leukemia, metastases) can cause a disruption in the skeletal remodeling process and result in osteoporosis. Patients with systemic mastocytosis have osteoidosis (accelerated bone remodeling) in the trabecular bone, peritrabecular fibrosis, increased numbers of osteoblasts and osteoclasts, and an increase in the osteoclastic resorbing surfaces *(53)*. In multiple myeloma, osteoclast-stimulating cytokines [interleukin-1 (IL-1), IL-6, tumor necrosis factor (TNF), and lymphotoxin] are produced that cause increased bone resorption. There also appears to be inhibition of osteoblast activity and bone formation in multiple myeloma *(37)*. Patients with multiple myeloma or monoclonal gammopathy of unknown significance (MGUS) have decreased concentrations of serum bone formation markers compared with healthy controls *(54)*.

GASTROINTESTINAL DISEASES

Disorders of the gastrointestinal tract can result in osteoporosis or osteomalacia. Common culprits are inflammatory bowel disease *(55,56)*, gluten-sensitive enteropathy *(57)*, postgastrectomy status *(58)*, and primary biliary cirrhosis

(PBC) *(59)*. The etiology of osteoporosis secondary to inflammatory bowel disease is usually considered to be chronic glucocorticoid treatment *(37)*. However, calcium malabsorption, altered sex hormone status, malnutrition, and vitamin D deficiency are additional hypothesized mechanisms for osteoporosis in inflammatory bowel disease *(56)*. Some authors suggest that osteoblast function is inhibited in PBC owing to the toxic effects of substances that are normally cleared by the liver *(59)*. Both gluten-sensitive enteropathy and postgastrectomy patients develop osteoporosis and osteomalacia *(57,58)*. Malabsorption of calcium, with or without vitamin D, may result in secondary hyperparathyroidism and osteoporosis, whereas malabsorption of vitamin D alone usually results in osteomalacia. Patients with gluten-sensitive enteropathy regain BMD after initiation of treatment with a gluten-free diet *(57)*. This finding suggests that treating the underlying etiology of malabsorption, or replacement with calcium and vitamin D if the disease cannot be fully reversed, should help to reverse or slow the process of bone loss.

CONNECTIVE TISSUE DISEASES

Connective tissue diseases are an independent risk factor for osteoporosis. The exact mechanisms are not known, but they are thought to be a combination of local disease-related inflammatory mediators and disuse osteoporosis. Goldring *(60)* describes three forms of bone loss in patients with rheumatoid arthritis. First, local erosions result from synovial inflammatory cells invading bone in the inflamed joint. Second, migration of inflammatory cells causes increased bone turnover and osteopenia in bones adjacent to inflamed joints. Last, systemic inflammatory mediators may cause overall reduced BMD. Patients with systemic lupus erythematosis, ankylosing spondylitis, and juvenile rheumatoid arthritis have also been reported to have a reduction in both cortical and cancellous bone *(60)*. The mechanism is felt to be similar to that seen in patients with rheumatoid arthritis. Many patients with connective tissue diseases are also on chronic steroids, methotrexate, and other immune modulators that can result in disordered bone metabolism.

CHRONIC OBSTRUCTIVE PULMONARY DISEASE

Osteoporosis is extremely common in patients with end-stage pulmonary disease *(61)*. Most patients with chronic obstructive pulmonary disease (COPD) have osteoporosis secondary to chronic glucocorticoid therapy. However, the degree of pulmonary impairment also affects bone density, independent of corticosteroid usage. Bone density of the spine is highly correlated with lung function *(62)*. This finding suggests that all patients with COPD should be assessed for osteoporosis, not just COPD patients on steroids. Furthermore, these patients should be given adequate calcium and vitamin D supplementation.

Anorexia Nervosa

Osteoporosis can be a very serious complication of anorexia nervosa. Individuals with anorexia develop profound osteopenia of cancellous and cortical bone and are at significantly increased risk of fractures *(63)*. More than 50% of women with anorexia have been reported to have a BMD less than 2 SD below normal *(64)*. The etiology of osteoporosis is thought to be multifactorial *(63)*. Virtually all women with anorexia nervosa are amenorrheic and hypogonadal. Therefore, hypogonadism was thought to play a major role in the etiology of osteoporosis in these women. However, estrogen/progestin administration along with calcium does not prevent bone loss or improve BMD in women with active disease *(64)*. Thus, estrogen deficiency and hypogonadism are not the sole etiologies for osteoporosis in these women. Nutritional status, calcium and vitamin D deficiency, excess physical activity resulting in stress fractures, hypercortisolemia, and low serum insulin-like growth factor-1 (IGF-1) levels are also thought to contribute to disordered bone metabolism *(63)*. At present, there is not an effective therapy for regaining bone losses during the time of active disease.

Organ Transplant

Bone loss may be severe and rapid after solid organ or bone marrow transplant. A major component of the bone loss is effects from glucocorticoid therapy used as part of the immunosuppressive regimen. However, both cyclosporine and tacrolimus independently cause increased bone resorption without adequate bone formation *(27,65)*. The occurrence of osteoporosis is best correlated with the cumulative dose of steroids and the duration of cyclosporine therapy in graft-versus-host disease *(65)*. Rapid bone loss (6% and 10% loss at the lumbar spine and femoral neck, respectively) occurs in the first 6 mo after heart transplantation *(66)*. Cancellous bone (lumbar spine and total hip) seems to stabilize at 6 mo after transplant, but there is continued loss in the cortical bone after 6 mo.

It is common for lung, renal, and bone marrow transplant patients to have evidence of osteoporosis prior to transplant *(27,61,65)*. The etiology of pretransplant osteoporosis in lung transplant patients is decreased lung function and chronic glucocorticoid therapy *(62)*. Etiologies of osteoporosis in end-stage renal patients awaiting transplant include secondary hyperparathyroidism, osteomalacia, and adynamic bone disease *(27)*. It is important to note that persistent hyperparathyroidism after renal transplant contributes to osteopenia and osteoporosis and may mandate parathyroidectomy.

Guidelines for Osteoporosis Screening

Every patient should have a comprehensive history and physical examination. The AACE recommends that certain populations be screened routinely for osteoporosis. These populations include all women aged 65 yr or older, all adult women with a history of fracture not caused by severe trauma, and younger

Table 2
Indications for Assessment of Bone Mineral Density[a]

For risk assessment in perimenopausal or postmenopausal women who have risk factors for fractures and are willing to consider available interventions

In men and women who have x-ray findings that suggest osteoporosis

In men and women who are receiving chronic glucocorticoid therapy of greater than physiologic replacement dose (prednisone 7.5 mg or equivalent daily) or who are receiving long-term therapy with other drugs associated with bone loss

In all adult women with hyperparathyroidism or other diseases or nutritional conditions associated with bone loss in whom evidence of bone loss would result in adjustment of management

For establishing skeletal stability and monitoring therapeutic response in men and women receiving treatment for osteoporosis (baseline measurements are made before intervention)

In all women 40 yr old or older who have sustained a fracture

In all women beyond 65 yr of age

Individuals who are candidates for solid organ or bone marrow transplantation

Individuals with chronic diseases known to be associated with osteoporosis, including malabsorptive gastrointestinal diseases

Individuals with Cushing's disease

Individuals with chronically suppressed thyroid-stimulating hormone related to thyroid hormone suppression therapy for thyroid cancer

[a]Based on the American Association of Clinical Endocrinologists 2001 clinical practice guidelines for osteoporosis (9) and our own practice.

postmenopausal women who have clinical risk factors for fractures (low body weight or strong family history of osteoporosis with vertebral or hip fractures) (9). The AACE recommendations for assessments of BMD are noted in Table 2.

The accepted screening and diagnostic test for osteoporosis is an assessment of BMD using the DXA scan. The criteria for the diagnosis of osteoporosis based on DXA BMD are listed in Table 3. There are other methods to measure BMD including quantitative computed tomography (CT) of the spine, forearm, or hip, quantitative ultrasound of the heel, forearm, tibia, phalanges, or metatarsals, and single-energy x-ray absorptiometry (9). However, the DXA remains the standard for assessment of BMD. Some studies have found heel ultrasound to be equal to DXA, when screening for osteoporosis, in renal transplant patients and children with rheumatic diseases (67,68). In these studies the authors recommend that, if the heel ultrasound is abnormal, then patients should be referred for DXA scan and more definitive evaluation. Heel ultrasound in at-risk patients may prove to be a less expensive, more available way of screening high-risk populations (such as patients with known secondary causes) for osteoporosis. However, comparative studies between heel ultrasound and hip or spine DXA in the general population undergoing BMD assessment have shown poor correlation (69). A

Table 3
WHO Criteria for Osteoporosis and Osteopenia

Osteoporosis:	BMD over 2.5 SD less than mean for young adults
Osteopenia:	BMD 1–2.5 SD less than mean for young adults
Normal:	BMD within 1 SD of the young adult reference
T-score:	BMD compared with healthy women at peak bone mass
	Osteoporosis: T < –2.5.
	Osteopenia: –1.0 > T-score > – 2.5
	Normal: T > –1.0
Z-score:	BMD compared with age-matched controls
	When the z-score is <–2.0, suspect osteoporosis from secondary causes

BMD, bone mineral density.
Data from refs. *1* and *123*.

definitive assessment of the role of heel ultrasound in the evaluation of bone density will have to await the results of further studies.

Primary osteoporosis is a diagnosis of exclusion. If a patient is found to have a BMD less than 2.5 SD below the young adult mean, all secondary causes should be considered and ruled out before primary osteoporosis can be diagnosed and treated. It is important to remember that patients should not begin treatment until the workup has been completed, as this may make certain laboratory values difficult to interpret.

The history and physical examination should include evaluation for the risk factors and predisposing medical or environmental conditions, as previously noted. Basic laboratory tests on initial evaluation should include a complete blood count, serum calcium, phosphorus, total protein, albumin, liver enzymes, alkaline phosphatase, creatinine, electrolytes, and urinary calcium excretion *(9)*. We also recommend obtaining 25-hydroxy vitamin D and TSH levels as part of the basic evaluation.

Subsequent testing should be guided by the results of the history, examination, and initial laboratory evaluations. Some of the more common tests for further evaluation of secondary causes of decreased BMD include:

- Erythrocyte sedimentation rate (ESR), to evaluate for rheumatic disorders or multiple myeloma
- PTH, to evaluate for hyperparathyroidism
- Urinary free cortisol, to evaluate for Cushing's syndrome or hypercortisolemia
- Acid base status (severe acidosis can cause increased phosphorous excretion)
- Serum and urine protein electrophoresis, to evaluate for multiple myeloma
- Bone marrow aspiration, to evaluate for hematologic malignancies or disorders.

Therapy

Recognizing risk factors for osteoporosis is the first step in prevention and treatment of the disorder. If osteopenia is identified on DXA scan, lifestyle modifications such as weight-bearing exercise and smoking cessation should be instituted, and adequate dietary intake of calcium and vitamin D should be ensured. We recommend a follow-up DXA scan after 1 yr of these measures. If osteopenia is unchanged, or worse, or if the patient has experienced fractures during that first year, we recommend careful review of the patient for contributing factors to bone loss and consideration of specific therapy to enhance bone density. All individuals who are identified with osteoporosis or osteoporosis-related fractures should undergo treatment (*see* specific therapies discussed in the following sections). Additionally, all persons with risk factors for osteoporosis should be evaluated for environmental factors that will add to their risk of falls and other osteoporosis-related complications.

LIFESTYLE MODIFICATION

Patients should be encouraged to start (or continue) an exercise program, emphasizing weight-bearing exercises. BMD decreases with inactivity, and age-associated loss in muscle mass leads to a decrease in the bone's ability to absorb shock. Lack of exercise also results in decreased flexibility and a less stable gait *(70)*. There are no absolute recommendations for exercise regimens. However, three 50-min exercise sessions (walking on the treadmill and stepping exercises) per week improved femoral neck and lumbar BMD in osteopenic postmenopausal women *(71)*.

Smoking cessation should be discussed with every patient. In addition, elderly persons who are at high risk for falls should undergo a home evaluation. Since falls are most common in the bathroom, grab bars should be installed near the toilet and shower, and a hand-held shower head or shower chair should be provided. Loose floor rugs should be removed or anchored, and nonskid mats should be used instead. Handrails should be installed in the halls and along the stairways. Hallways, stairwells, and entrances should be well lit. Loose wires should be removed, and clutter should be minimized. Lastly, patients should be encouraged to wear sturdy, low-heeled shoes.

CURRENT PHARMACOLOGIC THERAPY

Osteoporosis is an imbalance of bone formation and bone resorption. Prevention and treatment strategies have been aimed at inhibition of bone resorption or increasing bone formation. However, therapies inhibiting bone resorption are the only treatments approved at this time. Treatment for postmenopausal osteoporosis primarily involves using the following agents to inhibit bone resorption: estrogen, bisphosphonates, selective estrogen receptor modulators (SERMs), and calcitonin. There are agents that augment bone modeling such as PTH *(45,72,73)* and fluoride *(74,75)*, but these are not currently approved by the Food and Drug Administration (FDA).

Estrogen. Estrogen therapy is approved for both prevention and treatment of postmenopausal osteoporosis. Estrogen acts by suppressing osteoclastic bone resorption. Postmenopausal women taking ERT or HRT were shown to have a 3.5–5% increase in spinal BMD and a 1.7% increase in hip BMD after 3 yr of therapy in the Postmenopausal Estrogen/Progestin Interventions (PEPI) trial *(76)*. Older women, women with low initial BMD, and those with no previous hormone use gained significantly more bone than younger women and women with initially higher BMD. If estrogen is given to a woman without a uterus, it is given as ERT alone. If a postmenopausal woman still has an intact uterus, then she is given daily or cyclical progesterone in addition to estrogen (HRT). There are contraindications to taking estrogen, including pregnancy, undiagnosed genital bleeding, breast cancer, estrogen-dependent neoplasm, active thrombophlebitis, or a history of thromboembolic disorder. Relative contraindications to estrogen use include severe hypertriglyceridemia, family history of breast cancer, and hormone-related symptoms not tolerated by the patient. If a patient has any of these conditions, she should use one of the alternative agents.

Selective Estrogen Receptor Modulators. Raloxifene is approved for the prevention and treatment of osteoporosis. It is a benzothiophene SERM. Raloxifene is an estrogen receptor agonist in the skeletal and cardiovascular systems and an estrogen receptor antagonist in the breast and uterus *(77)*. The Multiple Outcomes of Raloxifene Evaluation (MORE) trial showed an increase in BMD at the lumbar spine and femoral neck and a reduction in vertebral fractures in the treatment group *(78)*. Currently, no data show that raloxifene reduces the incidence of peripheral fractures. Raloxifene does not have a proliferative effect on the endometrium, it reduces the risk of breast cancer, and it has a beneficial effect on serum lipids. However, it does increase the risk of venous thromboembolism. At a dosage of 60 mg per d, it is often given to patients who cannot, or will not, take estrogen and who do not have a history of thromboembolic disease *(77)*.

Bisphosphonates. Bisphosphonates inhibit pathologic bone resorption but not normal bone remodeling *(79)*. In the Fracture Intervention Trial (FIT), 3 yr of therapy with alendronate resulted in an 8% increase in spinal BMD and a 50% reduction in new vertebral, hip, and wrist fractures in postmenopausal women with at least one preexisting fracture. In osteoporotic postmenopausal women without fractures, there was a 36% decline in fracture rate *(80,81)*. Oral risedronate and oral alendronate are the only bisphosphonates that are FDA-approved for the prevention and treatment of osteoporosis. Risedronate increased spinal BMD by 1.4% and 4% with the 2.5- and 5-mg doses, respectively, over 24 mo. Increases in femoral neck BMD were also seen *(82)*. Risedronate was also shown to have beneficial effects on BMD for all postmenopausal women regardless of the time since menopause. There are no studies on risedronate and fracture incidence to date. Oral alendronate and intermittent intravenous etidronate or pamidronate have all been shown to be effective in prevention and treatment of glucocorticoid-induced osteoporosis (83–85).

Contraindications to oral bisphosphonates include active gastrointestinal reflux symptoms, esophageal strictures, achalasia or severe esophageal dysmotility, and renal insufficiency with a creatinine clearance of less than 35 mL/min. If patients have any of the contraindications (except renal insufficiency), some practitioners administer cyclical pamidronate intravenously. This treatment is not currently FDA-approved for the indication of osteoporosis. The alendronate dose for prevention of osteoporosis is 5 mg orally per d, or 35 mg orally once per wk. The treatment dosage of alendronate is 10 mg orally per d, or 70 mg orally per wk. Prevention and treatment dosages for risedronate are 5 mg orally per d.

Calcium and Vitamin D. Calcium and vitamin D are essential for bone formation. Unfortunately, it is becoming increasingly common for people to have inadequate dietary intake of calcium and vitamin D. Supplemental calcium and vitamin D have been shown to increase bone density and reduce the incidence of nonvertebral fractures (86). The AACE recommends that all persons older than 50 yr have at least 1200 mg of elemental calcium per d (9). Individuals between 19 and 50 yr should have at least 1000 mg elemental calcium per d. Supplemental vitamin D should also be used with calcium. It is recommended that 800 IU vitamin D per d be given to older adults with comorbid medical conditions that decrease vitamin D intake, production, or absorption. Younger, healthier adults may take 400 IU per d (9). The standard multivitamin with vitamin D contains 400 IU of vitamin D. Therefore, individuals should take 1–2 tablets per d depending on their requirements.

Calcitonin. Calcitonin is FDA-approved for the treatment of late postmenopausal osteoporosis. It has not been shown to be beneficial for prophylaxis in early menopause. Calcitonin decreases osteoclast formation, osteoclast attachment, and bone resorption. Use of nasal salmon calcitonin spray, 200 IU per d, resulted in a 33% reduction in new vertebral fractures in postmenopausal women with established osteoporosis (87). Calcitonin has also been noted to have an analgesic benefit, but the mechanism of its effect is unknown (88). Historically, the chronic use of calcitonin resulted in tolerance to calcitonin at initial doses (89). However, recent studies have shown calcitonin to have a sustained effect for up to 5 yr (87). The recommended dose is 200 IU by nasal spray or 100 IU subcutaneously or intramuscularly per d.

Combination Treatment. Combination therapy with different antiresorptive agents has not been routinely recommended for patients with osteoporosis. However, a recent study demonstrated a greater increase in BMD with combined estrogen and alendronate than with either agent alone *(90)*. This is not yet the standard of care, but it provides promise for future treatments. Furthermore, the combination of antiresorptive agents with anabolic agents may show a much stronger synergy than combinations of antiresorptive agents alone. Studies of these important issues are ongoing.

OTHER PHARMACOLOGIC TREATMENTS

Parathyroid Hormone. PTH is not currently approved for the prevention or treatment of osteoporosis; however, it has shown some promise in early clinical trials. PTH increases cancellous bone density by stimulating bone remodeling and formation. Vertebral BMD has been shown to increase by 10% after 2 yr of treatment *(72)*. PTH (1–34) monotherapy has also been shown to reduce the risk of vertebral and nonvertebral fractures *(73)*. The beneficial effects of PTH on BMD decline within a year of stopping the medication. PTH followed by antiresorptive therapy may, however, sustain the improvement in femoral and lumbar BMD *(45)*. Administration is once daily by subcutaneous injection *(73)*. Definitive recommendations regarding the role of PTH therapy for osteoporosis must await further studies.

Fluoride. Fluoride has been studied for many years, but to date it is not an approved therapy for osteoporosis *(74,75,91)* Fluoride enhances the recruitment of osteoblasts, resulting in increased bone remodeling and increased BMD. However, in multiple studies, it has failed to reduce vertebral and peripheral fractures. Furthermore, fluoride has been implicated in increased fracture rates and osteomalacia, when given at high doses. Current studies with slow-release, low-dose sodium fluoride are ongoing *(91)*.

Phytoestrogens. Many women have been interested in an herbal or nutritional alternative to conventional treatments for osteoporosis. Phytoestrogens, particularly soy isoflavones, are compounds that have estrogenic activity on several tissues in the body. These have been proposed as alternatives to ERT or HRT. However, results of studies have been conflicting. One study showed no clinically significant difference in serum and urine markers of bone remodeling after 3 mo of treatment with low-, medium- or high-dose soy isoflavones *(92)*. Studies of soy isoflavones in rats have shown a reduction in bone turnover markers but no clinically significant change in BMD *(93)*. Although the possible role of soy isoflavone therapy needs further evaluation, it is not currently recommended for prevention or treatment of osteoporosis.

Special Treatment Considerations

ANOREXIA NERVOSA

Estrogen and progesterone therapy for women with anorexia nervosa does not prevent progressive osteopenia in women with active disease *(64)*. However, patients do have improved BMD with recovery from anorexia. It is recommended that all patients with anorexia should receive at least 1500 mg of calcium along with a multivitamin containing 400 IU of vitamin D daily *(63)*. Estrogen therapy should be individualized to each patient, since it has not been proved to be beneficial for osteoporosis in active anorexia. BMD should be monitored every 6 mo to 1 yr *(63)*. Treatment of anorexia, weight gain, and restoration of menses still remain the most beneficial events for improving BMD.

Chronic Glucocorticoid Therapy

Alendronate (35 or 70 mg per wk), intermittent etidronate, and intermittent pamidronate have all been shown to increase BMD at the spine and hip in patients on glucocorticoids *(83–85)*. Therefore, individuals requiring more than 7.5 mg of prednisone (or its equivalent) per d for at least 3 wk, should take a bisphosphonate (alendronate or risedronate orally) in addition to calcium and vitamin D supplementation *(9)*.

Thyroid Disorders

Hyperthyroidism, either as a primary disorder or iatrogenic from over-replacement with thyroid hormone, can cause accelerated bone loss *(49–51)*. Thyroid function should be monitored (by TSH levels) and the hormone dose adjusted to achieve a normal TSH concentration in all individuals receiving thyroid hormone replacement therapy for nonmalignant conditions. Furthermore, patients with thyroid cancer on suppressive doses of thyroid hormone should have frequent evaluation of thyroid function and a baseline and repeat BMD every 1–2 yr until they are stable, and then again with clinical change. The monitoring of free thyroxine and TSH is to ensure that the lowest dose of thyroid replacement required to give adequate suppression of TSH is used.

Hyperparathyroidism

Patients with primary hyperparathyroidism usually undergo surgical removal of the adenoma unless there is a medical contraindication. The increase in fracture risk prior to parathyroidectomy disappears less than a year after surgery, suggesting that there is a rapid postsurgical restoration of bone biomechanical competence *(47)*. Additionally, the BMD has been shown to increase following parathyroidectomy. This suggests that parathyroidectomy, if possible, is the treatment of choice for hyperparathyroid-related osteopenia.

OSTEOMALACIA: *EARLY DIAGNOSIS AND MANAGEMENT*

Introduction

Osteomalacia and rickets are both disorders of the mineralization of osteoid, or bone matrix *(94)*. Osteomalacia occurs in adults after the cessation of bone growth and does not involve the growth plate. Rickets occurs in children and is a disorder of mineralization of growing bone. Therefore, in rickets, the growth plate and newly formed cancellous and cortical bone are both affected. If the disease starts in childhood, rickets and subsequent osteomalacia can represent a spectrum of the same disease. The causes of osteomalacia and rickets include nutritional deficiency of vitamin D or calcium, genetic causes of disordered vitamin D and phosphorous metabolism, lack of sunlight exposure, tumor-induced renal phosphate wasting, and drug effects *(94)*.

Osteomalacia presents relatively infrequently in a general medical practice, so it is important to have a high clinical index of suspicion for patients who present with subtle signs and symptoms consistent with rickets or osteomalacia. It is essential to understand aspects of vitamin D, calcium, and phosphorous metabolism to understand the pathophysiology of rickets and osteomalacia fully. This section reviews vitamin D, calcium, and phosphorous metabolism and discusses the etiology, clinical manifestations, diagnosis, and treatment of rickets and osteomalacia.

Vitamin D, Calcium, and Phosphorous Metabolism

VITAMIN D

Vitamin D2 (ergocalciferol) comes from yeasts and plants *(95)*. Vitamin D3 (cholecalciferol) is a steroid that is either made in the skin by the action of sunlight or found in fatty fish or cod liver *(95)*. Both are biologically inert and must undergo two successive hydroxylations, in the liver and kidney, respectively, to become the biologically active 1,25-dihydroxy vitamin D [$1,25(OH)_2D$]. The main function of $1,25(OH)_2D$ is to maintain serum calcium and phosphorous levels within the normal range and ensure mineralization of the skeleton. Calcium and phosphate absorption from the small intestine are enhanced by $1,25(OH)_2D$ *(94)*. The vitamin then promotes the mineralization of osteoid laid down by osteoblasts, by maintaining serum calcium and phosphorous levels. This results in the deposition of calcium hydroxyapatite into the bone matrix *(95)* and subsequent mineralization of bone.

Low serum vitamin D results in decreased intestinal calcium and phosphate absorption and subsequent hypocalcemia and hypophosphatemia. Hypocalcemia increases serum PTH. This secondary hyperparathyroidism activates osteoclasts and results in increases in calcium and phosphorous resorption from bone. Simultaneously, PTH promotes renal tubular calcium resorption, increased phosphate excretion, and renal conversion of 25-hydroxy vitamin D [$25(OH)D$] to $1,25(OH)_2D$.

A deficiency in active vitamin D can result from a combination of factors. These include a lack of sunlight exposure, poor dietary intake, gastrointestinal malabsorption, and liver or kidney defects impairing the hydroxylation of vitamin D. Impairment of 1α-hydroxylase can be seen in renal insufficiency/failure or vitamin D-dependent rickets, type II. Liver failure impairs the body's ability to make $25(OH)D$ *(96)*. Many drugs impair the metabolism of vitamin D, especially antiepileptics, which increase microsomal enzymatic degradation of vitamin D *(34)*.

CALCIUM

The action of calcium on bone is similar to that described in the Vitamin D section above. Hypocalcemia causes an increase in serum PTH and results in secondary hyperparathyroidism, which increases bone resorption and accelerates the conversion of 25(OH)D to 1,25(OH)$_2$D. Rarely, hypocalcemia in children has been reported to cause rickets *(94,97)*, but usually a deficiency in calcium in adults results in osteoporosis rather than osteomalacia. Deficiency of calcium can result from poor dietary intake, gastrointestinal malabsorption, or calcium-poor total parenteral nutrition (TPN) solutions.

PHOSPHORUS

Phosphorous is an important regulator of bone metabolism. Hypophosphatemia increases renal production of 1,25(OH)$_2$D and causes a subsequent increase in phosphorous absorption from the small intestine. Hypophosphatemia can result from nutritional deficiency of phosphorous. This can be seen in some breastfed babies without adequate supplementation and in patients receiving TPN without an adequate amount of phosphorous. It can also be seen in genetic disorders that cause disordered phosphorous metabolism such as hypophosphatemic rickets *(96)* and hypophosphatasia *(98)*. Some tumors have paraneoplastic properties that can result in phosphorous wasting and disordered bone metabolism *(99)*. This is termed oncogenic osteomalacia and should be suspected when a patient presents with hypophosphatemia, phosphaturia, decreased serum 1,25(OH)$_2$D, normal calcium, normal PTH, and osteomalacia. Hypophosphatemia secondary to aluminum-containing antacids was historically a common cause of osteomalacia in renal failure patients on dialysis and patients receiving long-term TPN.

Specific Disorders

LACK OF SUNLIGHT

Vitamin D3 is synthesized in the human skin by photoconversion of 7-dehydrocholesterol to previtamin D3, which is isomerized to vitamin D3 *(100)*. This form of vitamin D accounts for most vitamin D in a healthy person. Populations that do not have adequate sunlight exposure, such as housebound elderly, inner city children without adequate sunlight exposure, institutionalized patients, and people who wear clothing covering their entire bodies, are at increased risk for vitamin D deficiency. In addition, darker skin pigment reduces the capacity of skin to synthesize vitamin D *(101)*. Darker skinned individuals require six times the dose of ultraviolet radiation, compared with Caucasians, to attain the same vitamin D level. Sunscreens also reduce the skin's capacity to synthesize vitamin

D. However, if some areas remain exposed (legs, forearms, and hands), there does not appear to be an appreciable difference in vitamin D levels *(102)*. It is recommended that elderly individuals, who are at risk for vitamin D deficiency, have their hands, face, and forearms exposed to sunlight two to three times a wk *(102)*.

DIETARY DEFICIENCY

Sunlight exposure is the main source of vitamin D for most persons. However, if vitamin D synthesis in the skin is minimal, then dietary intake of vitamin D and calcium becomes much more important in preventing rickets and osteomalacia. The etiology of nutritional rickets in Nigerian children is related to low intake of both vitamin D and calcium, and supplementation with calcium alone or in combination with vitamin D is more effective than supplementation with vitamin D alone in healing active rickets *(97)*. Although the age of onset of nutritional rickets is usually maximal at 4–12 mo, the peak age of disease may be up to 25 mo *(97)*. Nutritional rickets is also seen in developed countries. In the United States, infants given rice or soymilk alternatives have developed rickets and kwashiorkor *(103)*.

HYPOPHOSPHATEMIC RICKETS

X-Linked Hypophosphatemia. The dominant disorder x-linked hypophosphatemia (XLH) usually presents with short stature, rickets with lower extremity deformities and enlargement of the wrists and knees, bone pain, tooth abscesses, premature cranial synostosis, and enthesopathy (calcification of tendons, ligaments, and joint capsules) *(104,105)*. Patients do not usually experience muscle weakness, unlike other forms of rickets. The clinical presentation can range from isolated hypophosphatemia to severe rickets and osteomalacia even within one family *(104,105)*. Affected persons have hypophosphatemia, elevated alkaline phosphatase, normal serum calcium and PTH, and an inappropriately normal serum 1,25(OH)$_2$D. Genetic mutations in the *PHEX* gene are the cause of XLH. There are many PHEX gene mutations, and none seem to be dominant *(105)*. The precise mechanism is not fully understood, but it is likely that the mutations inactivate *PHEX*, causing a failure to clear the hormone phosphatonin from the circulation *(104)*. It is postulated that phosphatonin is a circulating factor that affects renal proximal tubule phosphate reabsorption *(104)*.

Autosomal Dominant Rickets. This is a much less common entity than XLH. It is autosomal dominant with variable and incomplete penetrance *(105)*. In small studies, affected persons seem to have a milder course and a delayed onset of clinically evident disease compared with XLH. The gene defect has been located to chromosome 12p13 *(105)*. Further studies are needed to understand the pathogenesis of this disorder better.

Autosomal Recessive Rickets. This is extremely rare, is usually associated with hypercalciuria, and is also called hereditary hypophosphatemic rickets with hypercalciuria.

HYPOPHOSPHATASIA

Hypophosphatasia is a rare metabolic bone disorder that results from mutations in the gene that encodes tissue nonspecific alkaline phosphatase (TNSALP) *(98)*. There are many different clinical types: perinatal, infantile, childhood, adult, odontohypophosphatasia, and pseudohypophosphatasia. Inheritance can be autosomal recessive or autosomal dominant depending on the type *(106)*. There can be great variability in clinical presentation between the different forms. The perinatal form is the most severe, and death may occur *in utero* from skeletal malformation owing to undermineralization of the skeleton. In the mildest (adult) form, there may be very minor or no skeletal defects *(98)*. In addition to skeletal defects, patients usually have low serum alkaline phosphatase and increased levels of serum pyridoxal 5'-phosphate, urinary phosphoethanolamine, and inorganic pyrophosphate *(98,106)*. DNA analysis for the TNSALP gene can be used to diagnose this condition.

ONCOGENIC OSTEOMALACIA

Oncogenic osteomalacia is a tumor-induced osteomalacia. This is a rare syndrome that is characterized by hypophosphatemia, hyperphosphaturia, low plasma $1,25(OH)_2D$ levels, normal calcium, normal PTH, increased alkaline phosphatase, and osteomalacia *(107,108)*. These tumors are usually of mesenchymal origin, but tumors of epidermal and endodermal origin such as breast carcinoma, prostate carcinoma, oat cell carcinoma, small cell carcinoma, multiple myeloma, and chronic lymphoblastic leukemia have also been reported *(107,109–111)*. Usually these tumors are small and difficult to locate because they present in obscure places *(112)*. Cases are reported of oncogenic osteomalacia related to a small soft tissue mass on the palm of the hand or a lesion in the maxillary sinus that was originally diagnosed as a mucus retention cyst *(108,111)*. When the tumors were removed, all biochemical and pathologic abnormalities disappeared *(107,108,110,111)*. Histologically, the tumors are extremely vascular and contain many multinucleated giant cells *(108)*.

The molecular basis of the disorder is poorly understood. These patients have impaired phosphate reabsorption in the proximal tubules and resultant hyperphosphaturia. This suggests that a tumor-derived humoral factor causes serum phosphate depletion by acting on the proximal tubule cells to increase urinary phosphate excretion *(109)*. Several low-molecular-weight molecules with the ability to inhibit phosphate transport have been identified in tumor extracts, but it is uncertain whether these are actually the molecules responsible *(109)*.

VITAMIN D-DEPENDENT RICKETS

Vitamin D-Dependent Rickets Type I. Vitamin D-dependent rickets type I has also been termed pseudo-vitamin D deficiency rickets and 1α-hydroxylase deficiency. It is an autosomal recessive gene mutation at chromosome 12q13.3

resulting in a deficiency of renal vitamin D 1α-hydroxylase activity *(113)*. Affected persons usually present with failure to thrive, muscle weakness, hypocalcemia, secondary hyperparathyroidism, and bony changes of rickets in the first 1–2 yr of life. They have normal serum 25(OH)D but very low serum 1,25(OH)$_2$D. Treatment is with physiologic replacement doses of 1,25(OH)$_2$D (calcitriol).

Vitamin D Dependent Rickets Type II. VDDR II is also an autosomal recessive disease. In contrast to VDDR I, this disorder involves a mutation of the vitamin D receptor in the proximal tubules of the kidney. These patients have high levels of 1,25(OH)$_2$D and low levels of 24,25(OH)$_2$D (also made in the proximal tubules), hypocalcemia, hypophosphatemia, and secondary hyperparathyroidism *(114)*. Treatment is difficult and often requires high doses of vitamin D supplementation.

DRUGS

In general, drugs that interfere with the action or availability of vitamin D or phosphorus, or that impair bone mineralization, may result in rickets or osteomalacia. Some of the more common agents associated with osteomalacia are listed in Table 4.

Screening and Diagnosis

Osteomalacia is diagnosed using a combination of clinical signs and symptoms and laboratory results.

CLINICAL MANIFESTATIONS

Patients often have diffuse bone pain affecting several sites simultaneously, especially the shoulder, pelvic girdle, rib cage, and lower back. A mild proximal myopathy may result in a waddling gate *(115)*. These features often lead to incorrect diagnoses of fibromyalgia, polymyalgia rheumatica, ankylosing spondylitis, or myositis. Recurrent pedal stress fractures *(116)*, oligoarticular joint effusions, synovitis, and pain secondary to pseudofractures can also be seen *(115)*. Patients who have hypophosphatemic rickets, hypophosphatasia, and secondary hyperparathyroidism can also develop chondrocalcinosis or calcific enthesopathies. Bone deformities such as kyphosis, scoliosis, protrusio acetabuli, and leg bowing owing to bone softening occur late in the disease *(115)*.

X-RAY FINDINGS

Plain x-ray findings can be variable in osteomalacia. Early in the disease, there are often no radiologic abnormalities. The first radiologic abnormalities are usually seen in the long bones. Characteristic x-ray findings include Looser's lines, which are thin cortical radiolucent lines at right angles to the bone shaft *(94)*. There may also be thinning of the cortex and rarefaction of the shaft with widening, fraying, and cupping of the distal ends of the shaft, and disappearance

Table 4
Causes of Drug-Induced Osteomalacia

Physiologic effects	Pharmacologic effects
Effects on vitamin D	
Vitamin D deficiency	Sunscreens, cholestyramine
Impaired metabolism of 25(OH)D	Phenobarbital, primidone, phenytoin, rifampin, isoniazid
Impaired production of 1,25(OH)$_2$D	Cadmium, ketoconazole
Target organ resistance	Resistance to 1,25(OH)$_2$D: phenytoin
Effects on phosphate	
Impaired phosphate absorption	Aluminum-containing antacids
Enhanced renal phosphate wasting	Cadmium, lead
Effects on bone mineralization	
Decreased bone mineralization	Aluminum, bisphosphonates (high-dose parenteral etidronate only), fluoride

Data from refs. *124* and *125*.

of the zone of provisional cartilaginous calcification *(94)*. DXA scan shows decreased BMD; however, the condition is indistinguishable from osteoporosis. Case reports and small studies have reported that bone scans and technetium scintigraphy show increased uptake at sites of fractures and pseudofractures *(117,118)*. This finding, however, can be confusing, especially in prostate cancer patients who develop osteomalacia. Bone scans often show "hot spots," which are interpreted as bone metastasis. If these findings occur with concurrent hypophosphatemia, phosphaturia, decreased 1,25(OH)$_2$D, and normal PTH, thay are more likely to represent osteomalacia than bone metastasis.

LABORATORY FINDINGS

There is significant variability in the biochemical presentation of individuals with osteomalacia. Although they classically show low or low-normal calcium, low phosphorous, and elevated alkaline phosphatase, only about 50% of patients have either low calcium or low phosphorous, and individuals with both hypocalcemia and hypophosphatemia are rare *(115)*. Elevated alkaline phosphatase can be seen in 23–94% of patients, but it can also be normal in the presence of obvious disease. Depending on the etiology, the vitamin D levels will vary. In vitamin D deficiency, serum 25(OH)D is low. Secondary hyperparathyroidism and hypophosphatemia stimulate renal production of 1,25(OH)$_2$D; hence, levels are usually normal or high *(94,115)*. Primary hyperparathyroidism and VDDR type II also result in increased serum 1,25(OH)$_2$D. Low serum 1,25(OH)$_2$D

Table 5
Pharmacologic Treatment of Osteomalacia

Disorder	Treatment[a]	Side effects/ complications
Dietary deficiency	D2 (ergocalciferol): 5,000 IU/d po *and* Ca: 1 g/d po for 4–6 wk or until bones are healed	Hypercalcemia
Malabsorption	D2 (ergocalciferol): 50,000 IU/d po *and* Ca: 1.5 g/d po Alternatives: D2 (ergocalciferol): 10,000 IU/d im *or* 25(OH)D (calcifediol): 30 μg/d po *or* 1,25(OH)$_2$D: 0.5 μg/d po	Hypercalcemia
Hypophosphatemic rickets	1,25(OH)$_2$D: 0.75–5 μg/d po *and* Phosphorous (as Na or K): 1–3 g/d po	Hypercalcemia, hypercalciuria, hyperparathyroidism, soft tissue calcification, nephrolithiasis, renal failure. GI upset and diarrhea, poor taste
Vitamin D-dependent rickets		
Type I	1,25(OH)$_2$D: 0.25–1.0 μg/d po	Hypercalcemia
Type II	1,25(OH)$_2$D: 30-60 μg/d po *and* Ca: 3 g/d po	Hypercalcemia

Ca doses refer to elemental calcium.

levels are seen in patients with VDRR type I. Often a bone biopsy may be necessary for definitive diagnosis *(115)*.

BONE BIOPSY

The bone biopsy is the gold standard for diagnosing osteomalacia. It is often necessary for diagnosis if the characteristic laboratory and x-ray finding are absent in a patient suspected of having rickets or osteomalacia. The biopsy should show increased osteoid surface (hyperosteoidosis) and a reduction of mineralization activity documented by tetracycline labeling.

Therapy

The etiology of osteomalacia is important when determining treatment (*see* Table 5).

DIETARY DEFICIENCY

If rickets or osteomalacia is secondary to poor nutrition, patients should receive 5,000 IU of vitamin D (ergocalciferol) and 1 g of elemental calcium every day for 4–6 wk, or until the bone findings are healed (which usually happens within 6 mo) *(115)*. If the dietary deficiency is secondary to malabsorption, patients should receive 50,000 IU of vitamin D and 1.5 g of elemental calcium per d, in addition to treatment of the underlying disorder. If treatment with oral vitamin D and calcium fails in these patients, they may need to receive 10,000 IU intramuscularly of vitamin D2 per day, oral 25(OH)D (calcifediol, 30 μg per d), or oral 1,25(OH)$_2$D (calcitriol, 0.5 μg per d) to attain adequate replacement. It is important to monitor serum calcium levels carefully in patients on the higher doses of vitamin D.

HYPOPHOSPHATEMIC RICKETS

Unfortunately, treatment of these patients is not curative. Goals of treatment include improvement in growth and reduction in the severity of bone disease, bowing defects, and activity limitations *(119)*. Despite close monitoring, it should also be noted that therapy often results in side effects such as hypervitaminosis D, hyperparathyroidism, and soft tissue and renal calcification (sometimes resulting in renal failure) *(119,120)*. Therapy should be started as early as possible in persons suspected of having this genetic defect. The therapy consists of replacement of both phosphorous and vitamin D. Recommendations for therapy vary from 0.75 up to 5 μg of 1,25(OH)$_2$D (calcitriol) and 1-3 g of phosphorous per d *(115,119)*. The most important issues are that therapy be started early, that serum calcium, phosphorous, PTH, creatinine, and urine calcium be carefully monitored, and that doses be adjusted accordingly.

HYPOPHOSPHATASIA

There is no medical therapy for hypophosphatasia *(121)*. Affected patients usually have normal serum calcium, 25(OH)D, and 1,25(OH)$_2$D; hence, they should not receive supplemental calcium and vitamin D, as it predisposes them to hypercalcemia and hypercalciuria. They should be referred early to orthopedic specialists and dentists. Often, patients with fractures have delayed healing, and specific intramedullary rods may be needed. Dentures are frequently necessary for the pediatric and adult patients with this disorder.

ONCOGENIC OSTEOMALACIA

The cause of the osteomalacia is related to the humoral effects of certain tumors. When these tumors are removed, all biochemical and pathologic abnormalities disappear *(107)*, and patients start to recover without additional medical treatment. However, adequate nutritional calcium and vitamin D should be provided during the healing phase.

VITAMIN D DEPENDENT RICKETS

VDDR I can be successfully treated with 0.25–1.0 μg per d of $1,25(OH)_2D$ (the usual starting dose is 0.25 μg BID). VDDR II is more difficult to treat. These patients are usually treated with high doses vitamin D (up to 6 μg/kg per d or a total of 30–60 μg per d) and calcium (up to 3 g of elemental calcium per d) *(122)*. The duration of therapy should be sufficient to mineralize depleted bones and allow recovery from the hypocalcemia induced by rapid mineralization of chronically undermineralized bones (hungry bones syndrome). This process generally takes about 3–5 mo *(122)*. These patients should also have frequent monitoring of urinary calcium, serum calcium, phosphorous, PTH, $1,25(OH)_2D$, and creatinine, and adjustments to therapy should be made based on those results.

REFERENCES

1. World Health Organization. Guidelines for Preclinical Evaluation and Clinical Trials in Osteoporosis. World Health Organization, Geneva, 1998 pp. 1–6.
2. Eastell R. Pathogenesis of perimenopausal osteoporosis. In: Favus M J, ed. Primer on the Metabolic Bone Diseases and Disorders of Mineral Metabolism, 4th ed. Lippincott-Raven, Philadelphia, 1999, pp. 260–262.
3. Riggs BL, Khosla S, Melton LJ 3rd. A unitary model for involutional osteoporosis: estrogen deficiency causes both type I and type II osteoporosis in postmenopausal women and contributes to bone loss in aging men. J Bone Miner Res 1998;13:763–773.
4. National Osteoporosis Foundation. Physicians's Guide to Prevention and Treatment of Osteoporosis. Excerpta Medica, Washington, DC, 1999.
5. Dennison E, Cooper C. Epidemiology of osteoporotic fractures. Horm Res 2000; 54:58–63.
6. Melton LJ 3rd, Chrischilles EA, Cooper C, Lane AW, Riggs BL. Perspective. How many women have osteoporosis? J Bone Miner Res 1992;7:1005–1010.
7. Barrett JA, Baron JA, Karagas MR, Beach ML. Fracture risk in the U.S. Medicare population. J Clin Epidemiol 1999;52:243–249.
8. Weinstein L, Ullery B. Identification of at-risk women for osteoporosis screening. Am J Obstet Gynecol 2000;183:547–549.
9. American Association of Clinical Endocrinologists. Medical guidelines for clinical practice for the prevention and management of postmenopausal osteoporosis. Endocr Pract 2001;7:293–312.
10. National Institutes of Health. Osteoporosis prevention, diagnosis, and therapy. NIH Consensus Statement. MIH, Bethesda, MD, 2000, pp 1–45.
11. Wasnich R. Epidemiology of osteoporosis. In: Favus MJ, ed. Primer on the Metabolic Bone Diseases and Disorders of Mineral Metabolism, 4th ed. Lippincott-Raven, 1999, Philadelphia, pp. 257–259.

12. Henry YM, Eastell R. Ethnic and gender differences in bone mineral density and bone turnover in young adults: effect of bone size. Osteoporosis Int 2000;11:512–517.
13. Nelson DA, Barondess DA, Hendrix SL, Beck TJ. Cross-sectional geometry, bone strength, and bone mass in the proximal femur in black and white postmenopausal women. J Bone Miner Res 2000; 15:1992–1997.
14. Eisman JA. Genetics of osteoporosis. Endocr Rev 1999;20:788–804.
15. Bjarnason NH, Christiansen C 2000 The influence of thinness and smoking on bone loss and response to hormone replacement therapy in early postmenopausal women. J Clin Endocrinol Metab 2000;85:590–596.
16. Kiel DP, Baron JA, Anderson JJ, Hannan MT, Felson DT. Smoking eliminates the protective effect of oral estrogens on the risk for hip fracture among women. Ann. Intern Med 1992;116:716–721.
17. Sabo D, Blaich S, Wenz W, Hohmann M, Loew M, Gerner HJ. Osteoporosis in patients with paralysis after spinal cord injury. A cross sectional study in 46 male patients with dual-energy X-ray absorptiometry. Arch Orthop Trauma Surg 2001;121:75–78.
18. Kiratli BJ, Smith AE, Nauenberg T, Kallfelz CF, Perkash I. Bone mineral and geometric changes through the femur with immobilization due to spinal cord injury. J Rehabil Res Dev 2000;37:225–233.
19. Frey-Rindova P, de Bruin ED, Stussi E, Dambacher MA, Dietz V. Bone mineral density in upper and lower extremities during 12 months after spinal cord injury measured by peripheral quantitative computed tomography. Spinal Cord 2000;38:26–32.
20. Bikle DD, Halloran BP, Morey-Holton E. Space flight and the skeleton: lessons for the earthbound. Endocrinologist 1997;7:10–22.
21. Garland DE, Adkins RH, Stewart CA, Ashford R, Vigil D. Regional osteoporosis in women who have a complete spinal cord injury. J Bone Joint Surg 2001;[AM]83-A:1195–1200.
22. de Bruin ED, Frey-Rindova P, Herzog RE, Dietz V, Dambacher MA, Stussi E. Changes of tibia bone properties after spinal cord injury: effects of early intervention. Arch Phys Med Rehabil 1999;80:214–220.
23. Klibanski A, Biller BM, Rosenthal DI, Schoenfeld DA, Saxe V. Effects of prolactin and estrogen deficiency in amenorrheic bone loss. J Clin Endocrinol Metab 1988;67:124–130.
24. Shore RM, Chesney RW, Mazess RB, Rose PG, Bargman GJ. Skeletal demineralization in Turner's syndrome. Calcif Tissue Int 1982;34:519–522.
25. Cooper GS, Sandler DP 1997 Long-term effects of reproductive-age menstrual cycle patterns on peri- and postmenopausal fracture risk. Am J Epidemiol 1997;145:804–809.
26. Lukert B. Glucocorticoid induced osteoporosis. In: Favus MJ, ed. Primer on the Metabolic Bone Diseases and Disorders of Mineral Metabolism, 4th ed. Lippincott-Raven, Philadelphia, 1999, pp. 292–296.
27. Silkensen JR 2000 Long-term complications in renal transplantation. J Am Soc Nephrol 2000;11:582–588.
28. Suzuki Y, Ichikawa Y, Saito E, Homma M. Importance of increased urinary calcium excretion in the development of secondary hyperparathyroidism of patients under glucocorticoid therapy. Metab Clin Exp 1983;32:151–156.
29. Gennari C, Imbimbo B, Montagnani M, Bernini M, Nardi P, Avioli LV. Effects of prednisone and deflazacort on mineral metabolism and parathyroid hormone activity in humans. Calcif Tissue Int 1984;36:245–252.
30. Muir JM, Hirsh J, Weitz JI, Andrew M, Young E, Shaughnessy SG. A histomorphometric comparison of the effects of heparin and low-molecular-weight heparin on cancellous bone in rats. Blood 1997;89:3236–3242.
31. Barbour LA, Kick SD, Steiner JF, et al. A prospective study of heparin-induced osteoporosis in pregnancy using bone densitometry. Am J Obstet Gynecol 1994;170:862–869.

32. Dahlman TC. Osteoporotic fractures and the recurrence of thromboembolism during pregnancy and the puerperium in 184 women undergoing thromboprophylaxis with heparin. Am J Obstet Gynecol 1993;168:1265–1270.
33. Nilsson OS, Lindholm TS, Elmstedt E, Lindback A, Lindholm TC. Fracture incidence and bone disease in epileptics receiving long-term anticonvulsant drug treatment. Arch Orthop Trauma Surg 1986;105:146–149.
34. Sheth RD, Wesolowski CA, Jacob JC, et al. Effect of carbamazepine and valproate on bone mineral density. J Pediatr 1995;127:256–262.
35. Crilly RG, Anderson C, Hogan D, Delaquerriere-Richardson L. Bone histomorphometry, bone mass, and related parameters in alcoholic males. Calcif Tissue Int 1988;43:269–276.
36. Klein RF 1997 Alcohol-induced bone disease: impact of ethanol on osteoblast proliferation. Alcohol Clin Exp Res 1997;21:392–399.
37. Harper KD, Weber TJ. Secondary osteoporosis. Diagnostic considerations. Endocrinol Metab Clin North Am 1998;27:325–348.
38. Pfeilschifter J, Diel IJ. Osteoporosis due to cancer treatment: pathogenesis and management. J Clin Oncol 2000;18:1570–1593.
39. Stoch SA, Parker RA, Chen L, et al. Bone loss in men with prostate cancer treated with gonadotropin-releasing hormone agonists. J Clin Endocrinol Metab 2001;86:2787–2791.
40. Finkelstein JS, Klibanski A, Neer RM, Greenspan SL, Rosenthal DI, Crowley WF Jr. Osteoporosis in men with idiopathic hypogonadotropic hypogonadism. Ann Intern Med 1987;106:354–361.
41. Greenspan SL, Oppenheim DS, Klibanski A. Importance of gonadal steroids to bone mass in men with hyperprolactinemic hypogonadism. Ann Intern Med 1989;110:526–531.
42. Amin S, Zhang Y, Sawin CT, et al. Association of hypogonadism and estradiol levels with bone mineral density in elderly men from the Framingham study. Ann Intern Med 2000;133:951–963.
43. Rochira V, Faustini-Fustini M, Balestrieri A, Carani C. Estrogen replacement therapy in a man with congenital aromatase deficiency: effects of different doses of transdermal estradiol on bone mineral density and hormonal parameters. J Clin Endocrinol Metab 2000;85:1841–1845.
44. Edwards CQ, Cartwright GE, Skolnick MH, Amos DB. Homozygosity for hemochromatosis: clinical manifestations. Ann Intern Med 1980;93:519–525.
45. Rittmaster RS, Bolognese M, Ettinger MP, et al. Enhancement of bone mass in osteoporotic women with parathyroid hormone followed by alendronate. J Clin Endocrinol Metab 2000;85:2129–2134.
46. Silverberg SJ, Shane E, de la Cruz L, et al. Skeletal disease in primary hyperparathyroidism. J Bone Miner Res 1989;4:283–291.
47. Vestergaard P, Mollerup CL, Frokjaer VG, Christiansen P, Blichert-Toft M, Mosekilde L. Cohort study of risk of fracture before and after surgery for primary hyperparathyroidism. BMJ 2000;321:598–602.
48. Freehill AK, Lenke LG. Severe kyphosis secondary to glucocorticoid-induced osteoporosis in a young adult with Cushing's disease. A case report and literature review. Spine 1999;24:189–193.
49. Adlin EV, Maurer AH, Marks AD, Channick BJ Bone mineral density in postmenopausal women treated with L-thyroxine. Am JMed 1991;90:360–366.
50. Stall GM, Harris S, Sokoll LJ, Dawson-Hughes B. Accelerated bone loss in hypothyroid patients overtreated with L-thyroxine. Ann Intern Med 1990;113:265–269.
51. Toh SH, Claunch BC, Brown PH. Effect of hyperthyroidism and its treatment on bone mineral content. Arch Intern Med 1985;145:883–836.
52. Rosen HN, Moses AC, Garber J, et al. Randomized trial of pamidronate in patients with thyroid cancer: bone density is not reduced by suppressive doses of thyroxine, but is increased by cyclic intravenous pamidronate. J Clin Endocrinol Metab 1998;83:2324–2330.

53. Fallon MD, Whyte MP, Teitelbaum SL. Systemic mastocytosis associated with generalized osteopenia. Histopathological characterization of the skeletal lesion using undecalcified bone from two patients. Hum Pathol 1981;12:813–820.

54. Woitge HW, Horn E, Keck AV, Auler B, Seibel MJ, Pecherstorfer M. Biochemical markers of bone formation in patients with plasma cell dyscrasias and benign osteoporosis. Clin Chem 2001;47:686–693.

55. Bernstein CN, Blanchard JF, Leslie W, Wajda A, Yu BN. The incidence of fracture among patients with inflammatory bowel disease. A population-based cohort study. Ann Intern Med 2000;133:795–799.

56. Compston JE, Judd D, Crawley EO, et al. Osteoporosis in patients with inflammatory bowel disease. Gut 1987;28:410–415.

57. Caraceni MP, Molteni N, Bardella MT, Ortolani S, Nogara A, Bianchi PA. Bone and mineral metabolism in adult celiac disease. Am J Gastroenterol 1988;83:274–277.

58. Bisballe S, Eriksen EF, Melsen F, Mosekilde L, Sorensen OH, Hessov I. Osteopenia and osteomalacia after gastrectomy: interrelations between biochemical markers of bone remodelling, vitamin D metabolites, and bone histomorphometry. Gut 1991;32:1303–1307.

59. Hodgson SF, Dickson ER, Wahner HW, Johnson KA, Mann KG, Riggs BL. Bone loss and reduced osteoblast function in primary biliary cirrhosis. Ann Intern Med 1985;103:855–860.

60. Goldring S. Osteoporosis and rheumatic diseases. In: Favus MJ, ed. Primer on the Metabolic Bone Diseases and Disorders of Mineral Metabolism, 4th ed. Lippincott-Raven, Philadelphia, 1999, pp. 313–315.

61. Schulman LL. Lung transplantation for chronic obstructive pulmonary disease. Clin Chest Med 2000;21:849–865.

62. Bikle DD, Halloran B, Fong L, Steinbach L, Shellito J. Elevated 1,25-dihydroxyvitamin D levels in patients with chronic obstructive pulmonary disease treated with prednisone. J Clin Endocrinol Metab 1993;76:456–461.

63. Grinspoon S, Herzog D, Klibanski A. Mechanisms and treatment options for bone loss in anorexia nervosa. Psychopharmacol Bull 1997;33:399–404.

64. Klibanski A, Biller BM, Schoenfeld DA, Herzog DB, Saxe VC. The effects of estrogen administration on trabecular bone loss in young women with anorexia nervosa. J Clin Endocrinol Metab 1995;80:898–904.

65. Ebeling PR, Thomas DM, Erbas B, Hopper JL, Szer J, Grigg AP. Mechanisms of bone loss following allogeneic and autologous hemopoietic stem cell transplantation. J Bone Min Res 1999;14:342–350

66. Berguer DG, Krieg MA, Thiebaud D, et al. Osteoporosis in heart transplant recipients: a longitudinal study. Transplant Proc 1994;26:2649–2651.

67. Mondry A, Hetzel GR, Willers R, Feldkamp J, Grabensee B. Quantitative heel ultrasound in assessment of bone structure in renal transplant recipients. Am J Kidney Dis 2001;37:932–937.

68. Falcini F, Bindi G, Ermini M, et al. Comparison of quantitative calcaneal ultrasound and dual energy X-ray absorptiometry in the evaluation of osteoporotic risk in children with chronic rheumatic diseases. Calcif Tissue Int 2000;67:19–23

69. Grampp S, Henk CB, Fuerst TP, et al. Diagnostic agreement of quantitative sonography of the calcaneus with dual X-ray absorptiometry of the spine and femur. AJR 1999;173:329–334

70. Miszko TA, Cress ME. A lifetime of fitness. Exercise in the perimenopausal and postmenopausal woman. Clin Sports Med 2000;19:215–232.

71. Chien MY, Wu YT, Hsu AT, Yang RS, Lai JS. Efficacy of a 24-week aerobic exercise program for osteopenic postmenopausal women. Calcif Tissue Int 2000;67:443–448.

72. Hodsman AB, Fraher LJ, Watson PH, et al. A randomized controlled trial to compare the efficacy of cyclical parathyroid hormone versus cyclical parathyroid hormone and sequential calcitonin to improve bone mass in postmenopausal women with osteoporosis. J Clin Endocrinol Metab 1997;82:620–628.

73. Neer RM, Arnaud CD, Zanchetta JR, et al. Effect of parathyroid hormone (1–34) on fractures and bone mineral density in postmenopausal women with osteoporosis. N Engl J Med 2001;344:1434–1441.
74. Kleerekoper M. The role of fluoride in the prevention of osteoporosis. Endocrinol Metab Clin North Am 1998;27:441–452
75. Rosen CJ, Bilezikian JP. Clinical review 123: Anabolic therapy for osteoporosis. J Clin Endocrinol Metab 2001;86:957–964.
76. Anonymous. Effects of hormone therapy on bone mineral density: results from the Postmenopausal Estrogen/Progestin Interventions (PEPI) trial. The Writing Group for the PEPI. JAMA 1996;276:1389–1396.
77. Lufkin EG, Wong M, Deal C. The role of selective estrogen receptor modulators in the prevention and treatment of osteoporosis. Rheum Dis Clin North Am 2001;27:163–185, vii.
78. Ettinger B, Black DM, Mitlak BH, et al. Reduction of vertebral fracture risk in postmenopausal women with osteoporosis treated with raloxifene: results from a 3-year randomized clinical trial. Multiple Outcomes of Raloxifene Evaluation (MORE) Investigators. JAMA 1999;282:637–645.
79. Parfitt AM, Mundy GR, Roodman GD, Hughes DE, Boyce BF. A new model for the regulation of bone resorption, with particular reference to the effects of bisphosphonates. J Bone Miner Res 1996;11:150–159.
80. Black DM, Cummings SR, Karpf DB, et al. Randomised trial of effect of alendronate on risk of fracture in women with existing vertebral fractures. Fracture Intervention Trial Research Group. Lancet 1996;348:1535–1541.
81. Cummings SR, Black DM, Thompson DE, et al. Effect of alendronate on risk of fracture in women with low bone density but without vertebral fractures: results from the Fracture Intervention Trial. JAMA 1998;280:2077–2082.
82. Fogelman I, Ribot C, Smith R, Ethgen D, Sod E, Reginster JY. Risedronate reverses bone loss in postmenopausal women with low bone mass: results from a multinational, double-blind, placebo-controlled trial. BMD-MN Study Group. J Clin Endocrinol Metab 2000;85:1895–1900.
83. Saag KG, Emkey R, Schnitzer TJ, et al. Alendronate for the prevention and treatment of glucocorticoid-induced osteoporosis. Glucocorticoid-Induced Osteoporosis Intervention Study Group. N Engl J Med 1998;339:292–299.
84. Adachi JD, Bensen WG, Brown J, et al. Intermittent etidronate therapy to prevent corticosteroid-induced osteoporosis. N Engl J Med 1997;337:382–387.
85. Boutsen Y, Jamart J, Esselinckx W, Stoffel M, Devogelaer JP. Primary prevention of glucocorticoid-induced osteoporosis with intermittent intravenous pamidronate: a randomized trial. Calcif Tissue Int 1997;61:266–271.
86. Dawson-Hughes B, Harris SS, Krall EA, Dallal GE. Effect of calcium and vitamin D supplementation on bone density in men and women 65 years of age or older. N Engl J Med 1997;337:670–676.
87. Chesnut CH, 3rd, Silverman S, Andriano K, et al. A randomized trial of nasal spray salmon calcitonin in postmenopausal women with established osteoporosis: the prevent recurrence of osteoporotic fractures study. PROOF Study Group. Am J Med 2000 109:267–276.
88. Ito A, Kumamoto E, Takeda M, Shibata K, Sagai H, Yoshimura M. Mechanisms for ovariectomy-induced hyperalgesia and its relief by calcitonin: participation of 5-HT1A-like receptor on C-afferent terminals in substantia gelatinosa of the rat spinal cord. J Neurosci 2000;20:6302–6308.
89. Silverman SL. Calcitonin. Rheum Dis Clin North Am 2001;27:187–196.
90. Bone HG, Greenspan SL, McKeever C, et al. Alendronate and estrogen effects in postmenopausal women with low bone mineral density. Alendronate/Estrogen Study Group. J Clin Endocrinol Metab 2000;85:720–726.

91. Pak CY, Sakhaee K, Adams-Huet B, Piziak V, Peterson RD, Poindexter JR. Treatment of postmenopausal osteoporosis with slow-release sodium fluoride. Final report of a randomized controlled trial. Ann Intern Med 1995;123:401–408.

92. Wangen KE, Duncan AM, Merz-Demlow BE, et al. Effects of soy isoflavones on markers of bone turnover in premenopausal and postmenopausal women. J Clin Endocrinol Metab 2000;85:3043–3048.

93. Picherit C, Bennetau-Pelissero C, Chanteranne B, et al. Soybean isoflavones dose-dependently reduce bone turnover but do not reverse established osteopenia in adult ovariectomized rats. J Nutr 2001;131:723–728.

94. Klein G. Nutritional rickets and osteomalacia. In: Favus MJ, ed. Primer on the Metabolic Bone Diseases and Disorders of Mineral Metabolism, 4th ed. Lippincott-Raven, Philadelphia, 1999, pp. 315–319.

95. Holick M. Vitamin D: photobiology, metabolism, mechanism of action and clinical applications. In: Favus MJ, ed. Primer on the Metabolic Bone Diseases and Disorders of Mineral Metabolism, 4th ed. Lippincott-Raven, Philadelphia, 1999, pp. 92–93.

96. Aurbach G, Marx S, Spiegel A. Rickets and osteomalacia. In: Wilson J, Foster D, eds. Williams Textbook of Endocrinology, 9th ed. WB Saunders, Philadelphia, 1998, pp. 1228–1230.

97. Thacher TD, Fischer PR, Pettifor JM, et al. A comparison of calcium, vitamin D, or both for nutritional rickets in Nigerian children. N Engl J Med 1999;341:563–568.

98. Iqbal SJ, Plaha DS, Linforth GH, Dalgleish R. Hypophosphatasia: diagnostic application of linked DNA markers in the dominantly inherited adult form. Clin Sci 1999;97:73–78.

99. Drezner MK. Tumor induced osteomalacia. In: Favus MJ, ed. Primer on the Metabolic Bone Diseases and Disorders of Mineral Metabolism, 4th ed. Lipincott-Raven, Philadelphia, 1999, pp. 331–337.

100. Holick MF, MacLaughlin JA, Clark MB, et al. Photosynthesis of previtamin D3 in human skin and the physiologic consequences. Science 1980;210:203–205.

101. Clemens TL, Adams JS, Henderson SL, Holick MF. Increased skin pigment reduces the capacity of skin to synthesise vitamin D3. Lancet 1982;1:74–76.

102. Holick MF, Matsuoka LY, Wortsman J. Regular use of sunscreen on vitamin D levels. Arch Dermatol 1995;131:1337–1339.

103. Carvalho NF, Kenney RD, Carrington PH, Hall DE. Severe nutritional deficiencies in toddlers resulting from health food milk alternatives. Pediatrics 2001;107:E46.

104. Drezner MK. PHEX gene and hypophosphatemia. Kidney Int 2000;57:9–18.

105. Econs MJ. New insights into the pathogenesis of inherited phosphate wasting disorders. Bone 1999;25:131–135.

106. Iqbal SJ, Davies T, Cole R, Whitaker P, Chapman C. Neutrophil alkaline phosphatase (NAP) score in the diagnosis of hypophosphatasia. Clin Chim Acta 2000;302:49–57.

107. Cai Q, Hodgson SF, Kao PC, et al. Brief report: inhibition of renal phosphate transport by a tumor product in a patient with oncogenic osteomalacia. N Engl J Med 1994;330:1645–1649.

108. Weidner N, Bar RS, Weiss D, Strottmann MP. Neoplastic pathology of oncogenic osteomalacia/rickets. Cancer 1985;55:1691–1705.

109. Jonsson KB, Mannstadt M, Miyauchi A, et al. Extracts from tumors causing oncogenic osteomalacia inhibit phosphate uptake in opossum kidney cells. J Endocrinol 2001;169:613–620.

110. Weiss D, Bar RS, Weidner N. Oncogenic osteomalacia. Ann Intern Med 1985;102:557.

111. Weiss D, Bar RS, Weidner N, Wener M, Lee F. Oncogenic osteomalacia: strange tumours in strange places. Postgrad Med J 1985;61:349–355.

112. Econs MJ, Drezner MK. Tumor-induced osteomalacia—unveiling a new hormone. N Engl J Med 1994;330:1679–1681.

113. Wang JT, Lin CJ, Burridge SM, et al. Genetics of vitamin D 1alpha-hydroxylase deficiency in 17 families. Am J Hum Genet 1998;63:1694–1702.

114. Tiosano D, Weisman Y, Hochberg Z. The role of the vitamin D receptor in regulating vitamin D metabolism: a study of vitamin D-dependent rickets, type II. J Clin Endocrinol Metab 2001;86:1908–1912.

115. Reginato AJ, Falasca GF, Pappu R, McKnight B, Agha A. Musculoskeletal manifestations of osteomalacia: report of 26 cases and literature review. Semin Arthritis Rheum 1999;28:287–304.

116. Linde R, Saxena A, Feldman D. Hypophosphatemic rickets presenting as recurring pedal stress fractures in a middle-aged woman. J Foot Ankle Surg 2001;40:101–104.

117. Akbunar AT, Orhan B, Alper E. Bone-scan-like pattern with 99Tcm(V)-DMSA scintigraphy in patients with osteomalacia and primary hyperparathyroidism. Nucl Med Commun 2000;21:181–185.

118. Sahin M, Basoglu T, Albayrak S, Canbaz F, Yapici O. Pentavalent technetium-99m DMSA uptake in pseudofractures of osteomalacia. Clin Nucl Med 2001;26:62–64.

119. Carpenter TO. New perspectives on the biology and treatment of X-linked hypophosphatemic rickets. Pediatr Clin North Am 1997;44:443–466.

120. Garg RK, Tandon N. Hypophosphatemic rickets: easy to diagnose, difficult to treat. Ind J Pediatr 1999;66:849–857.

121. Whyte MP. Hypophosphatasia. In: Favus MJ, ed. Primer on the Metabolic Bone Diseases and Disorders of Mineral Metabolism, 4th ed. Lippincott-Raven, Philadelphia, 1999, pp. 337–339.

122. Liberman RA, Marx SJ. Vitamin D dependent rickets. In: Favus MJ, ed. Primer on the Metabolic Bone Diseases and Disorders of Mineral Metabolism, 4th ed. Lippincott-Raven, Philadelphia, 1999, pp. 323–327

123. Miller R, Bonnick S. Clinical application of bone densitometry. In: Favus MJ, ed. Primer on the Metabolic Bone Diseases and Disorders of Mineral Metabolism, 4th ed. Lippincott-Raven, Philadelphia, 1999; pp. 152–159.

124. Bikle DD. Drug induced osteomalacia. In: Favus MJ, ed. Primer on the Metabolic Bone Diseases and Disorders of Mineral Metabolism, 4th ed. Lippincott-Raven, Philadelphia, 1999, pp. 343–345.

125. Thomas MK, Demay MB. Vitamin D deficiency and disorders of vitamin D metabolism. Endocrinol Metab Clin North Am 2000;29:611–627, viii.

INDEX

From: *Contemporary Endocrinology: Early Diagnosis and Treatment of Endocrine Disorders*
Edited by: R. S. Bar © Humana Press, Totowa, NJ